CLINICAL DERMATOLOGY

FOR RUTH, PATRICIA AND ARLENE

CLINICAL DERMATOLOGY

J. A. A. HUNTER
BA MD FRCP Edin
Grant Professor of Dermatology
University of Edinburgh
The Royal Infirmary
Edinburgh

J. A. SAVIN
MA MD FRCP DIH
Consultant Dermatologist
The Royal Infirmary
Edinburgh

M. V. DAHL
MD
Professor of Dermatology
University of Minnesota
Minneapolis

PRESENTED BY THE
DERMATOLOGY BUSINESS UNIT

GLAXO LABORATORIES LIMITED

BLACKWELL SCIENTIFIC PUBLICATIONS
OXFORD LONDON EDINBURGH
BOSTON MELBOURNE

© 1989 by
Blackwell Scientific Publications
Editorial offices:
Osney Mead, Oxford OX2 0EL
8 John Street, London WC1N 2ES
23 Ainslie Place, Edinburgh EH3 6AJ
3 Cambridge Center, Suite 208
   Cambridge, Massachusetts 02142, USA
107 Barry Street, Carlton
   Victoria 3053, Australia

First published 1989

Set, printed and bound by
Gorenjski tisk, Yugoslavia

DISTRIBUTORS

Marston Book Services Ltd
PO Box 87
Oxford OX2 0DT
(*Orders:* Tel. 0865 791155
         Fax: 0865 791927
         Telex: 837515)

USA
   Year Book Medical Publishers
   200 North LaSalle Street
   Chicago, Illinois 60601
   (*Orders:* Tel. (312) 726-9733)

Canada
   The C. V. Mosby Company
   5240 Finch Avenue East
   Scarborough, Ontario
   (*Orders:* Tel. (416) 298-1588)

Australia
   Blackwell Scientific Publications
   (Australia) Pty Ltd
   107 Barry Street
   Carlton, Victoria 3053
   (*Orders:* Tel. (03) 347-0300)

British Library
Cataloguing in Publication Data

Hunter, J. A. A.
   Clinical dermatology
   1. Man. Skin. Diseases
   I. Title   II. Savin, J. A. (John A.)
   III. Dahl, Mark V.
   616.5

ISBN 0-632-01955-7

CONTENTS

Preface, vi

1 Skin Disease in Perspective, 1

2 The Function and Structure of the Skin, 4

3 Immunology of the Skin, 19

4 Diagnosis of Skin Disorders, 27

5 Disorders of Keratinization, 36

6 Psoriasis, 42

7 Other Papulosquamous Disorders, 54

8 The Hair and Nails, 60

9 Eczema and Dermatitis, 71

10 Reactive Erythemas and Vasculitis, 85

11 Bullous Diseases, 96

12 Connective Tissue Disorders, 103

13 Disorders of Blood Vessels and Lymphatics, 113

14 Sebaceous and Sweat Gland Disorders, 125

15 Infections, 136

16 Infestations, 165

17 Skin Reactions to Light, 173

18 Disorders of Pigmentation, 180

19 Skin Tumours, 188

20 The Skin in Systemic Disease, 212

21 The Skin and the Psyche, 221

22 Other Genetic Disorders, 225

23 Drug Eruptions, 231

24 Dermatological Therapy, 236

Formulary: 1. Topical Treatments, 245

Formulary: 2. Systemic Medication, 255

Index, 265

PREFACE

Some 10% of those who go to their family doctors do so with skin problems. We have seen an improvement in the way these have been managed over the last few years, but the subject still baffles many medical students — on both sides of the Atlantic. They find it hard to get a grip on the soggy mass of facts served up by some textbooks. For them we have tried to create an easily-read text with enough detail to clarify the subject but not enough to obscure it.

There are many doctors too who are puzzled by dermatology, even after years in practice. They have still to learn how to look at the skin with a trained eye. Anyone who denies that clinical dermatology is a visual specialty can never have practised it. In this book we have marked out the route to diagnostic success with a simple scheme for recognising primary skin lesions using many diagrams and coloured plates.

We hope that this book will help both groups — students and doctors, including some in general medicine and some starting to train as dermatologists — and of course their patients. We make no apologies for our emphasis on diagnosis and management, and accept that we cannot include every remedy. Here, we mention only those preparations we have found to be useful and, to avoid too many trade names, we have tabulated those used in the U.K. and the U.S.A. in a Formulary at the back of the book.

We have decided not to break up the text by quoting lists of references. For those who want to know more there are many large and excellent textbooks on the shelves of all medical libraries.

While every effort has been made to ensure that the doses mentioned here are correct, the authors and publishers cannot accept responsibility for any errors in dosage which may have inadvertently entered this book. The reader is advised to check dosages, adverse effects, drug interactions, and contra-indications in the *British National Formulary* or *Drug Information 1989* (American Society of Hospital Pharmacists) which are issued regularly.

Acknowledgements

The clinical photographs come from our departmental collections and we wish to thank all those who presented them. We are also most grateful to Moira Gray for typing and retyping the manuscript, to Mrs Angela McQuillin for preparing the diagrams and to the staff of Blackwell Scientific Publications for help and encouragement in preparing this book.

CHAPTER 1

SKIN DISEASE IN PERSPECTIVE

Many doctors admit that they panic when faced with a rash. They may have had only a brief glimpse of dermatology during their training: all too often the subject has been squeezed out of its place in the curriculum. The result is a growing number of visually illiterate doctors who quail before the skin and its reputed 2000 conditions, each with its own diverse presentations. They can see the eruptions clearly enough, but cannot identify them. There are no machines to help them. Patients quickly spot their weaknesses and show little sympathy.

The first sections of this book are designed to help medical students and doctors over these difficulties.

First they must understand something of the anatomy and physiology of the skin (Chapter 2). They will then be able to follow the simple steps which lead to a sensible working diagnosis. The sequence starts with the identification of primary skin lesions (p. 29) and the patterns that these can take up on the skin surface (p. 31). At that stage investigations can be directed along reasonable lines until a firm diagnosis is reached. Then, and only then, will the correct line of treatment snap into place.

But another cloud of mystery has settled here, over the subject of topical treatment. We attempt to blow this away in Chapter 24 with a few simple rules governing the choice of the right active ingredient (p. 237) and of the right vehicle in which it should be put up (p. 239). Correct choices here will be followed by good results. Patients are quick to complain if they are not doing well: equally they are delighted if their eruptions can be seen to melt rapidly away.

The arrangement of this book

The classification of skin diseases has never been easy. Early attempts, for example by Robert Willan (1757–1812), the founder of modern British dermatology, brought some order into a subject which was then in chaos, but have left us with an unfortunate legacy of cumbersome latin names (e.g. lichen planus), based on a defunct botanical classification. Many of these names are too well entrenched to be discarded, but in this book we have tried to limit their use, and to eliminate synonyms.

In addition, the early practice of grouping conditions which share physical characteristics (e.g. papules or blisters) is unsound, and has brought together some strange bedfellows. Even so, in some parts of this book we have still had to use such groupings, e.g. for the papulosquamous diseases (Chapter 7) and the bullous diseases (Chapter 11). Elsewhere we have tried, wherever possible, to present together conditions which have the same cause, e.g. fungal infections (Chapter 15) and drug reactions (Chapter 23).

Failing this, some chapters are based on shared physiology, e.g. disorders of keratinization (Chapter 5); others on a shared anatomy, e.g. hair and nails (Chapter 8), or micro-anatomy, e.g. disorders of blood vessels (Chapter 13) or sweat glands (Chapter 14). Such an arrangement, though not perfect, is inevitable while the causes of so many skin diseases have still to be discovered.

Overall our main aims in this book have been to deal in detail with the commonest conditions which make up the bulk of dermatology in developed countries, and to mention some others which may be rare but which illustrate important general principles.

Prevalence

No one who has worked in any branch of medicine will doubt the importance of diseases of the skin. In the U.K. they account for about 10% of all consultations in general practice; but this is only the tip of an iceberg of skin disease in the community. Indeed many people with skin problems never go to their doctors, preferring to deal with matters in their own way.

As an example of this, an estimate of the iceberg of psoriasis in the community in the U.K. is shown in Figure 1.1. In the course of a single year most of those with psoriasis see no doctor, and only a few see a dermatologist.

Several large studies have confirmed that this is the case with other skin diseases too:
- 31.2% of a large representative sample of the U.S. population were found to have significant skin disease which deserved medical attention. Scaled up, these figures would suggest that some 60 million of the U.S. population have significant skin diseases.
- A community study of adults in the U.K. found 22.5% to have a skin disease needing medical attention: only one in five of these had seen a doctor within the preceding six months. Self-medication was far more common than any treatment prescribed by doctors.

- Preparations used to treat skin disease can be found in about one half of homes in the U.K.: the ratio of non-prescribed to prescribed remedies is about six to one.

Morbidity

The pattern of skin disease in a community depends on many factors, both genetic and enviromental. Some of these are listed in Table 1.1. In addition, within each community, different age groups suffer from different skin conditions. In the U.S. for example, diseases of the sebaceous glands (mainly acne) peak at the age of about 20 and then decline, while the prevalence of skin tumours steadily mounts with age (Fig. 1.2).

Table 1.1 Some factors influencing the pattern of skin diseases in a community.

High level of:	High incidence of:
Ultraviolet radiation	Skin malignancy in Caucasians
Heat and humidity	Fungal and bacterial infections
Industrialization	Contact dermatitis
Underdevelopment	Infestations Bacterial and fungal infections

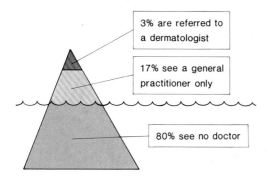

Fig. 1.1 The iceberg of psoriasis in the U.K. during a single year.

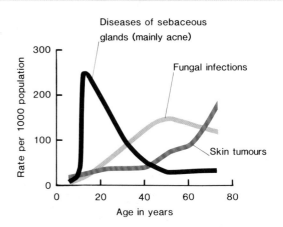

Fig. 1.2 The age-dependent prevalence of some skin conditions.

Deaths from skin disease may be few, but much of this book is taken up with ways in which skin diseases can harm affected individuals:
- Discomfort — itching (e.g. eczema, Chapter 9), pain (e.g. shingles, p. 150).
- Disfigurement, e.g. port-wine stains (p. 205).
- Embarrassment, e.g. psoriasis (Chapter 6).
- Leper complex, e.g. psoriasis (Chapter 6).
- Loss of work/wages — an average psoriatic in the U.S. has been estimated to lose more than $5000 per annum because of this disease.

At national level, the impact of skin diseases is equally devastating. In the U.S. for example, skin diseases account for almost half of all cases of occupational illness, and cause an estimated 52 million days to be lost from work each year.

Causes

The skin is the boundary between ourselves and what is around us. It reflects internal changes (Chapter 20), and reacts to changes in the environment.

Figure 1.3 shows some of the internal and external factors which are important causes of skin diseases. Often several factors will be operating at the same time: just as often no obvious cause for the condition can be found, and here lies much of the difficulty of dermatology.

LEARNING POINTS

1 The *prevalence* of a disease is the proportion of a defined population affected by it at a particular point in time.
2 The *incidence rate* is the proportion of a particular population developing the disease within a specific period of time.
3 Now that you can distinguish prevalence from incidence, read on.

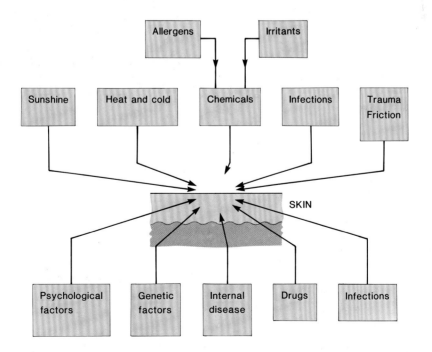

Fig. 1.3 Some internal and external factors causing skin diseases.

CHAPTER 2

THE FUNCTION AND STRUCTURE OF THE SKIN

The skin — the interface between man and his environment — is the largest organ in the body. It weighs an average of 4 kg and covers an area of $2\,m^2$. A death from loss of skin, as in a burn, or in toxic epidermal necrolysis (p. 102), and the misery of unpleasant acne, remind us of its many important functions which range from the vital to the cosmetic (Table 2.1).

The skin has two layers. The outer is epithelial, the *epidermis*, which is firmly attached to, and supported by, connective tissue in the underlying *dermis*. Beneath the dermis is loose connective tissue, the *hypodermis*, which usually contains abundant fat (Fig. 2.1).

Epidermis

The epidermis is formed from many layers of closely packed cells, the most superficial of which are flattened and filled with keratin; it is therefore a stratified squamous epithelium. It adheres to the dermis partly by the interlocking of its downward projections (*epidermal ridges* or pegs) with upward projections of the dermis (*dermal papillae*) (Fig. 2.2).

The epidermis contains no blood vessels. It varies in thickness, from less than 0.1 mm on the eyelids to nearly 1 mm on the palms and soles. As dead surface squames are shed (accounting for some of the dust in our houses), the thickness is kept constant by cells dividing in the deepest (*basal* or germinative) layer. A generated cell moves, or is pushed by underlying mitotic activity, to the surface, passing through the *prickle* and *granular cell layers* before dying in the *horny layer*. The journey from the basal layer to the

Table 2.1 Functions of the skin.

Function	Structure/cell involved
Protection against:	
Chemicals, Particles	Horny layer
Ultraviolet radiaton	Melanocytes
Antigens, Haptens	Langerhans cells
Microbes	Langerhans cells
	Horny layer
Preservation of a balanced internal environment	
Prevents loss of water, electrolytes and macromolecules	Horny layer
Shock absorber	
Strong, yet elastic and compliant	Dermis and subcutaneous fat covering
Temperature regulation	Blood vessels
	Eccrine sweat glands
Insulation	Subcutaneous fat
Sensation	Specialized nerve endings
Lubrication and waterproofing	Sebaceous glands
Protection and prising	Nails
Calorie reserve	Subcutaneous fat
Vitamin D synthesis	Keratinocytes
Body odour	Apocrine sweat glands
Psychosocial	Hair
	Nails

Fig. 2.1 Layers of the skin.

Epidermis — Keratinized, stratified, squamous epithelium

Papillary dermis

Reticular dermis — Collagenous and elastic connective tissue

Hypodermis (superficial fascia) — Adipose tissue

Fig. 2.2 The interlocking of epidermis and dermis.

Epidermis

Dermis

Dermal papillae

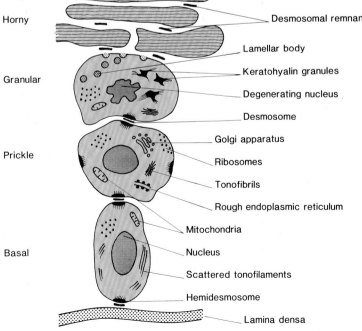

Fig. 2.3 Changes occurring during keratinization.

LAYER   ORGANELLE

Horny — Desmosomal remnants

— Lamellar body

Granular — Keratohyalin granules

— Degenerating nucleus

— Desmosome

— Golgi apparatus

Prickle — Ribosomes

— Tonofibrils

— Rough endoplasmic reticulum

— Mitochondria

Basal — Nucleus

— Scattered tonofilaments

— Hemidesmosome

— Lamina densa

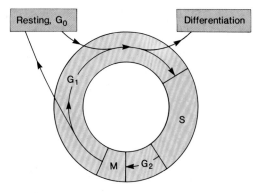

Fig. 2.4 The cell cycle.

surface takes normally about four weeks. During this time the cell's appearance changes. A vertical section through the epidermis summarizes the life history of a single epidermal cell (Fig. 2.3).

The *basal layer*, the deepest layer, rests on a basement membrane which attaches it to the dermis. It is a single layer of columnar cells, whose basal surfaces sprout many fine processes and hemidesmosomes, anchoring them to the *lamina densa* of the basement membrane.

In normal skin some 30% of basal cells are preparing for division (growth fraction). Following mitosis, a cell enters the G_1 phase, synthesizes RNA and protein, and grows in size (Fig. 2.4). Later, something triggers the cell to divide. DNA is then synthesized (S phase) and chromosomal DNA is replicated. A short post-synthetic (G_2) phase of further growth occurs before mitosis (M). DNA synthesis continues through the S and G_2 phases, but not during mitosis. The G_1 phase is then repeated, and one of the daughter cells moves into the suprabasal layer. Having lost the capacity to divide, it then differentiates into a keratinocyte (Fig. 2.3) and synthesizes keratin. The cell cycle time in normal human skin is about 300 hours.

The *spinous* or *prickle* cell layer is composed of such *keratinocytes*, which are firmly attached to each other by small interlocking cytoplasmic processes, abundant desmosomes and an intercellular cement of glycoproteins and lipoproteins. Under the light microscope, the desmosomes appear as 'prickles'.

Cytoplasmic continuity between keratinocytes occurs at *gap junctions*, specialized areas on opposing cell walls. Tonofilaments are more numerous in cells of this layer than in the basal layer, and are packed into bundles called *tonofibrils*. Many *lamellar bodies* (Odland bodies, keratinosomes) are seen in the superficial keratinocytes of this layer. They contain polysaccharides, free sterols, lipids and hydrolytic enzymes, and their contents are discharged into the intercellular space of the granular cell layer.

Differentiation continues in the *granular layer*, which normally has two or three layers of cells which are flatter than those in the spinous layer and have more tonofibrils. Granular layer cells contain lamellar bodies and large, irregular basophilic granules of *keratohyalin* which merge with tonofibrils (Fig. 2.5). Hydrolytic and degrading enzymes found in the lysosomes of granular cells destroy the cells' nuclei and intracytoplasmic organelles, as the granular cells become horny cells.

The *horny layer* (stratum corneum) is made of piled-up layers of flattened dead cells. Their cytoplasm is packed with keratin filaments embedded in a matrix probably derived from the keratohyalin granules. In normal skin these cells have no nuclei or intracytoplasmic organelles. The horny cell membrane is much thicker than that of the underlying keratinocytes. Cells of the horny layer stick tightly together but flake off at the surface.

Keratinization

The main structural protein of the epidermis is the fibrous protein, keratin, a triple-stranded helical mole-

Fig. 2.5 Ultrastructure of the epidermis. (a) Horny and granular layer. HL, horny layer; white asterisk, keratohyalin granule; broad arrows, lamellar bodies; fine arrows, desmosomes. (b) Dermo-epidermal junction. Fine arrows, tonofilaments; open arrow, melanosome; closed broad arrow, lamina densa; CO, collagen. (c) Part of melanocyte (M). Open arrows, melanosomes; K, part of keratinocyte. (d) Part of Langerhans cell. Broad arrows, Langerhans cell granules; G, Golgi apparatus.

cule. The synthesis of keratin starts in the basal or suprabasal layers, and continues in the spinous layer.
Keratin in the horny layer contains cystine, which is
responsible for the intra- and inter-chain disulphide
cross-links which give the epidermis strength to with-
stand tearing. Keratohyalin granules have two components, one of which is the precursor of the cell wall of
the horny cell. The other gives rise to the matrix in
which keratin filaments are aggregated.

Cell cohesion

Firm cohesion in the spinous layer is ensured by
'stick and grip' mechanisms. The glycoprotein intercellular substance acts as a cement, sticking the cells
together, and the intertwining of the small cytoplasmic processes of the prickle cells, together with their
desmosomal attachments, accounts for the grip. The
cytoskeleton of tonofibrils also rigidly maintains the
cell shape. Lipids and sterol sulphates form electro-
chemical bonds, the rupture of which by sterol sulphatase, present in the horny layer, may account for
the shedding of keratinized squames. One type of
ichthyosis (p. 37) is characterized by a deficiency of
sterol sulphatase; shedding then occurs in large
scales.

The epidermal barrier

The horny layer prevents the loss of interstitial fluid
from inside, and prevents the penetration of potentially harmful substances from outside. This *barrier
function* is impaired when the horny layer is removed, experimentally by successive strippings with
adhesive tape, or clinically by injury or skin disease.
It is also decreased by excessive hydration or dehydration of the horny layer, and by detergents or lipid
solvents.

The rate of penetration of a substance is propor-
tional to its concentration difference across the layer.
A rise in skin temperature aids penetration. The normal horny layer is slightly permeable to water but
relatively impermeable to ions, such as sodium and
potassium. Covalent substances (e.g. glucose and

urea) also penetrate poorly, whilst some aliphatic al-
cohols pass through easily. In general the penetration of a solute dissolved in an organic liquid is that
of the solvent.

Epidermal cell proliferation

Both external and internal factors affect this. External
factors that increase epidermal tumors are those that
injure the skin, such as ultraviolet irradiation and
wounding.

Epidermal growth factor, a polypeptide, stimulates
epidermal proliferation, while adrenocorticoids de-
press epidermal mitotic activity. Chalone, a tissue-
specific glycoprotein produced by keratinocytes,
inhibits basal cell mitosis and provides a negative
feedback control for cell division.

At molecular level, the ratio of cyclic AMP to cyclic GMP probably regulates epidermal proliferation.

Vitamin D synthesis

The steroid 7-dehydrocholesterol, found in keratinocytes, is converted by irradiation with sunlight to
cholecalciferol. The vitamin becomes active after
25-hydroxylation in the kidney. Lack of sun and kidney disease may both cause vitamin D deficiency,
and hence rickets.

Other cells in the epidermis

Keratinocytes make up about 85% of cells in the epidermis but three other types of cell are also found
there: melanocytes, Langerhans cells and Merkel
cells.

Melanocytes
Melanocytes are the only cells which can synthesize
melanin. They migrate into the basal layer of the ec-
toderm from the neural crest. They are also found in
hair bulbs, the retina and pia arachnoid. Each dendritic melanocyte associates with a number of keratinocytes, forming an 'epidermal–melanin unit' (Fig. 2.6).

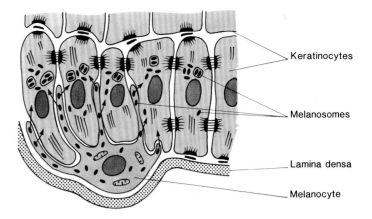

Fig. 2.6 The epidermal melanin unit. Arrows indicate transfer of melanosomes.

Keratinocytes

Melanosomes

Lamina densa

Melanocyte

The dendritic processes of melanocytes wind between the epidermal cells and end as discs in contact with them. Their cytoplasm contains discrete organelles, the *melanosomes*, containing varying amounts of the pigment melanin.

Melanogenesis

Melanocytes are the only cells in the epidermis to contain *tyrosinase* (dopa oxidase), the rate-limiting enzyme in melanogenesis. Tyrosinase, a copper-dependent enzyme, converts the substrate, tyrosine (derived from the essential amino acid phenylalanine), to melanin (Fig. 2.7). Dopa is formed by the oxidation of tyrosine, and further enzymic action leads to the formation of dopaquinone. Eumelanin, a brown or black pigment, is then formed by polymerization. Phaeomelanin, the pigment in red hair, is synthesized in the same way as eumelanin, except that cysteine reacts with dopaquinone. Phaeomelanin and eumelanins intermesh to form mixed melanin polymers (Fig. 2.7).

Eumelanin and phaeomelanin differ from neuro-melanin, the pigment found in the substantia nigra and in cells of the chromaffin system (adrenal medulla, sympathetic ganglia, etc.), which is derived from tyrosine by the enzyme tyrosine hydroxylase.

Melanin is made within melanosomes. These tiny particles, about 0.1 μm x 0.7 μm, are shaped like either American footballs (eumelanosomes, containing eumelanin) or British soccer balls (phaeomelanosomes, containing phaeomelanin). Eventually, fully

melanized organelles pass into the dendritic processes of the melanocyte and are then injected into neighbouring keratinocytes. Once there, melanosomes are distributed throughout the cytoplasm.

Negroids are black, not because they have more

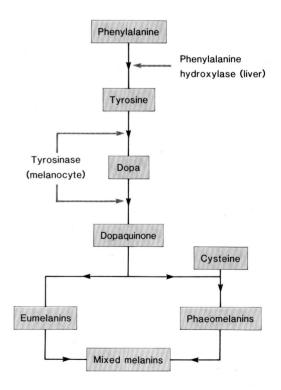

Fig. 2.7 Melanin synthetic pathway.

melanocytes, but because their melanocytes produce more and larger melanosomes, which are broken down less rapidly than those of Caucasoids.

The control of melanogenesis

Melanogenesis is increased by a variety of stimuli, the most important of which is ultraviolet radiation. Tanning involves two distinct reactions.

The first, the immediate reaction, happens within five minutes of exposure to long-wave ultraviolet (UVA: 320–400 nm) and may be due to photo-oxidation of pre-formed melanin. This pigment-darkening reaction, which lasts about 15 minutes, is responsible for the well-known phenomenon of a 'false tan'.

The production of *new* pigment is delayed for some 24 hours after exposure to medium-wave ultraviolet (UVB: 290–320 nm) and UVA. It depends on the proliferation of melanocytes, an increase in tyrosinase activity and melanosome production, and an increased transfer of new melanosomes to their surrounding keratinocytes.

A neat control mechanism involving glutathione has been postulated. Reduced glutathione in the epidermis, produced by the action of glutathione reductase on glutathione, inhibits tyrosinase. UVR and some inflammatory skin conditions may induce pigmentation by oxidizing glutathione and so blocking its inhibition of melanogenesis.

Melanocytes are also influenced by melanocyte stimulating hormone (MSH) peptides from the pituitary (Fig. 2.8). Their melanocyte stimulating activity is due to a common heptapeptide sequence. However MSH peptides are not involved in the physiological control of pigmentation. Hypophysectomy does not cause black skin to lighten and only large doses of ACTH, in pathological states (Chapter 18), will increase skin pigmentation. The role of melatonin from the pineal gland in skin lightening has yet to be established.

Animal experiments indicate that oestrogens, progestogens, and possibly testosterone, may, in some circumstances, stimulate melanogenesis either directly or by increasing the release of MSH peptides from the pituitary.

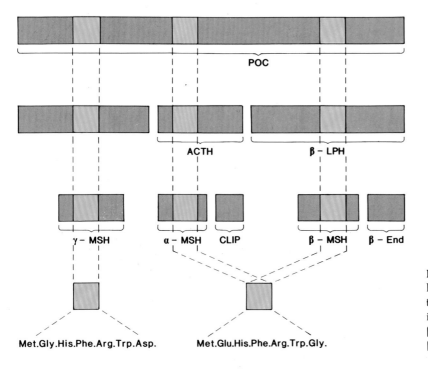

Fig. 2.8 Melanocyte stimulating hormone peptides. Abbreviations as in text. CLIP, corticotrophin-like intermediate lobe peptide; β-end, β-endorphin; POC, pro-opiocortin; βLPH, β-lipotrophin.

Genetics and skin pigmentation

Genetic differences determine the pigmentation of the different races. The Negroid in Britain, and the Caucasoid in Africa, remain respectively black and white. Nonetheless, there is some phenotypic variation in skin colour, for example tanning after sun exposure. Some genodermatoses with abnormal pigmentation are described in Chapter 22.

Langerhans cells

The Langerhans cell is a dendritic cell, like the melanocyte, which also lacks desmosomes and tonofibrils but which has a lobulated nucleus. The specific granules within the cell look like sycamore seeds — plate-like structures with a rounded bleb protruding from their surface, which appear rod- or racquet-shaped on electron microscopy (Fig. 2.5).

Langerhans cells come from a mobile pool of precursors originating in the bone marrow. There are approximately 800 Langerhans cells per square mm in human skin and their dendritic processes fan out to form a striking network seen best in epidermal sheets (Fig. 2.9). Langerhans cells are alone among epidermal cells in possessing surface receptors for the Fc portion of IgG, and C3b, and in bearing class II major histocompatibility complex antigens (HLA-DR, -DP and -DQ).

Langerhans cells play a key role in many immune reactions. They take up exogenous antigen, process it and present it to T lymphocytes either in the skin or in the local lymph nodes (p. 19). They probably play a part in immunosurveillance of viral and tumour antigens. In addition, ultraviolet radiation may induce skin tumours not only by causing mutations in the epidermal cells, but also by damaging Langerhans cells, so that cells bearing altered antigens are not recognized and destroyed by the immune system. The Langerhans cell is the principal cell in skin allografts to which the T lymphocytes of the host react during rejection.

Merkel cells

Merkel cells are also found in normal epidermis and may act as transducers for fine touch. These nondendritic cells, lying in or near the basal layer, are the same size as keratinocytes and are concentrated in localized thickenings of the epidermis near hair

Fig. 2.9 Network of Langerhans cells in an epidermal sheet.

follicles (hair discs). They contain membrane-bound spherical granules, 80–100 nm in diameter, which have a core of varying density, separated from the membrane by a clear halo. Sparse desmosomes connect these cells with neighbouring keratinocytes. Fine unmyelinated nerve endings are often associated with Merkel cells and the granules in the cell contain a neurotransmitter.

Epidermal appendages

The skin appendages are derived from epithelial germs during embryogenesis and, except for the nails, lie in the dermis. They include hair, nails, and the sweat and sebaceous glands.

The hair

The hair germ, a solid cylinder of cells, grows obliquely down into the dermis where it is met by a cluster of mesenchymal cells, bulging into the lower part of the hair germ to form the hair papilla. Eventually the papilla contains blood vessels bringing nutrients to the hair matrix. The sebaceous gland is an outgrowth at the side of the hair germ, establishing early the two parts of the pilosebaceous unit. The hair matrix, the germinative part of the follicle, is equivalent to the basal cells of the epidermis. Melanocytes migrate into the matrix and are responsible for the different colours of hair (eumelanin: brown; phae-omelanin: red). Grey or white hair is due to low pigment production, and the filling of the cells in the hair medulla with minute air bubbles which reflect light. The anatomy of an adult hair follicle is shown in Figure 2.10.

Hairs are classified into three main types:

1 *Lanugo hairs.* Fine long hairs covering the fetus, but shed about one month before birth.

2 *Vellus hairs.* Fine short unmedullated hairs covering much of the body surface. They replace the lanugo hairs just before birth.

3 *Terminal hairs.* Long, coarse medullated hairs seen, for example, in the scalp or pubic regions. Their growth is often influenced by circulating androgen levels.

Terminal hairs convert to vellus hairs in male-pattern alopecia and vellus hairs convert to terminal hairs in hirsutism (Chapter 8). The lips, glans penis, labia minora, palms and soles remain free of hair.

The hair cycle

Each follicle passes, independently of its neighbours, through regular cycles of growth and shedding. The three phases of follicular activity (Fig. 2.11) are known as:

1 *Anagen.* The active phase of hair production.

2 *Catagen.* A short phase of conversion from active growth to the resting phase. Growth stops, and the end of the hair becomes club-shaped.

3 *Telogen.* A resting phase at the end of which the club hair is shed.

The duration of each of these stages varies from region to region of the body. On the scalp, said to contain an average of 100 000 hairs, anagen lasts for up to five years, catagen for only a few days, and telogen for about three months. As many as 100 hairs may be shed from the normal scalp every day as a normal consequence of cycling. The proportion of hairs in the growing and resting stages can be estimated by looking at plucked hairs (a trichogram). On the scalp, about 85% are normally in anagen and 15% in telogen.

The cycle of alternating growth and rest is not synchronized in man. There is no moulting period. However, some diseases (*see* Telogen effluvium, Chapter 8) and drugs may synchronize catagen so that large numbers of hairs are lost at the same time.

There are important racial differences in hair. Asians tend to have straight hair, Negroids to have woolly hair and Europeans to have wavy hair. These differences are due to different cross-sectional shapes (round, flattened, etc.). Mongoloids have sparse facial and body hair when compared with Mediterranean people who also have more hair than northern Europeans.

The nail

The structure of the nail and nail bed is shown in Figure 2.12. The hard keratin of the nail plate is formed in the nail matrix, which lies in an invagination of the epidermis (the nail fold) on the back of the terminal phalanx of each digit. The matrix runs from the proximal end of the floor of the nail fold to

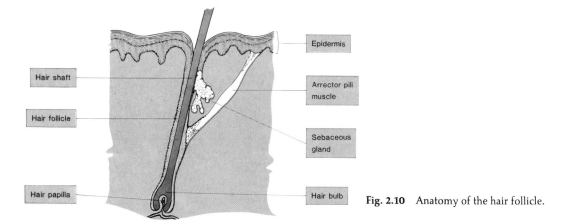

Fig. 2.10   Anatomy of the hair follicle.

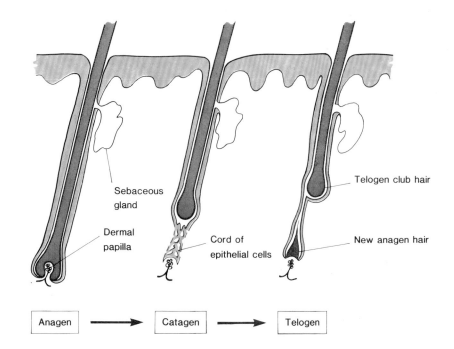

Fig. 2.11 The hair cycle.

| Anagen | → | Catagen | → | Telogen |

the distal margin of the lunule. From this area the nail plate grows forward over the nail bed, ending in a free margin at the tip of the digit. Longitudinal ridges and grooves on the under surface of the nail plate dovetail with similar ones on the upper surface of the nail bed. The cuticle acts as a seal to protect the potential space of the nail fold from chemicals and from infection.

The rate at which nails grow varies from person to person: finger nails average between 0.5 and 1.2 mm per week, while toe nails grow more slowly. Nails grow faster in youth and in the summer. The nails provide strength and protection for the terminal phalanx. Their presence helps with fine touch and with the handling of small objects.

Eccrine sweat glands

Two to three million sweat glands are present all over the body, being most numerous on the palms, soles and axillae. The tightly coiled glands lie deep in the dermis, and the emerging duct passes to the surface by penetrating the epidermis in a corkscrew fashion. Sweat is formed in the coiled gland by active secretion, involving the sodium pump. Some

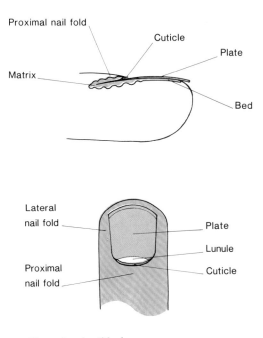

Fig. 2.12 The nail and nail bed.

damage occurs to the membrane of the secretory cells during sweating. Initially sweat is isotonic with plasma but, under normal conditions, it becomes hypotonic by the time it is discharged at the surface after the tubular resorption of electrolytes and water under the influence of aldosterone and antidiuretic hormone.

In some ways the eccrine sweat duct is like a renal tubule. Sweat contains sodium, potassium chloride, lactate, urea and ammonia. The concentration of sodium chloride in sweat is increased in cystic fibrosis, and sweat is analysed when this is suspected.

Sweat glands play an important role in temperature control, the skin surface being cooled by evaporation. Up to 10 litres of sweat may be excreted per day. Three stimuli induce sweating:

- *Thermal sweating* as a reflex response to a raised environmental temperature occurs all over the body, especially the chest, back, forehead, scalp and axillae.
- *Emotional sweating*, provoked mostly by fear and anxiety, is seen mainly on the palms, soles and axillae.
- *Gustatory sweating* is provoked by hot, spicy foods and affects the face.

The eccrine sweat glands are innervated by cholinergic fibres of the sympathetic nervous system. Sweating can therefore be induced by cholinergic, and blocked by anticholinergic, drugs. Central control of sweating resides in the pre-optic hypothalamic sweat centre.

Apocrine sweat glands

The apocrine glands in the adult are limited to the axillae, nipples, peri-umbilical area, perineum and genitalia. The coiled tubular glands (larger than those of eccrine glands) lie deep in the dermis, and during sweating the luminal part of their cells is lost (decapitation secretion). Apocrine sweat passes via the duct into the mid-portion of the hair follicle. The action of bacteria on apocrine sweat is responsible for body odour. The glands are innervated by adrenergic fibres of the sympathetic nervous system.

Sebaceous glands

Most sebaceous glands develop from hair germs, but a few free glands arise from the epidermis. The sebaceous glands associated with hair lie in the obtuse angle between the follicle and the epidermis. The gland itself is multilobed and contains cells full of lipid which, during secretion, are shed whole (holocrine secretion) so that sebum contains their remnants in a complex mixture of triglycerides, fatty acids, wax esters, squalene and cholesterol. Sebum is discharged into the upper part of the hair follicle (Fig. 2.10). It lubricates and waterproofs the skin and protects it from drying; it is also mildly bacteriocidal and fungistatic. Free sebaceous glands may be found in the eyelid (meibomian glands), mucous membranes (Fordyce spots), nipple, peri-anal region and genitalia.

Sebaceous glands are stimulated by androgenic hormones, especially dihydrotestosterone. Human sebaceous glands contain 5α-reductase, 3β- and 17β-hydroxysteroid dehydrogenase, which convert weaker androgens to dihydrotestosterone. The sebaceous glands are stimulated by maternal androgens for a short time after birth, and then lie dormant until puberty when a surge of androgens stimulates a sudden increase in sebum excretion and sets the stage for acne (Chapter 14).

The dermo-epidermal junction

At the interface between the epidermis and dermis lies the basement membrane zone. With light microscopy it may be highlighted using a PAS stain, due to its abundance of neutral mucopolysaccharides. Electron microscopy (Fig. 2.13) shows that the *lamina densa* (rich in type IV collagen) is separated from the basal cells by an electron-lucent area, the *lamina lucida*. The plasma membrane of basal cells has *hemidesmosomes* (cf. desmosomes above). Fine *anchoring filaments* cross the lamina lucida and connect the lamina densa to the plasma membrane of the basal cells. *Anchoring fibrils* (of type VII collagen), dermal microfibril bundles, and single small collagen fibres (types I and III), extend from the papillary dermis to the deep part of the lamina. The lamina lucida contains at least three distinct macromolecules, laminin, fibronectin, and the bullous pemphigoid antigen.

Tonofilaments

Attachment plaque
of hemidesmosome

Sub-basal dense plate
of hemidesmosome

Anchoring filaments

Anchoring fibrils

Collagen fibril

Basal keratinocyte

Lamina lucida

Lamina densa

Dermal microfibril bundle

Fig. 2.13   Structure of the dermo-epidermal
junction.

Laminin, a non-collagen glycoprotein (MW 90 kD) produced by keratinocytes, promotes adhesion between epithelial cells and type IV collagen, the main constituent of the lamina densa. The bullous pemphigoid antigen (MW 220 kD) is synthesized by basal cells and occurs in close association with the hemidesmosomes and laminin; its function is unknown but antibodies to it are found in the subepidermal blistering condition of pemphigoid (p. 99).

The structures of the dermo-epidermal junction provide mechanical support, encouraging adhesion, growth, differentiation and migration of the overlying basal cells, and also act as a semipermeable filter which regulates the transfer of nutrients and cells from dermis to epidermis.

Dermis

The dermis lies between the epidermis and the subcutaneous fat. It supports the epidermis structurally and nutritionally. Its thickness varies, being greatest in the palms and soles and least in the eyelids and penis. In old age the dermis is thinned and loses its elasticity.

The dermis interdigitates with the epidermis (Fig. 2.2) so that upward projections of the dermis, the dermal papillae, interlock with downward ridges of

the epidermis, the rete pegs. This interdigitation is responsible for the ridges seen most readily on the fingertips (fingerprints); it is important in the adhesion between epidermis and dermis, and increases the area of contact between them.

Like all connective tissues the dermis has three components: cells, fibres and amorphous ground substance.

Cells of the dermis

The main cells of the dermis are fibroblasts, but there are also small numbers of mononuclear phagocytes, lymphocytes, Langerhans cells and mast cells. Other blood cells, for example polymorphs, are seen during inflammation. The function of the resident dermal cells is summarized in Table 2.2 and their role in immunological reactions is discussed in Chapter 3.

Fibres of the dermis

The bulk of the dermis consists of interwoven fibres, principally of *collagen*, packed in bundles. Those in the papillary dermis are finer than those in the deeper, reticular dermis. When the skin is stretched,

Table 2.2 Functions of some resident dermal cells.

Fibroblast	Synthesis of collagen, reticulin, elastin, fibronectin, glycosaminoglycans, collagenase
Mononuclear phagocyte	Mobile; phagocytose and destroy bacteria Secrete mediators
Lymphocyte	Immunosurveillance
Langerhans cell	In transit between local lymph node and epidermis Antigen presentation
Mast cell	Stimulated by antigens, complement components, and other substances to release many mediators including histamine, heparin, prostaglandins, leukotrienes, tryptase and chemotactic factors for eosinophils and neutrophils

Table 2.3 Distribution of some types of collagen.

Collagen type	Tissue distribution
I	Most connective tissues including tendon and bone Accounts for approx. 85% of skin collagen
II	Cartilage
III	Accounts for about 15% of skin collagen Blood vessels
IV	Skin (lamina densa) and basement membranes of other tissues
V	Ubiquitous including placenta
VII	Skin (anchoring fibrils) Fetal membranes

collagen, with its high tensile strength, prevents tearing, and the elastic fibres, intermingled with the collagen, return it to the unstretched state.

Collagen makes up 70–80% of the dry weight of the dermis. Its fibres are composed of thinner fibrils, which are, in their turn, made up of microfibrils built from individual collagen molecules. These molecules consist of three polypeptide chains (MW 95 kD) forming a triple helix with a non-helical segment at both ends. The alignment of the chains is stabilized by covalent cross-links involving lysine and hydroxylysine. Collagen is an exceptional protein in that it contains a high proportion of proline and hydroxyproline and many glycine residues; the spacing of glycine as every third amino acid is a prerequisite for the formation of a triple helix. Defects in the enzymes needed for collagen synthesis are responsible for some skin diseases, including the Ehlers–Danlos syndrome (Chapter 22) and conditions involving other systems including lathyrism (fragility of skin and other connective tissues), and osteogenesis imperfecta (fragility of bones).

There are many, genetically distinct, collagen proteins, all with triple helical molecules, and all rich in hydroxyproline and hydroxylysine. The distribution of some is summarized in Table 2.3.

Reticulin fibres are fine collagen fibres seen in fetal skin, and around the blood vessels and appendages of adult skin.

Elastic fibres account for about 2% of the dry weight of adult dermis. They have two distinct protein components: the amorphous elastin core and a surrounding 'elastic tissue microfibrillar component'. Elastin (MW 72 kD) is made up of polypeptides (rich in glycine, desmosine and valine) linked to the microfibrillar component through their desmosine residues. Defects in elastic tissue cause cutis laxa (sagging inelastic skin) and pseudoxanthoma elasticum (Chapter 22).

Ground substance of the dermis

The amorphous ground substance of the dermis

consists largely of two glycosaminoglycans, hyaluronic acid and dermatan sulphate, with smaller amounts of heparan sulphate and chondroitin sulphate.

It has several important functions:

- It binds water, allowing nutrients, hormones and waste products to pass through the dermis.
- It is a lubricant between the collagen and elastic fibre networks during skin movement.
- It provides bulk, allowing the dermis to act as a shock absorber.

Cutaneous muscles

Both smooth and striated muscle are found in the skin. The arrector pili muscles are used by animals to raise their fur, and so to protect them from the cold. They are vestigial in man, but may help to express sebum. Smooth muscle is also responsible for 'goose pimples (bumps)' from cold and nipple erection, and the dartos muscle raises the scrotum. Striated fibres, for example the platysma, and some of the muscles of facial expression, are also found in the dermis.

Blood vessels

Although skin consumes little oxygen, it has an abundant blood supply to regulate body temperature. The blood vessels lie in two main horizontal layers (Fig. 2.14). The deep plexus is just above the subcutaneous fat, and its arterioles supply the sweat glands and hair papillae. The superficial plexus is in the papillary dermis and arterioles from it become capillary loops in the dermal papillae. An arteriole from the deep dermis supplies an inverted cone of tissue, with its base at the epidermis.

Cutaneous lymphatics

An afferent lymphatic begins as a blind-ended capillary in the dermal papilla and passes to a superficial lymphatic plexus in the papillary dermis. There are also two deeper horizontal plexuses, and collecting lymphatics from the deeper one run with the veins in the superficial fascia.

Innervation

The skin is liberally supplied with sensory nerves: some end as free nerve endings, others in special end organs such as the Paccinian and Meissner corpuscles, and Merkel cells. The free nerve endings respond to the potentially damaging stimuli of heat and trauma (nociceptors), while the specialized endings register deformation of the skin (mechanoreceptors).

Itching is an important feature of many skin diseases. It follows the stimulation of fine free nerve endings lying close to the dermo-epidermal junction. Areas with a high density of such endings (itch spots) are especially sensitive to itch-provoking

Arterial capillary

Venous capillary

Superficial vascular plexus

Descending collecting venule

Ascending arteriole

Deep vascular plexus

Fig. 2.14 Blood vessels of the skin.

stimuli. Impulses from these free endings pass centrally in two ways: quickly along myelinated A fibres, and more slowly along non-myelinated C fibres. As a result, itch has two components — a quick, localized, pricking sensation followed by a slow, burning, diffuse itching.

Many stimuli can induce itching (electrical, chemical and mechanical). In itchy skin diseases, pruritogenic chemicals such as histamine and proteolytic enzymes are liberated close to the dermo-epidermal junction. The detailed pharmacology of individual diseases is still poorly understood but prostaglandins potentiate chemically induced itching in inflammatory skin diseases.

LEARNING POINT

More and more diseases are being classified according to the abnormality of function and structure which they display rather than by their appearance.

CHAPTER 3

IMMUNOLOGY OF THE SKIN

The immune system works in the skin just as it does in other tissues, but certain reactions tend to occur there and are readily seen as skin disease. The immune system reacts to foreign antigens and finds many in the skin, at the interface of the body with its environment.

This chapter outlines the intricate mechanisms by which antigens are recognized by specialized skin cells (mainly Langerhans cells) and the ways in which antibodies, lymphocytes, macrophages, and polymorphs elicit inflammation.

The skin as an immunological organ

The epidermis contains Langerhans cells (p.11) which are antigen-presenting cells. Their dendrites ramify between the keratinocytes and interact with chemicals or organisms coming through the epidermal barrier. To induce an immune response, Langerhans cells process antigen and present it to appropriate T helper lymphocytes, in either the epidermis or the dermis (Fig. 3.1). During apposition between the Langerhans cell and the T cell the Langerhans cell releases interleukin 1 (IL-1) to trigger the T cell to secrete interleukin 2 (IL-2/T cell growth factor) and to express receptors on the T cell surface for interleukin 2. Keratinocytes also secrete mediators which aid this response, including epidermal T cell activating factor (ETAF), which appears to be identical to IL-1. This process of induction (sensitization) takes place in the skin or in the lymph nodes and results in the generation of a clone of lymphocytes which are specifically sensitized to a particular antigen (i.e. which specifically recognize the antigen).

On further challenge with the antigen, an inflammatory response is elicited in the skin. The antigen, again processed and presented by the Langerhans cell, stimulates antigen-specific T cells to produce lymphokines which bring other inflammatory cells into the area (see Fig. 3.6). The soluble factors recruit other, non-specific, lymphocytes into the area and they too produce lymphokines, i.e. there is augmentation by recruitment. Indeed only a few of the lymphocytes (less than 5%) in an immunological inflammatory reaction in the skin actually recognize the specific antigen. The rest are uncommitted lymphocytes recruited to the site by the committed ones.

Types of reactions in the skin

There are four basic types of immunological reaction (Table 3.1).

Type I: immediate hypersensitivity reactions

These are characterized by vasodilation and an outpouring of fluid from blood vessels. Such reactions can be mimicked by drugs or toxins, which act directly, but immunological reactions are mediated by antibodies, and are manifestations of allergy. IgE and IgG4 antibodies, produced by plasma cells in organs other than the skin, attach themselves to mast cells in the dermis. Mast cells contain inflammatory mediators, either in their granules or in their cytoplasm. The IgE antibody is attached to the mast cell by its Fc end, so that the antigen combining site dangles from the mast cell like a hand on an arm

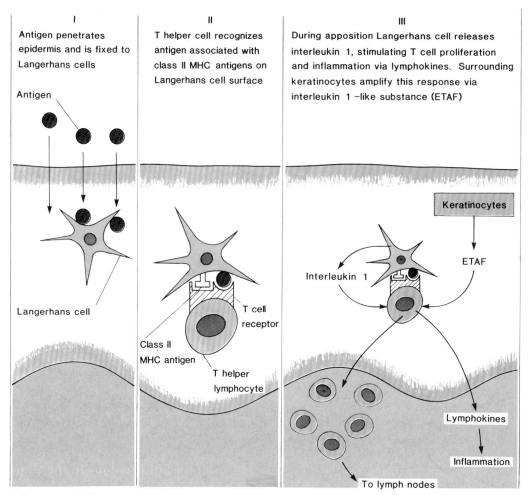

Fig. 3.1 Antigen presentation in the skin.

(Fig. 3.2). When specific antigen combines with the hand parts of the immunoglobulin (the antigen binding site or Fab end), the mast cell liberates its mediators into the surrounding tissue. Of these mediators, histamine (from the granules) and leukotrienes (from the cell membrane) induce vasodilatation, and endothelial cells retract allowing transudation into the extravascular space. The vasodilatation causes a pink colour and the transudation causes swelling. Urticaria (p. 85) and angioedema (p. 87) are examples of immediate hypersensitivity reactions occurring in the skin.

Antigen can be delivered to the skin from outside. A bee sting, for example, will induce swelling by direct pharmacological activity. However, some people, with IgE antibodies against bee venom, swell even more at the site of the sting as the result of a specific immunological reaction. If they are extremely sensitive, they may develop wheezing, wheals, and anaphylactic shock (p. 233; Fig. 23.4), due to a massive release of histamine into the circulation.

Antigens can also reach mast cells from inside the body. A person who is allergic to shellfish, for example, may develop urticaria within seconds, minutes, or hours of eating one. Antigenic material is absorbed from the gut, passes to tissue mast cells via the circulation, and elicits an urticarial reaction after binding to specific IgE on mast cells in the skin.

Table 3.1 Some immunological reactions in the skin.

Type I
Immediate hypersensitivity reactions (mediated by IgE and mast cells)
　anaphylaxis
　wheal-flare reactions
　angioedema

Type II
Humoral cytotoxic reactions (mediated by IgG, IgM and complement)
　complement-mediated cytolysis
　immunologically mediated hormone-like reactions

Type III
Immune complex diseases
Arthus reactions
Serum sickness
Vasculitis

Type IV
Cell-mediated reactions (mediated by lymphocytes and lymphokines)
　delayed hypersensitivity
　cell-mediated cytotoxicity
　antibody-dependent cellular cytotoxicity
　granulomatous reactions

Type II: humoral cytotoxic reactions

In the main, these involve IgG and IgM antibodies which, like IgE, are produced by plasma cells and are present in the interstitial fluid of the skin. When they meet an antigen, they fix and activate complement through a series of enzymatic reactions which generate mediator and cytotoxic proteins (Fig. 3.3), e.g. if bacteria enter the skin, IgG and IgM antibodies bind to antigens on them. Complement is activated through the classical pathway and a number of mediators are generated. Amongst these are the chemotactic factor, C5a, which attracts polymorphs to the area of bacterial invasion, and the opsonin, C3b, which coats the bacteria so that they can be ingested and killed by the polymorphs when these arrive (Fig. 3.4). In certain circumstances, activation of complement can kill cells or organisms directly by the 'membrane attack complex' (C5b6789) in the terminal complement pathway (Fig. 3.3). Complement can also be activated by bacteria directly through the alternative pathway (Fig. 3.3). Antibody is not required. The bacterial cell wall causes more C3b to be produced by the alternative pathway factors B, D, and P (properdin). Aggregated IgA can also activate the alternative pathway.

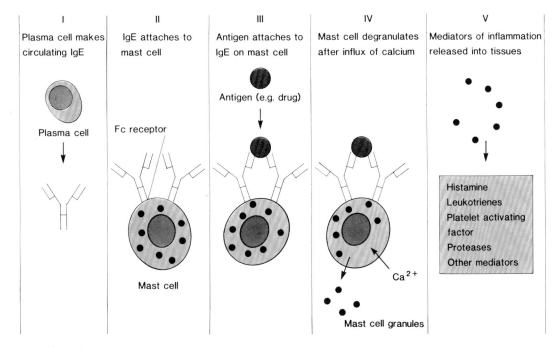

Fig. 3.2 Anaphylactic (type I) reaction.

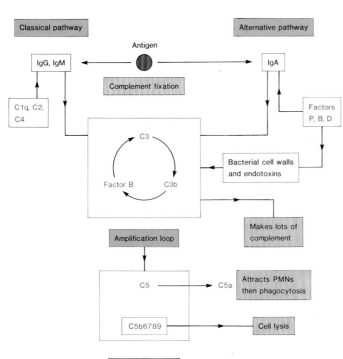

Fig. 3.3   Scheme of complement activation.

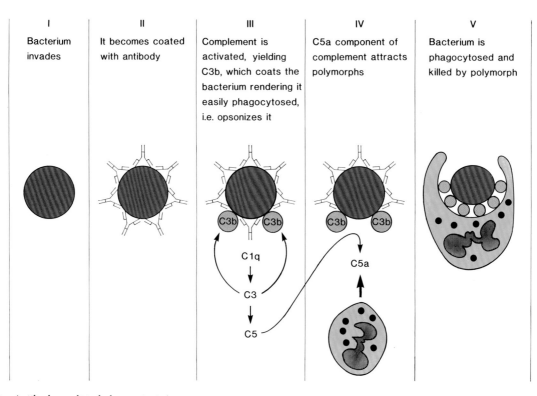

Fig. 3.4   Antibody-mediated phagocytosis (type II reaction).

Activation of either pathway produces C3b, the pivotal component of the complement system. Through the amplification loop, a single reaction can flood the area with C3b, C5a, and other amplification loop and terminal pathway components. Complement is the mediator of humoral reactions.

Humoral cytotoxic reactions are typical of defence against infectious agents such as bacteria. However, they also mediate certain auto-immune diseases such as pemphigoid (Chapter 13).

Occasionally antibodies bind to the surface of a cell and make it active without causing its death or activating complement. Instead, the cell is stimulated to produce a hormone-like substance which may mediate disease. Pemphigus (Chapter 13) is a blistering disease of skin in which this type of reaction is important. IgG antibodies react with an antigen on epidermal cells and induce them to release a proteolytic enzyme which dissolves the intercellular glue sticking the cells together. The keratinocytes fall apart from each other and the patient develops bullae and erosions.

Type III: immune complex disease

Antigen may combine with antibodies near vital tissues so that the ensuing inflammatory response damages them. When an antigen is injected intradermally, it combines with appropriate antibodies on the walls of blood vessels, complement is activated, and polymorphonuclear leucocytes are brought to the area (an Arthus reaction). Degranulation of polymorphs liberates lysosomal enzymes which damage the vessel walls.

Antigen–antibody complexes may also be formed in the circulation, move to the small vessels in the skin, and lodge there (Fig. 3.5). Complement will then be activated and inflammatory cells will injure

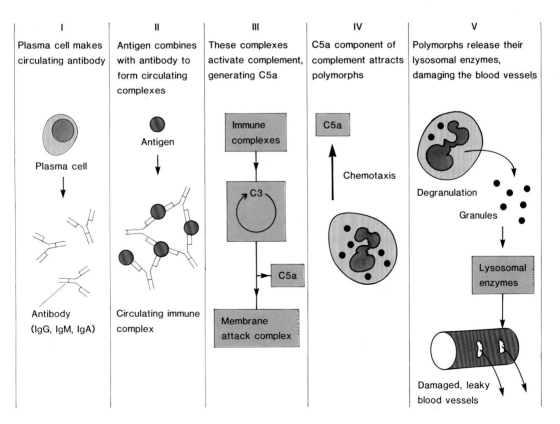

Fig. 3.5   Immune complex-mediated vasculitis (type III reaction).

THE PROCESS OF SENSITIZATION (AFFERENT LIMB OF IMMUNE RESPONSE)

I	II	III
Antigen is processed by an antigen–presenting cell, e.g. macrophage or Langerhans cell	Antigen associates with class II MHC antigen and is presented to T helper lymphocyte. Interleukin 1 is released by antigen–presenting cell and the immune response has now been triggered	T helper lymphocyte now secretes interleukin 2, expresses surface IL–2 receptors and proliferates. Daughter T cells, including memory cells, are generated

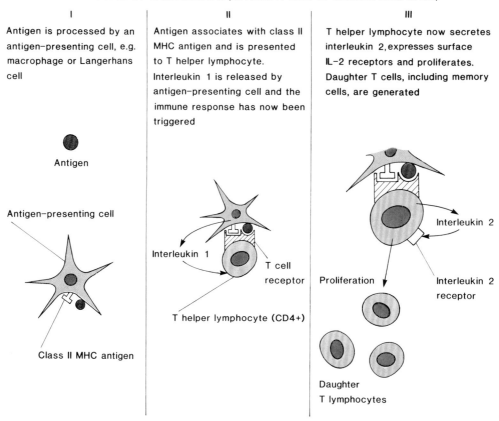

THE RESPONSE TO FURTHER ANTIGENIC CHALLENGE (EFFERENT LIMB)

IV

The memory T cell recognizes this antigen on re-exposure to it, but only after antigen has been processed and presented as in columns I and II. The memory T cell becomes activated and secretes lymphokines which induce the vascular and cellular components of inflammation

Activated T lymphocyte

Lymphokines
e.g. γ–Interferon
Migration inhibition factor
Chemotactic factors
Skin reactive factor
Interleukins 2 and 3
Macrophage activation factor

Recruited inflammatory cells

Fig. 3.6 Cell-mediated immune reaction (type IV reaction).

the vessels as in the Arthus reaction. This causes oedema and the extravasation of red blood cells — the palpable purpura which characterizes vasculitis (Chapter 12).

Type IV: cell-mediated immunity

As its name implies, this is mediated by lymphocytes rather than by antibodies. Sensitized lymphocytes entering the skin interact with antigens processed by antigen-presenting cells, such as macrophages and Langerhans cells (Fig. 3.6). The lymphocytes are stimulated to enlarge, divide, and to secrete soluble chemicals called lymphokines which can injure tissues directly and kill cells or microbes. Other lymphokines bring other inflammatory cells into the area. For example, macrophage activating factor (MAF) encourages macrophages to increase their phagocytic capacity, and macrophage migration inhibitory factor (MIF) immobilizes phagocytes at the site of inflammation.

Cell-mediated immune reactions are common in the defence against fungal and viral infections of the skin. They are also important in granulomatous reactions, delayed hypersensitivity reactions, and allergic contact dermatitis. They probably play a role in some photosensitive disorders, in protecting against cancer, and in mediating reactions to the bites of hostile or hungry insects.

In certain circumstances, some mononuclear cells can kill other cells directly. The cytotoxic/suppressor class of lymphocytes can attack cells bearing class I major histocompatibility antigens (*see below*) on their surfaces (e.g. as in some viral infections and graft rejection). K cells are a subset of lymphocytes which kill by antibody-dependent cellular cytotoxicity (Fig. 3.7). In this reaction, antibody binds to antigen on the surface of a target cell: the K cell binds to the antibody at its other (Fc) end. The antibody acts as a receptor for the K cell, which then kills its target. Natural killer cells (NK cells) are large granular lymphocytes which can kill tumour cells in the absence of specific antibodies or sensitization.

Granulomas are formed when cell-mediated immunity fails to eliminate antigen. Foreign body granulomas occur because a material remains undigested.

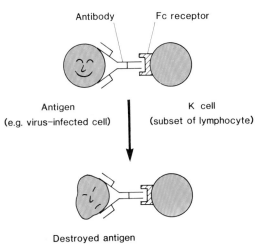

Fig. 3.7   Antibody-mediated cellular cytotoxicity.

Immunological granulomas require persistence of antigen, but the response is augmented by a cell-mediated immune reaction. Lymphokines, released by lymphocytes sensitized to the antigen, cause macrophages to differentiate into epithelioid cells and giant cells. These cells secrete other cytokines which influence inflammatory events. Immunological granulomas of the skin are characterized by Langhans giant cells (not to be confused with Langerhans cells; p. 11), epithelioid cells, and a surrounding mantle of lymphocytes.

Granulomatous reactions in the skin also arise when infectious organisms cannot be destroyed (e.g. in tuberculosis, leprosy, leishmaniasis), or when a chemical cannot be eliminated (e.g. zirconium or beryllium). Similar reactions are also seen in persisting inflammation of undetermined cause (e.g. in rosacea, granuloma annulare, sarcoidosis, and certain forms of panniculitis).

Histocompatibility

Like other cells in the body, those in the skin express surface antigens directed by genes of the major histocompatibility complex (HLA) on human chromosome 6. In particular, HLA A, B and C antigens (the class I antigens) are expressed on all nucleated cells including keratinocytes, Langerhans cells, and cells of the dermis. HLA-DR, -DP and -DQ antigens (the class II antigens) are expressed only on some cells. For example, they are poorly expressed on keratinocytes except during certain reactions (e.g. allergic contact dermatitis) or diseases (e.g. lichen planus). T cells recognize antigens only in the presence of cells bearing class II antigens. Class II antigens are also important for certain cell–cell interactions. On the other hand, class I antigens mark target cells for cell-mediated cytotoxic reactions such as the rejection of skin allografts and the destruction of cells infected by viruses.

Immunodeficiency

The immune system defends the host against infectious agents which threaten it; hence immunodeficiency often leads to cutaneous infection.

Immunodeficiency should be considered in the following circumstances:
- Recurrent infections, particularly when severe, extensive or of several organs.
- Failure to respond to appropriate antibiotics.
- Infection with ordinary organisms in unusual sites, especially when resistant to treatment.
- Infections with opportunistic organisms in any site.

- Prolonged infection with weight loss, failure to thrive, severe diarrhoea, or graft-versus-host reaction.
- Atypical syndromes mimicking lupus erythematosus.

Many chronic infections of the skin are due to favourable local conditions rather than to immunodeficiency. For example, fungal infections of the toe webs become chronic because the skin there is moist and ideal for fungal growth. Recurrent infection in many organs, however, is the hallmark of an immunodeficient state.

LEARNING POINTS

1 Many skin reactions are good examples of immune mechanisms at work.
2 However, beware of accepting that immunological events are the prime cause of any disorder. If *Treponema pallidum* had not been discovered, some immunologists would have included syphilis amongst the auto-immune disorders.

CHAPTER 4
DIAGNOSIS OF SKIN DISORDERS

The key to successful treatment is accurate diagnosis. This requires a careful history, a thorough physical examination, and the intelligent use of the laboratory.

Dermatology is different from other specialties because the diseases can easily be seen. Keen eyes, aided sometimes by a magnifying glass, are all that are needed for a complete examination of the skin. Often it is best to examine the patient briefly before obtaining a full history. A quick look will prompt the right questions.

History

The key points in the history are listed in Table 4.1 and should include a description of the events surrounding the onset of the skin lesions, and the progression of individual lesions and of the disease in general, including any responses to treatment. Many patients try a few salves before seeing a physician. Some try all the medications in their medicine cabinets, many of which can aggravate the problem. A careful inquiry into drugs taken for other conditions is often useful. Ask also about previous skin disorders, occupation, hobbies, and disorders in the family.

Examination

To examine the skin properly, the lighting must be uniform and bright. The patient should undress. Do not be put off this too easily by the elderly, the stub-

Table 4.1 Outline of dermatological history.

History of present skin condition ● Duration ● Site at onset, details of spread ● Itch ● Burning ● Pain ● Wet, dry, blisters	*General health at present*
Past history of skin disorders	*Past general medical history* ● Enquire specifically about asthma and hay fever
Family history of skin disorders	*Family history of other medical disorders*
Social and occupational history Should include details of: ● Hobbies ● Travels abroad	
Drugs used to treat present skin condition ● Topical ● Systemic ● Physician prescribed ● Patient initiated	*Drugs prescribed for other disorders* (including those taken before onset of skin

born, the shy, or the surroundings. Sometimes make-up must be washed off or wigs removed. There is nothing more embarrassing than missing the right diagnosis because clothing or make-up has obscured an important sign.

Distribution

Diagnosis in dermatology is based both on the distribution of lesions and on their morphology and configuration. For example, on inspection, an area of seborrhoeic dermatitis may look very like one of atopic dermatitis; but the key to diagnosis lies in their location. Seborrhoeic dermatitis affects the scalp, forehead, eyebrows, nasolabial folds, and central chest; atopic dermatitis typically affects the antecubital and popliteal fossae.

Determine if the skin disease is localized, universal, or symmetrical. Depending on the disease, or group of diseases, suggested by the morphology, you may want to check special areas, like the feet in a patient with hand eczema, or the gluteal cleft in a patient you think might have psoriasis. Examine as much of the skin as possible. Remember the old adage that if you do not look in the mouth, you will put your foot in it. Note negative as well as positive findings, for example the way the shielded areas are

spared in a photosensitive dermatitis. Always keep your eyes open for incidental skin cancers which the patient may have ignored.

Morphology

After the distribution has been noted, next define the morphology of the primary lesions. Many skin diseases have a characteristic morphology, but scratch marks, ulceration, and other events may later change this appearance. The rule is to find an early or 'primary' lesion and to inspect it closely. What is its shape? What is its size? What is its colour? What are its margins like? What are the surface characteristics?

Most types of primary lesion have one name if small, and a different one if large. The scheme is summarized in Table 4.2.

There are many reasons why you should describe skin diseases properly:
- Skin disorders are often grouped by their morphology. Once the morphology is clear, a differential diagnosis comes easily to mind.
- If you have to describe a condition accurately, you will have to look at it carefully.
- You can paint a verbal picture if you have to refer the patient for another opinion.

Table 4.2 Terminology of primary lesions.

	Small (less than 0.5 cm)	Large (greater than 0.5 cm)
Elevated solid lesions	Papule	Nodule (greater than 0.5 cm in both width and depth) Plaque (greater than 2 cm in width but without substantial depth)
Flat area of altered colour or texture	Macule	Large macule (patch)
Fluid-filled blister	Vesicle	Bulla
Pus-filled lesion	Pustule	Abscess
Extravasation of blood into skin	Petechia (pinhead size) Purpura (up to 2 mm in diameter)	Ecchymosis Haematoma
Accumulation of dermal oedema	Wheal (can be any size)	Angioedema

- You will sound like a physician and not a homoeopath.
- You will be able to understand the terminology of this book.

Terminology of lesions (Fig. 4.1)

Primary lesions

A *papule* is a small solid elevation of skin, less than 0.5 cm in diameter.

A *plaque* is an elevated area of skin greater than 2 cm in diameter but without substantial depth.

A *macule* is a small flat area of altered colour or texture.

A *vesicle* is a circumscribed elevation of skin, less than 0.5 cm in diameter, and containing fluid.

A *bulla* is a circumscribed elevation of skin over 0.5 cm in diameter and containing fluid.

A *pustule* is a visible accumulation of pus in the skin.

An *abscess* is a localized collection of pus in a cavity, more than 1 cm in diameter. Usually abscesses are nodules, and the term 'purulent bulla' is sometimes used to describe a pus-filled blister which is situated on top of the skin surface rather than in it.

A *wheal* is an elevated white compressible, evanescent area produced by dermal oedema. It is often surrounded by a red, axon-mediated flare. Although usually less than 2 cm in diameter, wheals may be huge.

Angioedema is a diffuse swelling of oedema which extends to the subcutaneous tissue.

A *nodule* is a solid mass in the skin, usually greater than 0.5 cm in diameter, which can be observed as an elevation or can be palpated.

A *tumour* is harder to define, as the term is based more correctly on microscopic pathology than on clinical morphology. We keep it here as a convenient term to describe an enlargement of the tissues by normal or pathological material or cells that form a mass, usually more than 1 cm in diameter. Because the word 'tumour' scares patients, tumours are courteously called 'large nodules', especially if they are not malignant.

A *papilloma* is a nipple-like mass projecting from the skin.

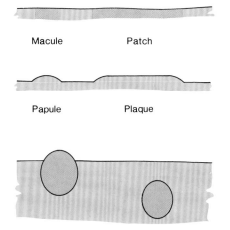

Macule   Patch

Papule   Plaque

Nodules may be exophytic (left) or endophytic (right)

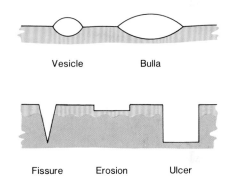

Vesicle   Bulla

Fissure   Erosion   Ulcer

Fig. 4.1   Terminology of skin lesions.

Petechiae are pinhead-sized macules of blood in the skin.

The term *purpura* describes a larger macule or papule of blood in the skin. Blood-filled lesions do not blanch if a glass lens is pushed against them (diascopy).

An *ecchymosis* is a larger extravasation of blood into the skin.

A *haematoma* is a swelling from gross bleeding.

A *burrow* is a linear or curvilinear papule, caused by a burrowing scabies mite.

A *comedo* is a plug of keratin and sebum wedged in a dilated pilosebaceous orifice. Open comedones are blackheads. The follicle opening of a closed comedo is nearly covered over by skin so that it looks like a pinhead-sized, ivory-coloured papule.

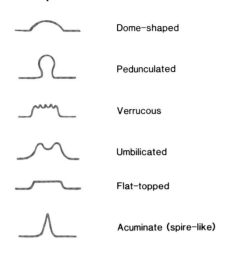

Dome-shaped

Pedunculated

Verrucous

Umbilicated

Flat-topped

Acuminate (spire-like)

Fig. 4.2 Surface contours of papules.

Telangiectasia is the visible dilatation of small cutaneous blood vessels.

Poikiloderma is a combination of atrophy, reticulate hyperpigmentation and telangiectasia.

Secondary lesions

These evolve from primary lesions.

A *scale* is a flake arising from the horny layer.

A *crust* may look like a scale, but is composed of dried blood or tissue fluid.

An *ulcer* is an area of skin from which the whole of the epidermis and at least the upper part of the dermis has been lost. Ulcers may extend into subcutaneous fat and heal with scarring.

An *excoriation* is an ulcer or erosion produced by scratching.

An *erosion* is an area of skin denuded by a complete or partial loss of the epidermis. Erosions heal without scarring.

A *fissure* is a slit in the skin.

A *sinus* is a cavity or channel that permits the escape of pus or fluid.

A *scar* is a result of healing, where normal structures are permanently replaced by fibrous tissue.

Atrophy is a thinning of skin due to diminution of the epidermis, dermis or subcutaneous fat. When the epidermis is atrophic it may crinkle like cigarette paper, appear thin and translucent, and lose normal surface markings. Blood vessels may be easy to see in both epidermal and dermal atrophy.

A *stria* is a streak-like, linear, atrophic, pink, purple or white lesion of the skin due to changes in the connective tissue.

Pigmentation, either more or less than surrounding skin, may develop after lesions heal.

Having identified the lesions as primary or secondary, adjectives can be used to describe them in terms of their:
- Colour (e.g. salmon-pink, lilac, violet).
- Sharpness of edge (e.g. well-defined, ill-defined).
- Surface contour (e.g. dome-shaped, umbilicated, spike-like) (Fig. 4.2).
- Geometric shape (e.g. nummular, oval, resembling the coast of Maine).
- Texture (e.g. rough, silky, smooth, hard).
- Smell (e.g. foul-smelling).
- Temperature (e.g. hot, warm).

Dermatologists also use a few special adjectives which warrant definition. *Nummular* means round or coin-like. *Annular* means ring-like. *Circinate* means circular. *Arcuate* means curved. *Discoid* means disc-like. *Gyrate* means wave-like. *Retiform* and *reticulate* mean net-like.

To describe a skin lesion, use the term for the primary lesion as the noun, and the adjectives mentioned above to define it. For example, the lesions of psoriasis may appear as 'salmon-pink, sharply demarcated, nummular plaques covered by large, silver, polygonal scales'.

Try not to use the term 'lesion'. Why say 'papular lesion' when you can say papule? It is almost as bad as the well worn 'skin rash'. By the way, there are very few diseases that are truly 'maculopapular'. The term is best avoided except to describe certain drug eruptions and viral exanthems. Even then, the terms 'scarlatiniform' (like scarlet fever — punctate, slightly elevated papules) or 'morbilliform' (like measles — a net-like, blotchy, slightly elevated, pink, exanthem) are more helpful.

Configuration

After unravelling the primary and secondary lesions, look for arrangements and configurations which are, for example, discrete, confluent, grouped, annular, arcuate, linear and dermatomal (Fig. 4.3). Note that

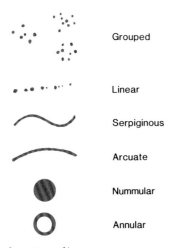

Grouped

Linear

Serpiginous

Arcuate

Nummular

Annular

Fig. 4.3 Configuration of lesions.

while individual lesions may be annular, several individual lesions may arrange themselves into an annular configuration. Terms like annular, and other adjectives discussed under the morphology of individual lesions, may therefore apply to their groupings too.

Special tools and techniques

A *magnifying lens* is a helpful aid to diagnosis because subtle changes in the skin become more apparent when enlarged.

Skin lesions can also be examined using long-wave ultraviolet radiation emitted by a *Wood's light*. By demonstrating fluorescence, Wood's light may help in the diagnosis of fungus infections (Chapter 15), subtle disorders of pigmentation, erythrasma (p. 136), *Pseudomonas* infections, and pityriasis versicolor (p. 162).

In *diascopy*, a glass slide or clear plastic spoon is used to blanch vascular lesions and so to unmask their true colour.

Assessment

Next try to put the disease into a general class. The titles of the chapters in this book are representative. Once classified, a differential diagnosis is usually forthcoming. Each diagnosis can then be considered on its merits, and laboratory tests may be used to

confirm or refute diagnoses in the differential list. *At this stage you must make a working diagnosis or formulate a plan to do so!*

Side-room and office tests

A number of tests can be performed in the practice or office with results immediately available:

Potassium hydroxide preparations for fungal infections

If a fungal infection is suspected, scales or hair pluckings can be dissolved in an aqueous solution of 20% potassium hydroxide (KOH) containing 40% dimethyl sulphoxide (DMSO). The scale from the edge of a scaling lesion is vigorously scraped with a No. 15 scalpel blade. Other samples can include nail clippings, the roofs from tops of blisters, hair pluckings and the contents of pustules when a candidal infection is suspected. The specimen is transferred to a slide and a drop or two of KOH solution is added before applying the coverslip. After 5–10 minutes, with the exception of nail clippings which take an hour or so to clear, the mount is examined under a microscope with the condenser lens lowered to increase contrast. With experience, fungal and candidal hyphae can be readily detected (Fig. 4.4). No heat is required if DMSO is included in the KOH solution.

Fig. 4.4 Fungal hyphae in a KOH preparation.

Detection of scabies mite

The finding of burrows in an itchy patient is diagnostic of scabies. The retrieval of a mite from the skin will confirm the diagnosis and convince a sceptical patient of the infestation. The burrow should be examined under a magnifying glass; the acarus may be seen as a tiny black or grey dot at the most recent, least scaly end. It can be removed by a sterile needle and placed on a slide within a marked circle. Alternatively, if mites are not seen, questionable burrows are vigorously scraped with a No. 15 scalpel blade, moistened with liquid paraffin or vegetable oil, and the scrapings transferred to a slide. Patients never argue the toss when confronted by a magnified mobile mite.

Cell cytology (Tzank smear)

Cell cytology can aid diagnosis of viral infections like herpes simplex and zoster, and bullous diseases such as pemphigus. A blister roof is removed and the cells from the base of the blister are scraped off with a curved surgical blade. The cells are smeared on to a microscope slide, air-dried and fixed with methanol. They are then stained with Giemsa, toludine blue, or Wright's stain. Acantholytic cells (Chapter 11) are seen in pemphigus and multinucleate giant cells are diagnostic of herpes simplex or varicella zoster infections (Chapter 15).

Patch tests

Patch tests are invaluable in detecting allergens responsible for allergic contact dermatitis (Chapter 9). Either suspected antigens or a battery of antigens which are common culprits are tested (Fig. 4.5). Standard dilutions of the common antigens in appropriate bases are available commercially. The test materials are applied to the back under aluminium discs or patches; the occlusion encourages penetration of the allergen. The patches are left in place for 48 hours and then, after careful marking, are removed. The sites are inspected then and again at 96 hours. The test detects type IV delayed hypersensitivity reactions (Chapter 3). The readings are scored according to the reaction seen:

Not tested	NT
No reaction	o
Doubtful (minimal/marginal) reaction	±
Weak (non-vesicular) reaction	+
Strong (vesicular or oedematous) reaction	+ +
Extreme reaction	+ + +
Irritant reaction	IR

A positive patch test does not prove that this substance is the cause of the current episode of contact dermatitis; the results must be interpreted in the light of the history and possible previous exposure to the allergen.

Patch testing requires attention to detail in applying the patches properly and skill and experience in interpreting the results.

Fig. 4.5 Patch testing equipment. Syringe contains commercially prepared antigen, to be applied in aluminium cups.

Prick testing

Prick testing is much less helpful in dermatology. It detects immediate (type I) hypersensitivity (Chapter 3). Commercially prepared diluted antigens and a control are placed as single drops on marked areas of the forearm. The skin is gently pricked through the drop and the drop removed with a tissue wipe. The prick should not cause bleeding. After 10 minutes the sites are inspected and the diameter of any wheal measured and recorded. Like patch testing, prick testing is not recommended for those without formal training in the procedure. The relevance of positive results to the cause of the condition under investigation (usually urticaria or atopic dermatitis) is often debatable.

Skin biopsy

Skin biopsy is easily performed. There are two main types, punch and scalpel biopsy.

Punch biopsy

The skin is sampled with a small (3 – 4 mm diameter) tissue punch. Xylocaine 1% is injected intradermally first, and a cylinder of skin is incised with the punch by rotating it back and forth. It is lifted up carefully with a needle or forceps and the base is cut off at the level of subcutaneous fat. The biopsy must not be crushed with the forceps or critical histological patterns may be squashed.

The tissue can be sent to the pathologist with a summary of the history, a differential diagnosis, and the patient's age. Close liaison with the pathologist is essential, because the diagnosis may only become apparent with knowledge of *both* the clinical and histological features.

Scalpel biopsy

This provides more tissue than a punch biopsy. This technique can be used routinely, but is especially useful for biopsying disorders of the subcutaneous fat and for obtaining specimens with both normal and abnormal skin for comparison. After selecting the lesion for biopsy, an elliptical piece of skin is excised. The specimen should include the subcutaneous fat. Removing the specimen with forceps may cause crush artefact; this can be avoided by lifting the specimen with either a Gillies hook or a syringe needle. The wound is then sutured; firm compression for five minutes stops oozing. 3/0 non-absorbable sutures are used for biopsies on the legs and back, 5/0 for the face, and 4/0 for elsewhere. Stitches are usually removed from the face in four days, from the anterior trunk and arms in seven days, and from the back and legs in ten days. Some guidelines for skin biopsies are listed in Table 4.3.

Table 4.3   Guidelines for skin biopsies.

- Sample a fresh lesion
- Obtain specimen from near the lesion's edge
- Avoid sites where a scar would be conspicuous
- Avoid the upper trunk or jawline where keloids are more likely to form
- Avoid the legs, where healing is slow
- Avoid lesions over bony prominences, where infection is more likely
- Use the scalpel technique for diagnosing scalp disorders and diseases of the subcutaneous fat or vessels
- Do not crush the tissue
- Place in proper fixative
- If two lesions are sampled, be sure they do not get mixed up or mislabelled. Label specimen containers *before* biopsy is placed in them
- Make sure that patient's name, age and sex is clearly indicated on the pathology form
- Provide the pathologist with a legible summary of the history, the site of the biopsy, and a differential diagnosis
- Discuss the results with the pathologist

Laboratory tests

The laboratory is vital for the accurate diagnosis of many skin disorders. Tests include various assays of blood and serum, bacterial, fungal and viral culture from skin and other specimens, immunofluorescent and immunohistological examinations (Figs. 4.6 and 4.7), X-radiology, and other methods of image intensification. Specific details will be discussed as each disease is presented.

Treatment

This is the easiest part, but only if the diagnosis is correct. You can look up treatments, but you cannot look up diagnoses. Without a diagnosis, you will be asking 'what's a good treatment for scaling feet?'

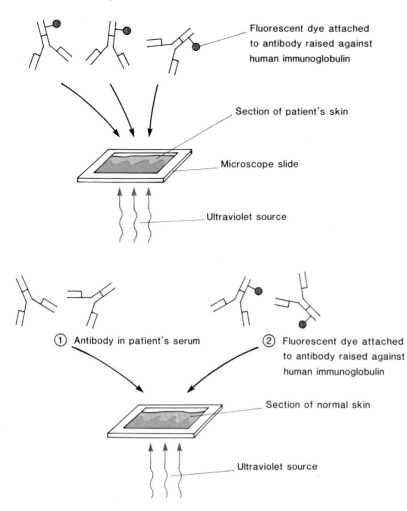

Fluorescent dye attached to antibody raised against human immunoglobulin

Section of patient's skin

Microscope slide

Ultraviolet source

Fig. 4.6 Direct immunofluorescence detects antibodies in patient's skin. Here IgG antibodies are detected by staining with a fluorescent dye attached to antihuman IgG.

① Antibody in patient's serum

② Fluorescent dye attached to antibody raised against human immunoglobulin

Section of normal skin

Ultraviolet source

Fig. 4.7 Indirect immunofluorescence detects antibodies in patient's serum. There are two steps:
1 Antibodies in this serum are made to bind to antigens in a section of normal skin.
2 Antibody raised against human immunoglobulin, conjugated with a fluorescent dye can then be used to stain these bound antibodies (as in the direct immunofluorescence test).

instead of 'what's good for tinea pedis?' (Would you ever ask yourself 'what's a good treatment for chest pain?') Once the diagnosis has been made, the treatment should take this into account, and also the age of the patient, the severity of the disorder, its extent, the disability it causes, the safety of the useful drugs, the cost of the drugs or treatments, and the likelihood of compliance with a treatment regimen. The patient's lifestyle should not be changed unless absolutely necessary.

Summary

Clinical dermatology is a visual specialty. You must see the disease and know what you see. Look closely and thoroughly. Take time. Examine the whole body. Locate primary lesions and check configuration and distribution. Ask appropriate questions, especially if the diagnosis is difficult. Classify the disorder and list the differential diagnosis. Use the history, examination, and laboratory tests to make a diagnosis. Then treat. Refer the patient if:
- You cannot make a diagnosis.
- The disorder does not respond to treatment.
- The disorder is unusual or severe.
- You are just not sure.

LEARNING POINTS

1 The term 'skin rash' is as bad as 'gastric stomach'.

2 Do not use long Latin descriptive names as a cloak for ignorance.

3 The history becomes more important when the diagnosis is difficult.

4 Undress patients and use a lens, even it it only gives you more time to think.

CHAPTER 5

DISORDERS OF KERATINIZATION

The complex but orderly process of keratinization has been described on p. 6. In it, the living cells of the deeper epidermis are transformed into the dead cornified cells of the stratum corneum, from which they are shed in such a way that the surface of the normal skin does not seem scaly to the naked eye. In addition, shedding balances production, so that the thickness of the stratum corneum does not alter. If, however, the process of keratinization is abnormal, the stratum corneum may become thick or the surface of the skin may become dry and scaly. Such changes may be localized or generalized.

In this chapter we describe several skin disorders, mostly unrelated, which have as their basis a disorder of keratinization.

The ichthyoses

The word ichthyosis comes from the Greek word for a fish. It is applied to disorders which share, as their main feature, marked scaling in the absence of inflammation. Strictly speaking the scales lack the overlapping pattern of those of a fish, but the term is usefully descriptive and too well entrenched to be discarded. There are several types.

Ichthyosis vulgaris

Cause
Inherited as an autosomal dominant, this condition is common and affects about one person in 300.

Presentation
The dryness is usually mild and symptoms are few.

The scales are small and branny, most obvious on the limbs and least obvious in the major flexures. The skin creases of the palm may be accentuated. Keratosis pilaris (p. 38) is often present on the limbs.

Clinical course
The skin changes are usually not present at birth but develop over the first few years of life. Some patients improve in adult life, particularly during warm weather, but the condition seldom clears fully.

Complications
The already dry skin tends to chap in the winter and to be easily irritated by degreasing agents. This should be taken into account in the choice of a career. This type of ichthyosis is apt to appear in a stubborn combination with atopic eczema.

Differential diagnosis
It can usually be distinguished from less common types of ichthyosis on the basis of the pattern of inheritance and of the type and distribution of the scaling.

Investigations
None are usually needed.

Treatment
This is palliative. The dryness can be helped by the regular use of emollients which are best applied after a shower or bath. Emulsifying ointment, soft white paraffin, E45 and unguentum merck are all quite suitable (Formulary, p. 245), and the selection depends on the patient's preference. Many find

proprietary bath oils and creams containing urea or lactic acid helpful also (Formulary, p. 245).

Sex-linked ichthyosis

Cause
This less common type of ichthyosis is inherited as a sex-linked recessive and therefore, in its complete form, is seen only in males, though some female carriers may show mild scaling. The condition affects some 1 in 6000 males in the U.K. and is associated with a deficiency of the enzyme aryl sulphatase which hydrolyses cholesterol sulphate.

Presentation and course
In contrast to the delayed onset of the dominantly inherited ichthyosis vulgaris, scaling appears early, often soon after birth, and always by the first birthday. The scales are larger and browner (Fig. 5.1), and involve the major flexures as well as the skin generally. There is no association with atopy or keratosis pilaris. The condition persists throughout life.

Complications
Corneal opacities may appear in adult life.

Differential diagnosis
As for ichthyosis vulgaris. It is helpful to remember that only males are affected.

Fig. 5.1 Ichthyosis: large rather dark scales suggest the less common type inherited as a sex-linked recessive, though the sparing of the axilla may be against this.

Investigations
None are usually needed. A few centres can measure aryl sulphatase in fibroblasts cultured from a skin biopsy and lipoprotein electrophoresis may disclose a fast-migrating sulphated beta-lipoprotein.

Treatment
Oral aromatic retinoids are probably best avoided. Topical measures are as for ichthyosis vulgaris.

Collodion baby
This is a description and not a diagnosis. The bizarre skin changes are seen at birth. At first the stratum corneum is smooth and shiny, and the skin looks as though it has been covered with cellophane or collodion. Its tightness may cause ectropion and feeding difficulties. The shiny outer surface is shed within a few days leaving behind, most often, a lamellar ichthyosis, less often an X-linked ichthyosis, and occasionally a normal skin.

Lamellar ichthyosis
This rare condition, affecting perhaps one person in 600 000, is probably inherited as an autosomal recessive. The skin changes at birth are those of a collodion baby (*see above*). After this phase the skin remains red (Fig. 5.2); later the redness tends to fade, but an ugly thickening and scaliness appears, particularly in the flexures. Ectropion is often present. Scalp hair may be absent. The condition lasts for life, and is often sufficiently disfiguring for the

Fig. 5.2 Lamellar ichthyosis in a neonate.

long-term use of etretinate to be justifiable (Formulary, p. 260).

Epidermolytic hyperkeratosis (bullous ichthyosiform erythroderma)
This rare condition is inherited as an autosomal dominant. Shortly after birth the baby's skin becomes generally red and shows numerous blisters. The redness fades over a few months, and the tendency to blister also lessens, but during childhood a gross brownish warty hyperkeratosis appears, sometimes in a roughly linear form and usually worst in the flexures. The histology is distinctive: a thickened granular cell layer contains large granules, and clefts may be seen in the upper epidermis. A few patients have localized areas of hyperkeratosis with the same histological features. Treatment is symptomatic and antibiotics may be needed if the blisters become infected. Etretinate (Formulary, p. 260) may be tried in severe cases.

Other ichthyosiform disorders
Sometimes ichthyotic skin changes are a minor part of a multisystem disease, but such associations are very rare. *Refsum's syndrome*, an autosomal recessive trait, is due to deficiency of a single enzyme concerned in the breakdown of phytanic acid, which accumulates in the tissues. The other features (retinal degeneration, peripheral neuropathy and ataxia) overshadow the minor dryness of the skin.

Rud's syndrome is an ichthyosiform erythroderma in association with mental retardation and epilepsy. In *Netherton's syndrome*, brittle hairs, with a so-called 'bamboo deformity', are present with a curious gyrate and erythematous hyperkeratotic eruption (ichthyosis linearis circumflexa).

Acquired ichthyosis
It is unusual for ichthyosis to appear for the first time in adult life: if it does, an underlying disease should be suspected. The most frequent is Hodgkin's disease. Other recorded causes include other lymphomata, leprosy, sarcoidosis, malabsorption and a poor diet. The skin may also appear dry in hypothyroidism.

Fig. 5.3 The distribution of keratosis pilaris lesions.

Other disorders of keratinization

Keratosis pilaris

Cause
This common condition is inherited as an autosomal dominant trait. The abnormality lies in the keratinization of hair follicles which become filled with horny plugs.

Presentation and course
The changes begin in childhood and tend to become less obvious in adult life. In the commonest type, the greyish horny follicular plugs are confined to the outer aspects of the thighs and upper arms, where the skin feels rough (Fig. 5.3). Less often the plugs affect the sides of the face and the eyebrows. There is an association with ichthyosis vulgaris.

Complications
Involvement of the cheeks may lead to an ugly pitted scarring. Rarely the follicles in the eyebrows may be damaged with subsequent loss of hair there.

Differential diagnosis

A rather similar pattern of widespread follicular keratosis (phrynoderma) can occur in severe vitamin deficiency. The lack is probably not just of vitamin A, as was once thought, but of several vitamins.

Investigations

None are needed.

Treatment

Keratolytics such as salicylic acid or urea in a cream base may be helpful though not curative (Formulary, p. 247).

Keratosis follicularis (Darier's disease)

Cause

This rare condition is inherited as an autosomal dominant trait. Fertility tends to be low and many cases represent new mutations. The basic defect is not fully understood but seems to involve tonofibrils and desmosomes.

Presentation

The first signs usually appear in the mid-teens, sometimes after overexposure to sunlight. The characteristic lesions are small, pink and brownish papules with a greasy scale. These tend to coalesce into warty plaques in a 'seborrhoeic' distribution (Fig. 5.4).

Fig. 5.4 Darier's disease.

Fig. 5.5 The nail in Darier's disease. One or more longitudinal, pale or pink stripes run over the lunula to the free margin where they end in a triangular nick.

The severity of the condition varies greatly from person to person: early lesions are often seen on the sternal and interscapular areas, and behind the ears. In severe cases the skin may be widely affected, and the abnormalities remain for life, often causing much embarrassment and discomfort.

Other changes include lesions looking like plane warts on the backs of the hands, punctate keratoses or pits on the palms and soles, and a distinctive nail dystrophy in which linear white or pinkish lines or ridges run longitudinally to the free edge of the nail where they end in triangular nicks (Fig. 5.5).

Complications

Some patients are stunted and of poor intelligence. An impairment of delayed hypersensitivity may be the basis for a tendency to develop widespread herpes simplex and bacterial infections. Bacterial overgrowth is responsible for the unpleasant smell of some severely affected patients.

Differential diagnosis

The distribution of the lesions may be similar to that of seborrhoeic eczema, but discrete warty papules are not seen in this condition. The distribution differs from that of acanthosis nigricans (mainly flexural) and of keratosis pilaris (favours the outer upper arms and thighs).

Investigations

The diagnosis should be confirmed by a skin biopsy which will show characteristic clefts in the epidermis, and dyskeratotic cells.

Treatment

Severe and disabling disease can be dramatically alleviated by long-term etretinate (Formulary, p. 260). Milder cases need only topical keratolytics, such as salicylic acid, and the control of local infection (Formulary, p. 247).

Fig. 5.7 Keratoderma climactericum — thickly keratotic skin, especially around the heels. Painful fissures are a problem.

> LEARNING POINTS
>
> 1 Life has been a living death for some patients with severe congenital disorders of keratinization. For them retinoids, used carefully, are the greatest advance in medicine.
> 2 The side effects of systemic retinoids preclude their use in minor disorders of keratinization.

Keratoderma of the palms and soles

Inherited types
Many genodermatoses share keratoderma of the palms and soles as their main feature. They cannot be described in detail here. The clinical patterns and modes of inheritance vary from family to family: punctate, striate, diffuse and mutilating varieties have been documented, sometimes in association with metabolic disorders such as tyrosinaemia, or with changes elsewhere.

The commonest pattern is a diffuse one, known also as tylosis (Fig. 5.6), which is inherited as an

autosomal dominant trait. In a few families these changes have been associated with carcinoma of the oesophagus, but in most families this is not the case.

Treatment tends to be unsatisfactory but keratolytics such as salicylic acid and urea can be used in higher concentrations on the palms and soles than elsewhere (Formulary, p. 247).

Acquired types
It is not uncommon for normal people to have a few inconspicuous punctate keratoses on their palms, but it is no longer thought that these relate to internal malignancy.

Keratoderma of the palms and soles may be part of the picture of some generalized skin diseases such as pityriasis rubra pilaris (p. 57) and lichen planus (p. 55).

A distinctive pattern (*keratoderma climactericum*) is sometimes seen in middle-aged women at about the time of the menopause. It is most marked around the borders of the heels where painful fissures form and may interfere with walking (Fig. 5.7). Regular paring and the use of keratolytic ointments is often more helpful than attempts at hormone replacement, and the condition tends to settle over a few years.

Knuckle pads

Cause
Sometimes these are familial; most often they are not. Trauma seems not to be important.

Fig. 5.6 Tylosis.

Presentation
Fibromatous and hyperkeratotic areas appear on the backs of many finger joints, usually beginning in late childhood and persisting thereafter. There may be an association with Dupuytren's contracture.

Differential diagnosis
Occupational callosities, granuloma annulare and viral warts should be considered.

Investigations
A biopsy may be helpful in the few cases of genuine clinical difficulty.

Treatment
None, including surgery, is satisfactory.

Callosities and corns
Both are responses to pressure. A callosity is a more diffuse type of thickening of the keratin layer which seems to be a protective response to widely applied repeated friction or pressure. Callosities are often occupational, for example they are seen on the hands of manual workers. Usually painless, they need no therapy.

Corns, on the other hand, have a central core of hard keratin which can hurt if forced inwards. They appear where there is high local pressure, often between bony prominences and shoes. Favourite areas include the backs of the toe joints, and the soles under prominent metatarsals. 'Soft corns' arise in the third or fourth toe clefts when the toes are squeezed together by tight shoes; such corns are often macerated.

The main differential is from hyperkeratotic warts, but these will show tiny bleeding points when pared down. A corn, however, has only its hard compacted avascular core surrounded by a more diffuse thickening of opalescent keratin.

The right treatment for corns is to eliminate the pressure which caused them, but patients may be slow to accept this. However, while regular paring may reduce the symptoms temporarily, well-fitting shoes are essential. Corns under the metatarsals may be helped by using soft spongy soles, but sometimes need orthopaedic alteration of weight bearing. Especial care is needed for corns on ischaemic or diabetic feet, which are at greater risk of infection and ulceration.

CHAPTER 6
PSORIASIS

Psoriasis is a chronic, non-infectious, inflammatory disease of the skin, characterized by well-defined erythematous plaques bearing large, adherent, silvery scales. One to three per cent of most populations have psoriasis, which may be most common in Europe and North America, and least common in black people. It may start at any age but is rare under 10 years, and commonest between 15 and 40. Its course is unpredictable but is usually chronic with exacerbations and remissions.

Cause and pathogenesis

The cause remains unknown. There is often a genetic predisposition, and the disease is sometimes triggered by an outside factor. Some biochemical abnormalities are described below under separate headings but undoubtedly interact.

1   Genetics
A child with one affected parent has a 25% chance of developing the disease, and this rises to 60% if both parents are affected. If non-psoriatic parents have a child with psoriasis, the risk for subsequent children is about 20%. Inheritance may be polygenic but an autosomal dominant trait with incomplete penetrance is also possible.

The idea of a 'psoriatic tendency' gained scientific merit when a strong association between the disease and certain antigens of the major histocompatibility complex was found, e.g. HLA-CW6 and those HLA antigens linked with CW6, e.g. B13, B16, B17, B27, B37 and DR7.

2   Epidermal cell kinetics
In psoriasis there is increased epidermal proliferation due both to an excessive number of geminative cells entering the cell cycle, and to a decrease in cell cycle time. The transit time of cells through the viable epidermis is greatly shortened, to two days as compared to 14 days in normal skin, and the epidermal turnover time falls from 28 days to five or six days. This epidermal hyperproliferation accounts for many of the metabolic abnormalities associated with psoriasis.

3   Altered epidermal maturation
During normal keratinization the molecular weights of keratins change as a cell moves from the basal layer (MW 55 and 60 kD) towards the surface (MW 70 kD). Some 30% of the keratin in a normal epidermis is of MW 70 kD but this falls to about 7% in psoriasis. This defect is secondary and non-specific, merely a result of increased epidermal proliferation.

4   Arachidonic acid metabolism (Fig. 6.1)
Arachidonic acid is bound to cell membranes and released from them by the activity of phospholipase A_2. Levels of arachidonic acid, and of its metabolites prostaglandin $E_2(PGE_2)$, leukotriene $B_4(LTB_4)$, 12-hydroxyeicosatetraenoic acid (12-HETE), and 15-HETE are elevated in the lesional skin of psoriasis. It is uncertain how these chemicals influence cell proliferation, though 12-HETE and other intermediates may inhibit adenylate cyclase and lower intracellular cyclic AMP (cAMP) (*see below*). LTB_4 attracts polymorphs strongly, and may be responsible for the micro-abscesses which are a feature of the histology (*see below*).

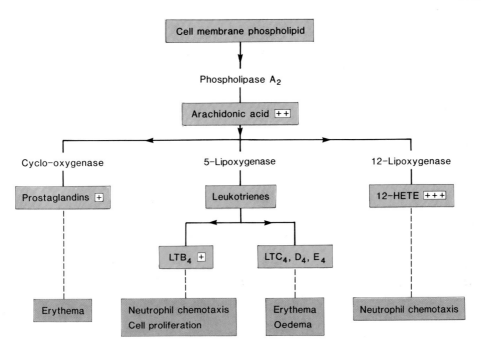

Fig. 6.1 Arachidonic acid and some of its metabolites in psoriasis. Arrows indicate those which are raised in lesional as compared with normal skin.

5 Cyclic nucleotides

There is some evidence that cAMP levels are decreased, while cyclic guanosine monophosphate (cGMP) levels are increased in the lesions of psoriasis. β-blockers, such as practolol and propanolol, may worsen psoriasis by decreasing cAMP levels. Similarly, lithium exacerbates psoriasis and inhibits cAMP formation.

6 Polyamines

The biosynthesis of the polyamines putrescine, spermidine and spermine is intimately associated with cellular proliferation. Levels of the enzyme ornithine decarboxylase, catalysing the reaction ornithine to putrescine, are raised in the lesions of psoriasis, and the levels of the above polyamines are therefore elevated in lesional skin.

7 Proteases and antiproteases

Proteases (e.g. plasminogen activator, cathepsins and certain complement components), and certain protease inhibitors (e.g. α_1-antitrypsin and B_2-macro-

globulin), regulate cell proliferation. Plasminogen activator is greatly increased in the lesions of psoriasis and parallels the mitotic rate; this increase may be due to deficiency of an inhibitor. Plasminogen activator is normally released following experimental injury, and in psoriasis its release could lead to the Koebner phenomenon.

8 Calmodulin

The level of the specific receptor protein for calcium, calmodulin, is greatly raised in lesions of psoriasis and falls with successful treatment. Interestingly, two drugs which help in psoriasis, dithranol and cyclosporin A, are calmodulin antagonists. The calcium–calmodulin complex, by influencing the activity of phospholipase A_2 (Fig. 6.1) and phosphodiesterase (catalyses cAMP to AMP), may regulate cell proliferation abnormally in psoriasis.

9 Immunopathology

Many immunological abnormalities have been found in psoriasis but it has still to be proven that immune events play a primary role in the disease. Circulating antibodies to the horny layer have been found in psoriatics, but can also be present in normal people. On the other hand, circulating antibodies to the basal cell nuclei of psoriatic lesions have been found only in psoriatics. Injury to the skin may unmask hidden antigens and cause circulating horny layer antibodies and circulating immune complexes to be deposited in the epidermis, thereby activating complement which would attract neutrophils to the area (p. 22). The dermal mononuclear infiltrate in psoriasis is mainly of T lymphocytes, most of which are of the helper type. The beneficial effect of cyclosporin A in psoriasis may be due to its anti-T helper cell effect, hinting at a significant role for T lymphocytes in the pathogenesis of the disease. While cyclosporin A helps psoriasis, AIDS worsens it.

10   The dermis
The dermis is abnormal in psoriasis. When psoriatic skin is grafted onto athymic mice, both epidermis and dermis must be present for the graft to sustain its psoriasis. The dermal capillary loops in psoriatic plaques are abnormally dilated and tortuous, and these changes come before epidermal hyperplasia. Fibroblasts from psoriatics replicate more rapidly *in vitro* and produce more glycosaminoglycans than do those from non-psoriatics.

Precipitating factors

These include:
1 Trauma — in active psoriasis, lesions appear in skin damaged by scratches or surgical wounds (Koebner phenomenon) (Fig. 6.2).
2 Infection — beta-haemolytic streptococcal tonsillitis often triggers guttate psoriasis.
3 Sunlight — most psoriatics improve but 10% become worse.
4 Drugs — antimalarials, β-blockers, and lithium may worsen psoriasis. Psoriasis may 'rebound' after treatment with systemic steroids or potent topical steroids.
5 Emotion — emotional upsets seem to cause some exacerbations.

Fig. 6.2   Koebner phenomenon. Linear plaques of psoriasis, following scratching due to previous scabies.

Histology (Fig. 6.3)

The main changes are:
1 Parakeratosis (nuclei retained in the horny layer).
2 Irregular thickening of the epidermis; but thinning over dermal papillae is apparent clinically when bleeding is caused by scratching and the removal of scales.
3 Polymorphonuclear leucocyte microabscesses (described originally by Munro).
4 Dilated and tortuous capillary loops in the dermal papillae.
5 T lymphocyte infiltrate in upper dermis.

Presentation

Common patterns

Plaque pattern
This is the most common type. Lesions are well demarcated and range from a few millimetres to several centimetres in diameter (Figs. 6.4 and 6.5). The lesions are pink or red with large, dry silvery-

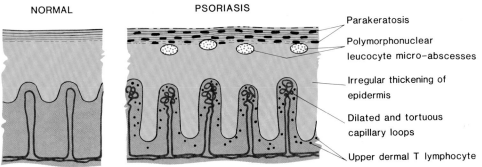

NORMAL   PSORIASIS

Parakeratosis

Polymorphonuclear
leucocyte micro-abscesses

Irregular thickening of
epidermis

Dilated and tortuous
capillary loops

Upper dermal T lymphocyte
infiltrate

Fig. 6.3   Histology of psoriasis compared with normal skin.

white scales (like candle grease). The elbows, knees, lower back, and scalp are sites of predilection (Fig. 6.6).

Guttate pattern
This is usually seen in children and adolescents and may be the first sign of the disease, often triggered by tonsillitis. Numerous small round red macules come up suddenly on the trunk and soon become scaly (Fig. 6.7). The rash often clears in a few months but plaque psoriasis may develop later.

Scalp
The scalp is often involved. Areas of scaling are interspersed with normal skin; their lumpiness is more

Fig. 6.5   Widespread plaques with coalescing lesions on chest.

Fig. 6.4   Extensive plaque psoriasis.

Fig. 6.6   Sharply defined plaques on elbows.

Fig. 6.7   Guttate lesions on trunk and plaques on elbow.

Fig. 6.8   Scalp psoriasis. The extent and associated marked hair loss are unusual.

Fig. 6.9   Psoriasis of scalp margin.

Fig. 6.10   Thimble-like pitting of nails with minor onycholysis.

Fig. 6.11   Onycholysis and coarse pitting of little finger nail.

Fig. 6.12   Gross subungual hyperkeratosis.

easily felt than seen (Fig. 6.8). Frequently there is an overflow just beyond the scalp margin (Fig. 6.9). Significant hair loss is rare.

Nails

Involvement of the nails is common, with 'thimble pitting' (Fig. 6.10), onycholysis (separation of the nail from the nail bed) (Fig 6.11) and sometimes sub-ungual hyperkeratosis (Fig. 6.12).

Flexures

Psoriasis of the submammary, axillary and anogenital folds is not scaly though the glistening sharply demarcated red plaques (Fig. 6.13), often with fissuring in the depth of the fold, are still readily recognizable. Flexural psoriasis is commonest in women and in the elderly.

Palms

Palmar psoriasis may be hard to recognize as its lesions are often poorly demarcated and barely erythematous.

Less common patterns

Napkin psoriasis

A psoriasiform spread outside the napkin (nappy/diaper) area may give the first clue to a psoriatic tendency in an infant (Fig. 6.14). Usually it clears quickly but there is an increased risk of ordinary psoriasis developing in later life.

Localized pustular psoriasis

This is a recalcitrant, often painful, condition which some regard as a separate entity. It affects the palms and soles which become studded with numerous sterile pustules, 3–10 mm in diameter, lying on an erythematous base. The pustules change to brown macules or scales (Fig. 6.15). Generalized pustular psoriasis is a rare but serious condition, with fever and recurrent episodes of pustulation within areas of erythema (Fig. 6.16).

Erythrodermic psoriasis

This is also rare and may be sparked off by the irritant effect of tar or dithranol, by a drug eruption or

Fig. 6.13 Sharply defined glistening erythematous patch of flexural psoriasis.

Fig. 6.14 Napkin psoriasis. Note constriction marks on thighs caused by polythene pants.

Fig. 6.15 Pustular psoriasis of right sole.

by the withdrawal of potent topical or systemic steroids. The skin becomes universally and uniformly red with variable scaling (Fig. 6.17). Malaise is accompanied by shivering and the skin feels hot and uncomfortable.

Complications

Psoriatic arthropathy

Arthritis occurs in about 5% of psoriatics. Several patterns are recognized. Distal arthritis involves the terminal interphalangeal joints of the toes and fingers, especially those with marked nail changes (Fig. 6.12). Other patterns include involvement of a single large joint; one which mimics rheumatoid arthritis and may become mutilating (Figs. 6.18 and 6.19); and one where the brunt is borne by the sacro-iliac joints and spine. Tests for rheumatoid factor are negative and nodules are absent. In patients with spondylitis and sacro-iliitis there is a strong correlation with the presence of HLA-B27.

Fig. 6.16 Generalized pustular psoriasis. Clusters of superficial pustules at edge of spreading erythema.

Fig. 6.17 Erythrodermic psoriasis.

Fig. 6.18 Fixed flexion deformity of distal interphalangeal joints following arthropathy. Same patient as in Figure 6.12.

Fig. 6.19 Rheumatoid-like changes associated with severe psoriasis of hands and marked nail changes.

Differential diagnosis

Discoid eczema (p. 80)
Lesions are less well defined and may be exudative, lack 'candle grease' scaling, and may be extremely itchy.

Pityriasis rosea (p. 54)
May be confused with guttate psoriasis but the lesions, which are oval rather than round, tend to run along rib lines. Scaling is of collarette type and a herald plaque may precede the rash.

Secondary syphilis (p. 140)
There is usually a history of a primary chancre. The scaly lesions are brownish and characteristically the palms and soles are involved. Oral changes, patchy alopecia and lymphadenopathy complete the picture.

Seborrhoeic eczema (p. 79)
Scalp involvement is more diffuse and less lumpy. Flexural plaques are less well defined and more exudative. There may be signs of seborrhoeic eczema elsewhere, such as on the chest.

Cutaneous T cell lymphoma (p. 208)
The lesions are not in typical locations and are often annular or arcuate. Atrophy or poikiloderma may be present.

Tinea unguium (p. 157)
This is often confused with psoriasis but is more asymmetrical and there may be obvious tinea of neighbouring skin. Uninvolved nails are common. Pitting is not seen and nails tend to be crumbly and discoloured at their free edge.

Investigations

1 Biopsy is seldom necessary.
2 Throat swabbing for beta-haemolytic streptococci is needed in guttate psoriasis.
3 Skin scrapings and nail clippings may be required to exclude tinea.
4 Radiology and tests for rheumatoid factor are helpful in assessing arthritis.

Treatment

General measures

Instruction of the patient is of great importance. Explanations and reassurances must be geared to the patient's or the parent's intelligence. The doctor as well as the patient should keep the disease in perspective, and treatment must never be allowed to be more troublesome than the disease itself.

Physical and mental rest help to back up the specific management of acute episodes. Concomitant anxiety and depression should be treated on their own merits. See Table 6.1 for appropriate treatments.

Local treatment

1 Coal tar preparations
Crude coal tar and its distillation products have been used to treat psoriasis for many years. Their precise mode of action is uncertain but they do inhibit DNA synthesis.

Many preparations are available but it is wise to become familiar with a few. The less refined tars are smelly, messy and stain clothes, but are more effective than the cleaner refined preparations. Tar emulsions can also be added to the bath. Suitable preparations are listed in the Formulary (p. 252). Surprisingly, no increase in skin cancer has been found in patients treated for prolonged periods with tar preparations; it has even been suggested that psoriatics are less likely than normal to develop skin cancer.

2 Dithranol
The use of dithranol (anthralin) has become popular in the last few decades. Like coal tar it inhibits DNA synthesis, but some of its benefits may be due to the formation of free radicals of oxygen.

Dithranol is more tricky to use than coal tar. It has to be applied carefully, to the plaques only, and, if left on for more than 30 minutes covered with gauze dressings. As it is irritant, one should start with a weak (0.1%) preparation and then step up the strength at weekly intervals. Dithranol stronger than 1% is seldom necessary. Irritation of the surrounding skin can be lessened by the application of a protec-

Table 6.1 Treatment options in psoriasis

Type of psoriasis	Treatment of choice	Alternative treatments
Stable plaque	Short-contact dithranol	Tar
Extensive stable plaque (>20% surface area)	PUVA + etretinate	Short-contact dithranol UVB Tar
Widespread small plaque	UVB	Tar
Guttate	Emollients while erupting; then UVB	Weak tar preparations Mild local steroids
Facial	Mild local steroids	
Flexural	Mild to moderately potent local steroids + antifungal	
Pustular psoriasis of hands and feet	Moderately potent or potent local steroid	Etretinate
Acute erythrodermic, unstable or generalized pustular	In-patient treatment with ichthammol paste, local steroids may be used initially	Etretinate Methotrexate

tive bland paste, e.g. zinc paste.

Dithranol stains normal skin, but the purple-brown discoloration peels off after a few days. It also stains bathtubs, clothes, and anything else it touches. One popular regimen is to apply dithranol daily for five days in the week, and many patients clear within a month.

Short contact therapy, in which dithranol is applied for no longer than 30 minutes, is also effective. Initially a test patch of psoriasis is treated with an 0.1% dithranol cream, left on for 20 minutes and then washed off. If there is no undue reaction the application can be extended the next day and if tolerated the duration of application increased to 30 minutes. After the cream is washed off, a bland application such as soft white paraffin or emulsifying ointment is applied. Depending on response, the strength of the dithranol may be increased from 0.1% to 2% over two or three weeks. Suitable preparations are listed in the Formulary (p. 252).

As dithranol is so irritant it should not be applied to the face, the inner thighs, genital region or skin folds. Special care should be taken to avoid contact with the eyes.

3   Topical corticosteroids

These are liked by patients, and by some doctors, because they are clean and seem effective at first. However, routine long-term use of potent or very potent topical steroids is not recommended as, on their withdrawal, psoriasis may relapse rapidly or even move into an unstable phase which is difficult to manage (Fig. 6.20). Their use should be restricted to:

1 'No choice' areas such as the face, ears, genitals and flexures where tar and dithranol are seldom tolerated.

2 Patients who cannot use tar or dithranol because of allergic or irritant reactions.

3 Unresponsive psoriasis on the scalp, palms and soles.

4 Patients with minor localized psoriasis.

Suitable preparations are mentioned in the Formulary (p. 248).

Only weak topical steroids should be used on the face but moderately potent ones can be used elsewhere. Combined tar–steroid preparations may be useful. The weekly ration for long-term use seldom exceeds 100 g of a moderately potent steroid.

Fig. 6.20 Unstable psoriasis following long-term topical steroid treatment. There is no scaling and numerous small lesions are erupting around ill-defined plaques.

Ultraviolet radiation

Most patients improve with natural sunlight and should be encouraged to sunbathe. During the winter, courses of artificial ultraviolet radiation (UVB) as an out-patient, or at home, may help (Fig. 6.21). Treatments, sufficient to produce a minimal erythema, should be given twice weekly for eight weeks. Goggles should be worn.

Combination therapy

Some of these treatments may be combined to clear chronic plaque psoriasis more quickly. For example, the Goeckerman regimen includes tar baths, crude coal tar and UVB therapy. The Ingram regimen combines tar baths, dithranol and UVB.

Special situations

1   Scalp psoriasis

This is often recalcitrant. Oily preparations containing 3% salicylic acid are useful (Formulary, p. 247). They should be rubbed into the scalp three times a week and washed out with a tar shampoo 4–6 hours later. If progress is slow they may be left on for one or two nights before shampooing. Salicylic acid and tar combinations are also effective.

2   Guttate psoriasis

A course of penicillin V or erythromycin is indicated for any associated streptococcal throat infection. Bland local treatment is often enough as the natural trend is towards remission. Suitable preparations include emulsifying ointment and zinc and ichthammol cream. Tar–steroid preparations are reasonable alternatives. A course of ultraviolet therapy (UVB) may be helpful after the eruptive phase is over.

3   Eruptive/unstable psoriasis

Bland treatment is needed and rest is important. Tar, dithranol and ultraviolet therapy are best avoided. Suitable preparations include emulsifying ointment and zinc and ichthammol cream.

Systemic treatment

A systemic approach should be considered if extensive psoriasis (> 20% of the body surface) fails to improve with prolonged courses of tar or dithranol. As the potential side effects are great, local measures should be given a good trial first. The most commonly used systemic treatments are photochemotherapy with PUVA (*P*soralen + *U*ltra*V*iolet *A* treatment), retinoids and methotrexate.

Fig. 6.21 Ultraviolet radiation therapy.

Photochemotherapy; PUVA

In this ingenious therapy, a drug is photo-activated in the skin by ultraviolet radiation. An oral dose of 8-methoxypsoralen is followed by exposure to long wave ultraviolet radiation (UVA: 320–400 nm). The psoralen reaches the skin and, in the presence of UVA, forms photo-adducts with DNA pyrimidine bases and cross-links between complementary DNA strands; this inhibits DNA synthesis and epidermal cell division.

The 8-methoxypsoralen (8-MOP) (0.6–0.8 mg/kg body weight) is taken 1–2 hours before exposure to a bank of UVA tubes mounted in a cabinet similar to that seen in Figure 6.20. The initial exposure is calculated either by determining the patient's minimal phototoxic dose (the least dose of UVA which after ingestion of 8-MOP produces a barely perceptible erythema 72 hours after testing) or by assessing skin colour and ability to tan. The usual starting dose is from 0.5 joules/cm^2 (skin type I: always burns and never tans) to 2.0 joules/cm^2 (skin type IV: never burns and always tans). Treatment is given two or three times a week with increasing doses of UVA, depending on erythema production and the therapeutic response. Protective goggles are worn during radiation and UVA opaque plastic glasses must be used after taking the tablets and for 24 hours after each treatment (*see below*).

Clearance takes 5–6 weeks. Thereafter it is often possible to keep the skin clear by PUVA once a fortnight or every three weeks. However, as the side effects of PUVA relate to its cumulative dose (*see below*) maintenance therapy is not generally used for the young.

Side effects

Erythema is the most common but is minimized by careful dosimetry. A quarter of patients itch during and immediately after radiation; fewer feel nauseated after taking 8-MOP. 5-Methoxypsoralen, not yet available in the U.S.A., is worth trying if these effects become intolerable. Long-term side effects include premature ageing of the skin (with mottled pigmentation, scattered lentigines, wrinkles and atrophy), cutaneous malignancies, and the possibility of cataract formation. The use of UVA blocking glasses (*see above*) for 24 hours after each treatment should pro-

tect against the latter. The long-term side effects relate to the total amount of UVA received over the years; this must be recorded and kept as low as possible without denying treatment when it is clearly needed.

Retinoids

Etretinate (0.25–0.5 mg/kg/day) (Formulary, p. 260), a recently introduced analogue of vitamin A, is one of the few drugs helpful in pustular psoriasis. It is also used to thin down thick hyperkeratotic plaques. Minor side effects are frequent and dose-related. They include dry lips, mouth, vagina and eyes, peeling of the skin, pruritus, thinning of the hair, and unpleasant paronychia. All settle on stopping or reducing the dose of the drug, but the use of emollients and artifical tears is often recommended.

Etretinate may be used on its own for long periods but regular blood tests are needed to exclude abnormal liver function, elevation of serum lipids (mainly triglycerides but also cholesterol). Yearly X-rays should help to detect ossification of ligaments especially the paraspinal ones (DISH syndrome — disseminated interstitial skeletal hyperostosis). Children, and those with persistently abnormal liver function tests or hyperlipidaemia, should not be treated.

The most important side effect is *teratogenicity* and etretinate should not normally be given to women of child-bearing age. If it has to be given, for unavoidable clinical reasons, effective oral contraceptive measures must be taken and these, in view of the long half-life of etretinate (70–100 days), should continue for *two years after treatment has ceased.* Fortunately etretin (the active metabolite of etretinate), with a much shorter half-life than etretinate, will soon be available.

Retinoids and PUVA act synergistically and are often used together in the so-called Re–PUVA regimen. This clears plaque psoriasis quicker than PUVA alone, and needs a smaller cumulative dose of UVA. The standard precautions for both PUVA and retinoid treatment should, of course, still be observed.

Methotrexate

This folic acid antagonist (Formulary, p. 259) inhibits DNA synthesis during the S phase of mitosis. After an initial trial dose of 2.5 mg, in an adult of average weight the drug is given orally once a week in a dose of 7.5–10 mg. This often controls even aggressive psoriasis. The drug is eliminated largely by the kidneys and so the dose must be reduced if renal function is poor. Aspirin and sulphonamides displace the drug from binding with plasma albumin, and frusemide may decrease its renal clearance; note must therefore be taken of concurrent drug therapy and the dose reduced accordingly. Minor and temporary side effects such as nausea and malaise are common in the 48 hours after administration. The most serious drawback to this treatment is hepatic fibrosis. Unfortunately routine liver function tests and scans cannot predict this reliably, and a pretreatment liver biopsy is needed to exclude active liver disease. This should be repeated after every cumulative dose of 1.5–2 g. Regular blood checks to exclude marrow suppression, and to monitor renal and liver function, should also be performed. This drug is also teratogenic and should not be given to females in their reproductive years. Oligospermia has been noted in men and their fertility may be lowered; however, a child fathered by a man on methotrexate can be expected to be normal.

Other systemic drugs

Antimetabolites such as azathioprine and hydroxyurea help psoriasis, but less than methotrexate; they tend to damage the marrow rather than the liver. Regular blood monitoring is again essential. Recently, low dose cyclosporin A has been reported to be highly effective. However, its nephrotoxicity makes it difficult to handle and a rebound of the psoriasis may occur after the drug is stopped; at present its use is experimental but under wide scrutiny.

LEARNING POINTS

1 Do not aggravate eruptive psoriasis.
2 Never use systemic steroids.
3 Avoid the long-term use of potent or very potent topical steroids.
4 Never promise a permanent cure, but be encouraging.
5 Great advances have been made over the last 20 years in the treatment of severe psoriasis.

CHAPTER 7

OTHER PAPULOSQUAMOUS DISORDERS

Like psoriasis, the rashes described in this chapter are raised, marginated, and scaly. Eczema may also be raised and scaly, but is usually poorly marginated and fissures, crusts, or lichenifies (Chapter 11). Psoriasis is discussed in Chapter 6. The differential diagnosis of the most common papulosquamous diseases is given in Table 7.1.

Pityriasis rosea

Cause
The cause of pityriasis rosea is not known. An infectious agent has been suspected but not proven; the disorder seems not to be contagious.

Presentation
Most patients develop one plaque (the herald plaque) before the others. It is larger (2–5 cm in diameter)

Table 7.1 The papulosquamous diseases.

Psoriasis
Pityriasis rosea
Lichen planus
Pityriasis rubra pilaris
Parapsoriasis
Mycosis fungoides
Pityriasis lichenoides
Discoid lupus erythematosus
Tinea
Secondary syphilis
Drug eruptions

than later lesions, and is rounder, redder, and more scaly. After several days many smaller plaques appear, mainly on the trunk, but some also occur on the neck and extremities (Fig. 7.1). An individual plaque is oval, salmon pink, and shows a delicate scaling, adherent peripherally (a collarette) (Figs. 7.2 and 7.3). The configuration of such plaques is often characteristic. Their longitudinal axes run down and out from the spine, along the lines of the ribs.

Course
The herald plaque precedes the generalized eruption by several days. Subsequent lesions enlarge over the first week or two. Itching is slight or moderate. The eruption lasts between two and 10 weeks and then resolves spontaneously, sometimes leaving hyperpigmented patches which fade more slowly.

Differential diagnosis
Although the herald plaque is often taken for ring-

Fig. 7.1. The herald plaque of pityriasis rosea is usually on the trunk and is larger then the other lesions. Its annular configuration is well shown here.

Fig. 7.2. The numerous small oval patches of pityriasis rosea showing collarettes of scales attached just inside the periphery of the lesions. The long axes of the lesions here lie transversely.

Fig. 7.3. Close-up of an unusually severe pityriasis rosea: numerous erythematous follicular papules are seen as well as the standard oval plaques.

worm, the three disorders most likely to be misdiagnosed early in the general eruption are guttate psoriasis, pityriasis versicolor, and secondary syphilis. Tinea corporis and pityriasis versicolor can be distinguished by the microscopical examination of scales (p. 31), and secondary syphilis by its other features (mouth lesions, papules at edges of orifices, palmar lesions, condyloma lata, lymphadenopathy, alopecia) and by serology. Gold and captopril are the drugs most likely to cause a pityriasis rosea-like drug reaction, but barbiturates, penicillamine, and other drugs may also do so.

Investigations
Because secondary syphilis can mimic pityriasis rosea so closely, testing for syphilis is usually wise.

Treatment
No treatment is curative and active treatment is seldom needed. A moderately potent topical steroid or calamine lotion may help the itching. One per cent salicylic acid in soft white paraffin or emulsifying ointment reduces scaling. Sunlight or artifical UVB often relieves pruritus and may hasten resolution.

LEARNING POINTS

1 Check serology for syphilis if in doubt about the diagnosis.
2 Revise the diagnosis if rash persists for longer than three months.

Lichen planus

Cause
The cause of lichen planus is unknown, but chronic graft-versus-host disease can cause an eruption like lichen planus, as can certain drugs (*see below*).

Presentation
Typical lesions are violaceous or lilac-coloured, intensely itchy, flat-topped papules which arise usually on the extremities, particularly on the volar aspects of the wrists and legs (Fig. 7.4). One must look closely to see a white lace-like pattern on the surface of these papules (Wickham's striae). White asymptomatic streaking is also found in the mouth, particularly inside the cheeks, in about 50% of patients (Fig. 7.5). Variants of the classical pattern are rare and often testing diagnostically (Table 7.2). Curiously, although the plaques are usually itchy, patients rub rather than scratch, so that excoriations are uncommon. As in psoriasis, the Koebner phenomenon may occur (Fig. 7.6). The nails are usually normal, but may be affected with changes ranging from fine longitudinal grooves to destruction of the entire nail fold and bed.

Fig. 7.4. Shiny, flat-topped papules of lichen planus. Note Wickham's striae.

Fig. 7.5. Classic white lacy network lying on the buccal mucosa.

Fig. 7.6. Lichen planus. Note Koebner phenomenon on the wrist and pseudovesicular appearance on the palm.

Table 7.2 Variants of lichen planus.

Annular
Atrophic
Bullous
Follicular
Hypertrophic
Ulcerative

Course

Individual lesions may last for many months and the eruption as a whole tends to last about one year. As the lesions resolve they become darker, flatter, and leave discrete brown or grey macules. About one in six patients will have a recurrence.

Complications

Essentially none, but nail or hair loss may be permanent. The ulcerative form of lichen planus in the mouth has led to squamous cell carcinoma. Ulceration, usually over bony prominences, may be disabling, especially if it is on the soles.

Differential diagnosis

Lichen planus should be differentiated from the other papulosquamous diseases listed in Table 7.1. Lichenoid drug reactions can mimic lichen planus. Gold and other heavy metals have often been implicated. Other drug causes include antimalarials, para-aminobenzoic acid, thiazide diuretics, and penicillamine. Contact with chemicals used to develop colour film may also produce similar lesions. It may be hard to tell lichen planus from generalized discoid lupus erythematosus if only a few large lesions are present or if the eruption is on the palms, soles, or scalp. Wickham's striae or oral lesions favour the diagnosis of lichen planus.

Investigations

The diagnosis is usually obvious clinically. The histology is also characteristic (Fig. 7.7), so a biopsy will confirm the diagnosis if this is needed.

Treatment

Treatment can be difficult. If drugs are suspected as the cause, they should be stopped and unrelated

— Prominent granular layer

— Basal cell degeneration

— Sawtooth dermo-epidermal junction

— Colloid bodies

— Band-like upper dermal infiltrate

Fig. 7.7. Histology of lichen planus.

ones substituted. Potent topical steroids will sometimes relieve symptoms and flatten the plaques. Systemic steroid courses work too, but are recommended only in special situations (e.g. nail destruction, or painful and erosive oral lichen planus). Treatment with PUVA (p. 52) may help reduce pruritus and help to clear up the skin lesions. Etretinate (Formulary, p. 260) has also helped some patients with stubborn lichen planus. Antihistamines may blunt the itch. Mucous membrane lesions are usually asymptomatic and do not require treatment.

LEARNING POINTS

1 A good diagnostic tip is to look for light reflected from shiny papules.
2 Always look in the mouth.
3 If you can recognize lichen planus you have pulled ahead of 75% of your colleagues.

Pityriasis rubra pilaris

Cause

This is unknown. A defect in vitamin A metabolism was once postulated but has been disproved. The familial type has an autosomal dominant inheritance.

Presentation

The familial type develops gradually in childhood and persists throughout life. The more common acquired type begins in adult life with redness and scaling of the face and scalp. Later, red or pink areas grow quickly and merge, so that patients with pityriasis rubra pilaris are often erythrodermic. Small islands of skin may be 'spared' from this general erythema, but even here the follicles may be red and plugged with keratin (Fig. 7.8). Similarly, the generalized plaques, although otherwise rather like psoriasis, may also show follicular plugging.

Course

The palms and soles become thick, smooth, and yellow. They often fissure rather than bend. The acquired form of pityriasis rubra pilaris generally lasts for 6–18 months, but may recur. Even when the plaques have gone, the skin may retain a rough, scaly texture with persistent, small, scattered, follicular plugs.

Fig. 7.8. Pityriasis rubra pilaris. Note the red plugged follicles, even in the 'spared' areas.

Complications
There are usually no complications. However, widespread erythroderma may cause patients to tolerate cold poorly.

Differential diagnosis
Psoriasis is the hardest disorder to tell from pityriasis rubra pilaris, but lacks its slightly orange colour. The thickening of the palms and soles, the follicular erythema in islands of uninvolved skin, and the follicular plugging within plaques, especially over the knuckles, are other features which help to separate them.

Investigations
Unfortunately, a biopsy seldom distinguishes psoriasis clearly from pityriasis rubra pilaris.

Treatment
The disorder responds slowly to systemic retinoids such as etretinate (in the adult, 25–50 mg/day for 6–8 months (p. 260)). Oral methotrexate in low doses, once a week may also help (p. 259). Topical steroids and keratolytics (e.g. 2% salicylic acid in soft white paraffin) reduce inflammation and scaling, but usually do not suppress the disorder completely. Systemic steroids are not indicated.

Parapsoriasis

Cause
The cause is unknown.

Presentation
Parapsoriasis en plaque typically develops as round, slightly pink patches usually on the buttocks, breasts, abdomen, or flexural skin. Scaling is not marked but epidermal atrophy may give the skin a cigarette paper-like texture. Some patients with parapsoriasis develop cutaneous T cell lymphomas (mycosis fungoides), but the majority do not. The lesions in the benign type tend to be smaller, or digitate (finger-like) (Fig. 7.9) and are not atrophic. In contrast, the premalignant types are usually asymmetrical, larger, slightly atrophic, and associated with areas of poikiloderma (reticulate pigmentation with atrophy and telangiectasia). Biopsies of this type may

Fig. 7.9. Parapsoriasis. The benign type with finger-like lesions on the sides of the trunk.

suggest early mycosis fungoides, with bizarre mononuclear cells both in the dermis and in microscopic abscesses within the epidermis.

Individual lesions change very little. Other patches may occur at other sites. In contrast to psoriasis and pityriasis rosea, the lesions are characteristically asymmetrical. Itching is variable.

Complications
Parapsoriasis en plaque may be lymphomatous from the start, but the development of cutaneous T cell lymphoma is usually not evident for many years. Patients with parapsoriasis en plaque should be followed up carefully with this in mind. If poikiloderma or induration develops, the diagnosis of mycosis fungoides becomes likely.

Differential diagnosis
This includes psoriasis itself, tinea, and nummular (discoid) eczema. Topical steroids may cause atrophy and confusion.

Investigations
Several biopsies should be taken, if possible from thick or atrophic, untreated areas. Electron microscopy may show abnormal lymphocytes with convoluted nuclei in the dermis or epidermis, though the finding of these cells, especially in the dermis, is non-specific. DNA probes can determine monoclonality of the T cells within the lymphoid infiltrate of mycosis fungoides based on rearrangements of the T

cell receptor genes. The use of these probes is currently being investigated as an early diagnostic test for cutaneous T cell lymphoma and to differentiate the benign from the malignant form of parapsoriasis.

Treatment

Because of the premalignant potential of parapsoriasis en plaque, its treatment is controversial. Less aggressive treatments are used for the benign types. Usually moderately potent steroids or ultraviolet radiation bring some resolution, but lesions tend to recur when these are stopped. For the premalignant type, treatment with PUVA (p. 52) or topical nitrogen mustard is advocated by some, but it is not clear if this slows down or prevents the development of a subsequent cutaneous T cell lymphoma.

Pityriasis lichenoides

Pityriasis lichenoides is uncommon; it occurs in two forms. The numerous small circular scaly macules and papules of the chronic type are commonly confused with guttate psoriasis (p. 45). However, their scaling is distinctive in that single, silver-grey scales surmount the lesions (mica scales). The acute type is characterized by papules which become necrotic and leave scars like those of chickenpox. More often than not there are a few lesions of the chronic type in the acute variant and vice versa. UVB radiation may reduce the number of lesions and spontaneous resolution occurs eventually.

Other papulosquamous diseases

Discoid lupus erythematosus is typically papulosquamous; this is discussed with subacute cutaneous lupus erythematosus in Chapter 12. Fungus infections are nummular and scaly and can appear papulosquamous or eczematous; these are covered in Chapter 15. Seborrhoeic and nummular (discoid) eczema are discussed in Chapter 9. Secondary syphilis is discussed in Chapter 15.

Erythroderma/exfoliative dermatitis

Sometimes the whole skin becomes red and scaly. The disorders which can cause this are listed in Table 7.3. The best clue to the underlying cause is a history of a previous skin disease. Most often the histology is non-specific. Erythroderma is the term used when the skin is red with little or no scaling, whereas exfoliative dermatitis is preferred when scaling predominates.

Most patients have lymphadenopathy, and many have hepatomegaly as well. Temperature regulation is impaired and heat loss through the skin usually makes the patient feel chilly and shiver. Oedema, high output cardiac failure, tachycardia, anaemia, failure to sweat, and dehydration may occur.

Table 7.3   Causes of erythroderma/exfoliative dermatitis.

Psoriasis

Pityriasis rubra pilaris

Ichthyosiform erythroderma

Pemphigus erythematosus

Contact, atopic, or seborrhoeic eczema

Reiter's syndrome

Lymphoma (including the Sézary syndrome)

Drug eruptions

LEARNING POINTS

The dangers of erythroderma are:
1 Poor temperature regulation.
2 High-output cardiac failure.
3 Protein deficiency.

CHAPTER 8

THE HAIR AND NAILS

The hair

To have too much hair is as bad as not having enough. These twin torments make sense only when seen against the background of the activity of normal hair follicles (Fig. 8.1).

Anatomy and physiology

The structure of a typical hair follicle has been described on p. 12.

Alopecia

The term means nothing more than loss of hair and this may have many causes and patterns. It is convenient for the clinician to subdivide alopecia into localized and diffuse types. In addition it is important to decide whether or not the hair follicles have been replaced by scar tissue: if they have, regrowth cannot occur. The presence of any disease of the skin itself should also be noted.

Localized alopecia

Some of the commonest causes are listed in Table 8.1; only a few can be dealt with in detail.

Alopecia areata

Cause
An immunological basis is suspected because of its association with thyroid disease, vitiligo and atopy. The condition runs in some families. A few cases

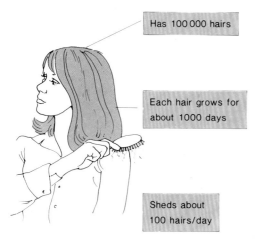

Fig. 8.1 An average scalp.

Has 100 000 hairs

Each hair grows for about 1000 days

Sheds about 100 hairs/day

Table 8.1 Some causes of localized alopecia.

Non-scarring	Scarring
Alopecia areata	Burns, radiodermatitis
Androgenic	Aplasia cutis
Hair-pulling habit	Result of kerion, carbuncle
Traction alopecia	Cicatricial basal cell carcinoma
	Lichen planus, lupus erythematosus
Scalp ringworm (human)	Necrobiosis, sarcoid, pseudopelade

Fig. 8.2   The characteristic uninflamed patches of alopecia areata. Already some early regrowth of pale hair can be seen.

Fig. 8.3   Exclamation-mark hairs: pathognomonic of alopecia areata.

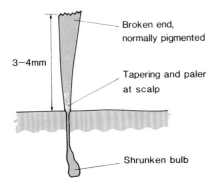

Fig. 8.4   An exclamation-mark hair.

Broken end, normally pigmented

3–4mm

Tapering and paler at scalp

Shrunken bulb

Fig. 8.5   Encouraging regrowth within a patch of alopecia areata.

seem to follow emotional trauma. It affects some 2% of new patients seen at skin clinics.

Presentation

The typical patch is uninflamed, with no scaling, but with easily seen empty hair follicles (Fig. 8.2). Pathognomonic 'exclamation-mark' hairs may be seen around the edge of enlarging areas; they are broken off about 4 mm from the scalp, and are narrower and less pigmented proximally (Figs. 8.3 and 8.4). Patches are most common in the scalp and beard but other areas, especially eyelashes and eyebrows, can be affected too. An uncommon diffuse pattern is recognized, with exclamation-mark hairs scattered widely over a diffusely thinned scalp. A few patients show fine pitting or wrinkling of the nails.

Course

The outcome is unpredictable. In a first attack, regrowth is usual within a few months. New hairs appear in the centre of patches as fine pale down and gradually regain their normal thickness and colour (Fig. 8.5), though the new hair may remain white in older patients. Subsequent episodes tend to have more patches and regrowth is slower. Hair loss in some areas may co-exist with regrowth in others. A minority of patients lose all the hair from their heads (alopecia totalis) or from the whole skin surface (alopecia universalis).

Regrowth is tiresomely erratic but the following suggest a poor prognosis:
1 Onset before puberty.
2 Association with atopy or mongolism.

3 Unusually widespread alopecia.
4 Involvement of the scalp margin.

Differential diagnosis

Patches are not scaly, in contrast to ringworm, and are usually uninflamed, in contrast to lupus erythematosus and lichen planus. In the hair-pulling habit of children, and in traction alopecia, broken hairs may be seen and true exclamation-mark hairs are absent. Secondary syphilis can cause a 'moth-eaten' patchy hair loss also.

Investigations

None are usually needed. Syphilis can be excluded with serological tests if necessary. Organ-specific auto-antibody screens provide interesting information but do not affect management.

Treatment

A patient with a first or minor attack can be reassured about the prospects for regrowth. Tranquillizers may be helpful at the start. Avoid giving systemic

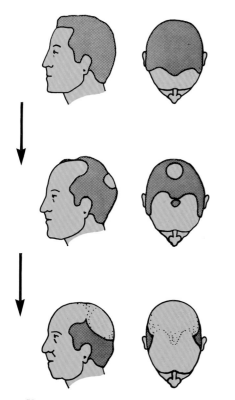

Fig. 8.6 Variations on male-pattern baldness.

Fig. 8.7 Androgenic alopecia most marked on the crown.

steroids but intralesional triamcinolone leads to localized tufts of regrowth while not affecting the overall outcome. This may be useful to re-establish eyebrows or to stimulate hope. Spirit-based steroid lotions are often used but with limited success. Ultraviolet radiation sometimes helps extensive cases. Irritants and contact sensitizers (e.g. diphencyprone) are used by a few doctors but topical minoxidil has failed to live up to its early promise. Wigs are necessary for extensive cases.

Androgenic alopecia (male-pattern baldness)

Cause

Although clearly familial, the exact mode of inheritance has not yet been clarified. Male-pattern baldness is androgen-dependent; in females, androgenic alopecia, with circulating levels of androgen within normal limits, is seen only in those who are strongly predisposed genetically.

Presentation

The common pattern (Fig. 8.6), in which hair is lost first from the temples and then from the crown, is too well known to need further description. However, hair loss in woman may be much more diffuse, particularly over the crown (Fig. 8.7). In bald areas, terminal hairs are replaced by finer vellus hairs.

Clinical course

Hair loss is relentless, tending to follow the family pattern with some losing hair quickly and others more slowly. The diffuse pattern seen in women tends to progress slowly.

Complications
Even minor hair loss may lead to great anxiety and monosymptomatic hypochondriasis (p. 222).

Differential diagnosis
The diagnosis is usually obvious in men, but other causes of diffuse hair loss have to be considered in women (p. 64).

Investigations
None are usually needed. In women virilization may have to be excluded.

Treatment
There is no effective treatment. Scalp surgery, hair transplants, and wigs are welcomed by some. Topical application of minoxidil lotions may slow hair loss and even stimulate new growth of hair in a minority of cases (Formulary, p. 253). Small and recently acquired patches respond best. When minoxidil treatment stops, the new hairs will fall out.

LEARNING POINTS

Androgenic alopecia:
1 Minoxidil lotion helps only if the areas of hair loss are small and recent.
2 Treatment with topical minoxidil must go on forever or else the new hairs will fall out.

Trichotillomania
This is dealt with on p. 224.

Traction alopecia

Cause
Hair can be pulled out by several procedures intended to beautify, including hot-combing to straighten kinky hair, styling hair tightly as with a pony tail, and rolling hair excessively or too tightly.

Presentation
The changes are usually seen in girls and young women, particularly those whose hair has always tended to be thin anyway. The bald areas show short broken hairs, folliculitis, and sometimes scarring. The pattern of hair loss is determined by the cosmetic procedure in use, hair being lost where there is maximal tug. The term 'marginal' alopecia is applied to one common pattern in which hair loss is mainly around the edge of the scalp — at the sides or at the front.

Clinical course
Patients are often slow to accept that they are responsible for the hair loss themselves, and notoriously slow to alter their cosmetic practices. Even if they do, regrowth is often disappointingly incomplete.

Differential diagnosis
The pattern of hair loss provides the main clue to the diagnosis, and if the possibility of traction alopecia is kept in mind there is usually no difficulty. The absence of exclamation-mark hairs distinguishes it from alopecia areata, and of scaling from tinea capitis.

Treatment
Patients have to stop doing whatever is causing their hair loss. Rollers which tug can be replaced by those which only heat.

Patchy hair loss due to skin disease

Scalp ringworm
Inflammation, often with pustulation, is a feature of infections derived from animals, and the resultant scarring can be severe. The classical scalp ringworm derived from human sources causes areas of scaling with broken hairs. The subject is covered in more detail on p. 157.

Psoriasis
The rough removal of adherent scales can also remove hairs, but regrowth is the rule.

Scarring alopecia
Hair follicles can be damaged in many ways. If the follicular openings can no longer be seen with a lens, regrowth of hair cannot be expected.

Sometimes the cause is obvious: a severe burn, trauma, a carbuncle, or an episode of inflammatory scalp ringworm. Discoid lupus erythematosus (p. 106), lichen planus (p. 55), and localized scleroderma (p. 108) can also lead to scarring alopecia. The term 'pseudopelade' is applied to a slowly progressive, non-inflamed type of scarring which leads to irregular areas of hair loss without any apparent preceding skin disease.

Diffuse hair loss

Hair is lost evenly from the whole scalp; this may, or may not, be accompanied by a thinning visible to others (Fig. 8.8). Some of the commonest causes are listed in Table 8.2, but often a simple explanation cannot be found.

Telogen effluvium

Cause
Each hair follicle goes through its growth cycles out of phase with its neighbours. However, if many pass into the resting phase (telogen) at the same time, then a correspondingly large number will be shed 2–3 months later. This process is known as telogen effluvium. It can be triggered by any severe illness, particularly if bouts of fever occur, and by childbirth.

Presentation and course
The diffuse hair fall, 2–3 months after the provoking illness, can be mild or severe. In the latter case Beau's lines (p. 68) may be seen on the nails. Regrowth, not always complete, usually occurs within a few months.

Differential diagnosis
This is from other types of diffuse hair loss (Table 8.2).

Treatment
This condition is unaffected by therapy.

Other causes of diffuse hair loss
The causes mentioned in Table 8.2 should be considered, and the exclamation-mark hairs seen in the dif-

Fig. 8.8 Diffuse hair loss causing much anxiety but with minor thinning only.

Table 8.2 Some causes of diffuse hair loss.

Telogen effluvium

Endocrine
    hypopituitarism, hypo- or hyperthyroidism,
    hypoparathyroidism

Drug-induced
    antimitotic agents, anticoagulants, vitamin A
    excess, oral contraceptives

Androgenic
Iron deficiency
Severe chronic illness
Malnutrition
Diffuse type of alopecia areata

fuse type of alopecia areata should be looked for. If no cause is obvious it is worth checking the haemoglobin, ESR, ANF, serum iron and thyroxine (Fig. 8.9). It is true to say that often no cause for diffuse alopecia can be found.

LEARNING POINTS

1 Be sympathetic even if the hair loss seems trivial to you.
2 Reassure your patient that total baldness is not imminent.

Fig. 8.9 Patient with hyperthyroidism, exophthalmos and diffuse hair loss most marked at the parting.

Hypotrichosis

The *ectodermal dysplasias* are a group of rare inherited disorders characterized by sparse hair, scanty sweat glands, and poor development of the nails and teeth. One type is inherited as a sex-linked recessive. Heat stroke may follow inadequate sweat production.

In other inherited disorders the hair may be beaded and brittle (*monilethrix*); flattened and twisted (*pili torti*); kinky (*Menke's syndrome* in association with abnormalities of copper metabolism); like bamboo (*Netherton's syndrome*); partly broken in many places (*trichorrhexis nodosa*); woolly or uncombable.

Hirsutism and hypertrichosis

Hirsutism is the growth of terminal hair in a female, but distributed in the pattern normally seen in a male. Hypertrichosis is an excessive growth of terminal hair but one which does not follow an androgen-induced pattern.

Hirsutism

Cause
Some degree of hirsutism may be a racial or familial trait, and some increase of facial hair is common af-

ter the menopause. In addition, some patients, without a family background of hirsutism, become hirsute in the absence of any demonstrable hormonal cause (idiopathic hirsutism). Finally, a few patients with hirsutism will have one of the disorders listed in Table 8.3.

Presentation
An excessive growth of hair may be seen in the beard area, on the chest and shoulder-tips, around the nipples, and in the male pattern of pubic hair. An androgenic alopecia may complete the picture.

Course
Familial, racial, or idiopathic hirsutism tends to start at puberty and to worsen with age.

Complications
Infertility will follow virilization; psychological disturbances are common.

Investigations
Significant hormonal abnormalities are not usually found in patients with a normal menstrual cycle. Investigations are needed:
- If hirsutism occurs in childhood.
- If there are other features of virilization.
- If the hirsutism is of sudden or recent onset.
- If there is menstrual irregularity or cessation.

The tests used will include measurement of the serum testosterone, sex-hormone-binding globulin, dehydroepiandrosterone sulphate and androstanedione. Ovarian ultrasound is a useful test when polycystic ovaries are suspected.

Table 8.3 Some causes of hirsutism.

1	Ovarian	Polycystic ovaries Arrhenoblastoma
2	Adrenal	Cushing's syndrome Virilizing tumours Adrenogenital syndromes
3	Pituitary	Acromegaly Hyperprolactinaemia
4	Iatrogenic	Anabolic steroids Progesterones

Treatment

Any underlying disorder must be treated on its merits. Otherwise the abnormally active follicles, if relatively few, may be destroyed by electrolysis. If the hairs are too numerous for this, the excess may be removed by waxing or shaving, or rendered less obvious by bleaching. Oral anti-androgens (e.g. cyproterone acetate, Formulary, p. 259) may sometimes be helpful, but will be needed long term. Spironolactone cannot now be recommended.

LEARNING POINTS

1 Full endocrinological assessment is needed for hirsutism plus virilization.
2 Significant hormonal abnormalities are rarely found in patients with a normal menstrual cycle.

Hypertrichosis

The localized type is most commonly seen over congenital melanocytic naevi. It can also affect the sacral area (a satyr's tuft) in some patients with spina bifida. Excessive amounts of hair may grow near chronically inflamed joints or under a plaster cast. Repeated shaving does not bring on hypertrichosis though occupational pressure may do so, for example from carrying weights on the shoulder.

Generalized hypertrichosis is much less common. Some causes are listed in Table 8.4.

Hair cosmetics

Hair may be made more attractive by dyeing, bleaching and waving, but there is often a price to be paid for beauty. Some hair dyes based on paraphenylene-diamine are allergens. Bleaches may weaken the hair shafts, and hair damaged in this way is especially susceptible to further damage by permanent waving.

Permanent waving solutions reduce disulphide bonds within hair keratin and so allow the hair to be deformed before being reset in a new position. The

Table 8.4 Some causes of generalized hypertrichosis.

Drug-induced (minoxidil, diazoxide)
Starvation, anorexia nervosa
Hepatic cutaneous porphyria
Fetal alcohol and fetal phenytoin syndromes
Hypertrichosis lanuginosa (congenital or acquired)
Some rare syndromes, e.g. Cornelia de Lange syndrome (hypertrichosis, microcephaly and mental deficiency)

thioglycollates used to dissolve disulphide bonds are also popular as chemical hair removers. If used incorrectly, either too strong or for too long a time, or on hair already damaged by excessive bleaching or waving, thioglycollate waving lotions can cause hair to break off flush with the scalp. Accompanying this hair loss, which may be severe though temporary, may be an irritant dermatitis of the scalp.

The nails

Congenital abnormalities

A few people are born with one or more nails missing. In addition there are many conditions, either inherited or associated with chromosomal abnormalities, and usually rare, in which nail changes form a minor part of the clinical picture. Most cannot be dealt with here.

In the rare *nail–patella syndrome*, thumb nails, and to a lesser extent those of the fingers, are smaller than normal. Rudimentary patellae complete the syndrome which is inherited as an autosomal dominant trait linked with the locus controlling ABO blood groups.

Pachyonychia congenita is also rare and inherited as an autosomal dominant. The nails are grossly thickened, especially peripherally, and have a curious triangular profile (Fig. 8.10). Hyperkeratosis may occur on areas of friction on the legs and feet.

Permanent loss of the nails may be seen with the dystrophic types of *epidermolysis bullosa*.

In the *yellow nail syndrome* the nail changes begin in adult life, against a background of hypoplasia of the lymphatic system. Peripheral oedema is usually present and pleural effusions may occur. The nails grow very slowly and become thickened and greenish-yellow; their surface is smooth but they are over-curved from side to side.

The *nail 'en racquette'* is a short broad nail (Fig. 8.10), usually a thumb nail, which is seen in some 1–2% of the population and may be inherited as an autosomal dominant trait. The basic abnormality is shortness of the underlying terminal phalanx.

Effects of trauma

Damage to the nail matrix may be followed by permanent ridges or splits in the nail plate. *Splinter haemorrhages*, the linear nature of which is determined by longitudinal ridges and grooves in the nail bed, are commonly seen under the nails of manual workers and are due to minor trauma. They may also be a feature of psoriasis of the nail and of subacute bacterial endocarditis. Larger *subungual haematomas* are usually easy to identify but trauma to nails may have escaped notice and dark areas of altered blood may raise worries about the presence of a subungual melanoma.

Chronic trauma from sport and from ill-fitting shoes contributes to haemorrhage under the nails of the big toes, to the gross thickening of toe nails known as *onychogryphosis*, and to *ingrowing nails*. *Onycholysis*, a separation of the nail plate from the nail bed (Fig. 8.10), may be due to minor trauma though it is also seen in nail psoriasis (Fig. 6.11), and possibly in thyroid disease.

Some nervous habits can damage the nails. *Bitten nails* are short and irregular; some also bite their cuticles and the skin around the nails. Viral warts can be seeded rapidly in this way. In the common *habit tic nail dystrophy*, the cuticle of the thumb nail is the target for picking or rubbing. This repetitive trauma causes a ladder pattern of transverse ridges and grooves to run up the centre of the nail plate (Fig. 8.10).

Lamellar splitting of the digital part of the finger nails, so commonly seen in housewives, has been attributed to repeated wetting and drying (Fig. 8.10).

The nail in systemic disease

The nails provide useful clues for general physicians.

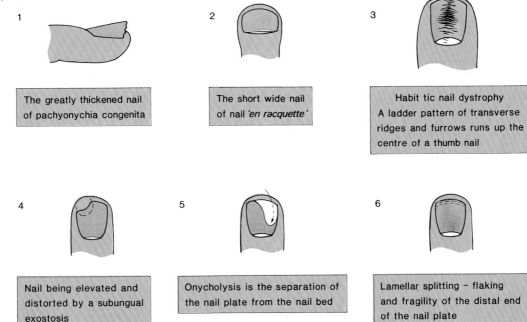

1 The greatly thickened nail of pachyonychia congenita

2 The short wide nail of nail *'en racquette'*

3 Habit tic nail dystrophy A ladder pattern of transverse ridges and furrows runs up the centre of a thumb nail

4 Nail being elevated and distorted by a subungual exostosis

5 Onycholysis is the separation of the nail plate from the nail bed

6 Lamellar splitting – flaking and fragility of the distal end of the nail plate

Fig. 8.10 Some nail plate abnormalities.

Clubbing is a bulbous enlargement of the terminal phalanx with an increase in the angle between the nail plate and the proximal fold to over 180° (Fig. 8.11). Its association with chronic lung disease and with cyanotic heart disease is well known. Rarely clubbing may be familial with no underlying cause. The mechanisms involved in its formation are still not known.

Koilonychia, a spooning and thinning of the nail plate, indicates iron deficiency (Fig. 8.12).

Colour changes: the 'half-and-half' nail, with a white proximal and red or brown distal half, is seen in a minority of patients with chronic renal failure. Whitening of the nail plates may be related to hypoalbuminaemia, as in cirrhosis of the liver. Some drugs, notably antimalarials, antibiotics and phenothiazines, may discolour the nails.

Beau's lines are transverse grooves which appear synchronously on all nails a few weeks after an acute illness, and which grow steadily out to the free margin (Fig. 8.12).

Connective tissue disorders: nail fold telangiectasia or erythema is a useful physical sign in dermatomyositis, systemic sclerosis and systemic lupus erythematosus (Figs. 8.12 and 12.7). In dermatomyositis the cuticles may become shaggy, and in systemic sclerosis loss of finger pulp may lead to over curvature of the nail plates. An impaired peripheral circulation, as in Raynaud's phenomenon, will lead to thinning and longitudinal ridging of the nail plate, sometimes with partial onycholysis.

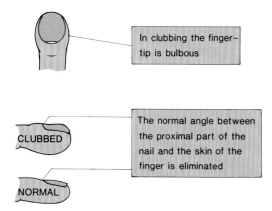

In clubbing the finger-tip is bulbous

CLUBBED

The normal angle between the proximal part of the nail and the skin of the finger is eliminated

NORMAL

Fig. 8.11 Clubbing.

Common dermatoses

Psoriasis

Most patients with psoriasis have nail changes at some stage: severe nail involvement correlates to some extent with the presence of arthritis. The best known nail change is pitting of the surface of the nail plate (Fig. 6.10). Almost as common is psoriasis under the nail plate, showing up as red or brown areas, often with onycholysis bordered by obvious discoloration (Fig. 6.11). There is no effective treatment for psoriasis of the nails.

Eczema

Patients with itchy chronic eczema may bring their nails to a high state of polish by scratching. In addition, eczema of the nail folds may lead to a coarse irregularity with transverse ridging of the adjacent nail plates.

Lichen planus

Some 10% of patients with lichen planus have nail changes, most often this is a reversible thinning of the nail plate with irregular longitudinal grooves and ridges. More severe involvement may lead to pterygium in which the cuticle grows forward over the base of the nail and attaches itself to the nail plate (Fig. 8.12). The threat of severe and permanent nail changes may rarely justify treatment with systemic steroids.

Alopecia areata

The more severe the hair loss, the more likely there is to be nail involvement. A roughness or fine pitting is seen on the surface of the nail plates and the lunulae may appear mottled.

Infections

Acute paronychia

The portal of entry for the organisms concerned, usually staphylococci, is a break in the skin or cuticle due to minor trauma. The acute inflammation, often with the formation of pus in the nail fold or under the nail, requires systemic antibiotics with flucloxacillin or erythromycin (Formulary, p. 256) and appropriate surgical drainage.

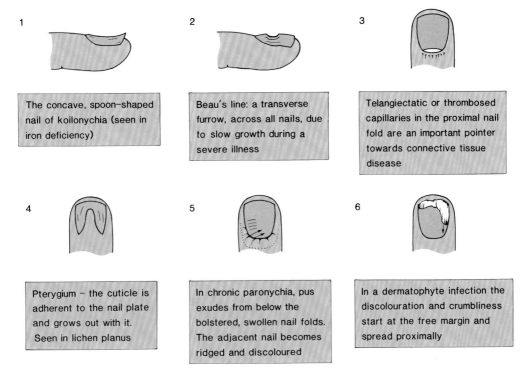

The concave, spoon–shaped nail of koilonychia (seen in iron deficiency)

Beau's line: a transverse furrow, across all nails, due to slow growth during a severe illness

Telangiectatic or thrombosed capillaries in the proximal nail fold are an important pointer towards connective tissue disease

Pterygium – the cuticle is adherent to the nail plate and grows out with it. Seen in lichen planus

In chronic paronychia, pus exudes from below the bolstered, swollen nail folds. The adjacent nail becomes ridged and discoloured

In a dermatophyte infection the discolouration and crumbliness start at the free margin and spread proximally

Fig. 8.12   Some other nail changes.

Chronic paronychia

Cause
A combination of circumstances allows a mixture of opportunistic pathogens (yeasts, Gram-positive cocci and Gram-negative rods) to colonize the space between the nail fold and nail plate. Predisposing factors include a poor peripheral circulation, wet work, working with flour, diabetes, vaginal candidosis, and overvigorous cutting back of the cuticles.

Presentation and course
The nail folds are tender and swollen (Fig. 8.12) and small amounts of pus are discharged at intervals. The cuticular seal is damaged and the adjacent nail plate becomes ridged and discoloured. The condition may last for many years.

Differential diagnosis
In atypical cases consider the outside chance of an amelanotic melanoma. Paronychia should not be confused with a dermatophyte infection in which the nail folds are not primarily affected.

Investigations
Test the urine for sugar, check for vaginal candidosis. Pus should be cultured.

Treatment
The hands should be kept as warm and as dry as possible, and the damaged nail folds may be packed several times a day with an imidazole cream (Formulary, p. 250).

Dermatophyte infections

Cause
The common dermatophytes which cause tinea pedis can also invade the nails (p. 157).

Presentation
Toe nail infection is common and associated with

tinea pedis. The early changes occur at the free edge of the nail and spread proximally. The nail plate becomes yellow, crumbly and thickened. Usually only a few nails are infected but occasionally all are. The finger nails are involved less often, and the changes, in contrast to those of psoriasis, are usually confined to one hand.

Clinical course
The condition seldom clears spontaneously.

Differential diagnosis
Psoriasis has been mentioned. Yeast infections of the nail plate, much more rare than dermatophyte infections, can look similar.

Investigations
Microscopic examination of a nail clipping is a simple procedure (p. 31). Cultures should be carried out in a mycology laboratory.

Treatment
Local therapy alone is not effective. Once the diagnosis has been confirmed by isolating an organism known to be sensitive to griseofulvin, this drug should be given at the dose of 500 mg daily as a single dose taken with the largest meal. For children the dose is 10 mg/kg body weight taken in two divided doses. The average duration for finger nail treatment is eight months, and for the toe nails 18 months. Not all cases can be cured in this way, and many relapse. Ketoconazole cannot now be recommended for the routine treatment of tinea unguium.

Tumours
Peri-ungual warts are common and differ in no way from warts elsewhere. Cryotherapy must be used carefully to avoid damage to the nail matrix; it is painful but effective.

Peri-ungual fibromas arise from the nail folds, usually in late childhood, in patients with tuberous sclerosis.

Glomus tumours may occur beneath the nail plate. The small red or bluish lesions are exquisitely tender and also hurt with changes in temperature. Treatment is surgical.

Subungual exostoses (Fig. 8.10) protrude painfully under the nail plate. Usually secondary to trauma to the terminal phalanx, the bony abnormality can be seen on X-ray and treatment is surgical.

Myxoid cysts occur on the proximal nail folds, usually of the fingers. The smooth domed swelling contains a clear jelly-like material which transilluminates well. A groove may form on the adjacent nail plate. Cryotherapy, injections of triamcinolone, and surgical excision all have their advocates.

Malignant melanoma should be suspected in any subungual pigmented lesion, particularly if the pigment spreads to the surrounding skin. Subungual haematomas may cause confusion but 'grow out' with the nail. The risk of misdiagnosis is highest with an amelanotic melanoma which may mimic chronic paronychia or a pyogenic granuloma.

LEARNING POINT

Do not let the nail stop you from biopsying suspicious lesions under it promptly.

CHAPTER 9
ECZEMA AND DERMATITIS

The conditions grouped under this heading are the most common to be referred to our clinics, making up some 20% of all new patients.

Terminology

Too much time has been devoted in the past to trying to distinguish between eczema and dermatitis. This exercise in hair-splitting semantics can be avoided by accepting that the two terms mean the same thing. Such an approach has now been adopted by most dermatologists, and will be used in this book. Contact eczema, therefore, is here the same as contact dermatitis; seborrhoeic eczema the same as seborrhoeic dermatitis, etc.

It may, however, be wise to stick to the term eczema when talking to patients as, to them, 'dermatitis' may carry industrial and compensation overtones which sometimes stir up unnecessary legal battles.

Classification of eczema

This remains difficult and unsatisfactory. Eczema is a reaction pattern which has many causes (Fig. 9.1). Some terms are based on the appearance of lesions, e.g. discoid eczema and hyperkeratotic eczema, while others reflect outmoded or unproven theories of causation, e.g. infective eczema and seborrhoeic eczema. Classification by site, e.g. flexural eczema and hand eczema, is equally unhelpful. Perhaps the most acceptable subdivision is into:

1 Exogenous (or contact) eczema.
2 Endogenous (or constitutional) eczema.

Any rational approach to therapy depends upon making this distinction, but even experienced dermatologists admit that they can only classify some two-thirds of the cases they see. Further confusion can occur when the groups overlap, e.g. when a contact eczema is superimposed on a stasis eczema. A convenient working classification is shown in Table 9.1.

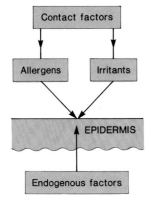

Fig. 9.1 The causes of eczema.

Table 9.1 Eczema — a working classification.

Exogenous (contact)	Irritant
	Allergic
	Photodermatitis (Chapter 17)
Endogenous (constitutional)	Atopic
	Seborrhoeic
	Discoid (nummular)
	Pompholyx
	Gravitational (stasis)
Unclassified	Asteatotic
	Neurodermatitis
	Juvenile plantar dermatosis

Clinical features common to most patterns of eczema

The different types of eczema have their own distinguishing marks, and these will be dealt with later; but most share certain general features which it is convenient to consider here.

Acute eczema

Acute eczema (Figs. 9.2 and 9.3) is recognized by its:
- Redness and swelling, usually with an ill-defined border.
- Papules, vesicles and, in fierce cases, large blisters (Fig. 9.4).
- Exudation and crusting.
- Scaling.

Chronic eczema

Chronic eczema may show all of the above changes but in general is:
- Less vesicular and exudative.
- More scaly, pigmented and thickened.
- More likely to be lichenified (Fig. 9.5) (a dry leathery thickened state, with increased skin markings, secondary to repeated scratching or rubbing).
- More likely to develop painful fissures.

Histology (Fig. 9.6)

The clinical appearance of the different stages of eczema mirrors their histology. In the acute stage, oedema in the epidermis (spongiosis) progresses to the formation of intra-epidermal vesicles, which may coalesce into larger blisters or rupture. The chronic stages of eczema show less spongiosis and vesication but more thickening of the prickle cell (acanthosis) and horny layers (hyperkeratosis and parakeratosis). These changes are accompanied by a variable degree of vasodilation and infiltration with lymphocytes.

Complications

1 Heavy bacterial colonization is common in all

Fig. 9.2 Acute vesicular contact eczema of the hand.

Fig. 9.3 Vesicular and crusted contact eczema of the face (cosmetic allergy).

Fig. 9.4 Acute bullous photodermatitis of plant origin.

Fig. 9.5 Lichenification behind the knee in chronic atopic eczema.

Vesication

Weeping

Crusting

Chronic lichenification

Fig. 9.6 The sequence of histological events in eczema.

types of eczema but overt infection is most troublesome in the seborrhoeic and atopic types.

2 Reactions to medicaments may provoke dissemination, especially in stasis eczema.

3 Anxiety states may develop with all severe forms of eczema.

Differential diagnosis

This falls into two halves. Eczema has first to be separated from other skin conditions which look like it:

- *Psoriasis* (Chapter 6). This presents problems on the scalp (neurodermatitis and seborrhoeic eczema), in the flexures (seborrhoeic eczema), on the hands (all chronic eczemas) and on the limbs (discoid eczema). Psoriasis tends to be less itchy and more marginated. One should look for signs of psoriasis elswhere, particularly on the nails, elbows and knees.

- *Fungal infections* (Chapter 15). These must be considered in any apparent eczema of the groin, feet and hands, particularly if assymetrical and not doing well with topical steroids. In addition tinea pedis can provoke a secondary pompholyx-like eruption of the hands. Pityriasis versicolor (p. 162) may look like seborrhoeic eczema of the trunk but is browner and depigments in the sun. In all of these instances examination of scales made transparent with potassium hydroxide solution should settle the issue.

- *Scabies* (Chapter 16). Beware of the patient with no past history of skin trouble who suddenly develops itchy lesions mimicking infected eczema, especially if there are also itchy contacts.

- Also consider the following:

  Head lice in infected eczema of the scalp.

  Angio-oedema and erysipelas in facial contact eczema.

  Lichen planus in palmar eczema.

  Pityriasis rosea and secondary syphilis in seborrhoeic eczema of the trunk.

  Drug reactions in photodermatitis.

  It is also important to try to distinguish between exogenous and endogenous eczema on clinical grounds, as this will determine both the need for investigation and the best line of treatment. Sometimes an eruption will follow one of the well-known patterns of eczema, and the distinction can then be made readily enough; often, however, this is not the case, and the history then becomes especially important. A contact element is more likely if:

- There is obvious contact with known irritants or allergens.
- The eruption clears when the patient goes on holiday, or at the weekends.
- The eczema is asymmetrical, or with a linear or rectilinear configuration.
- The rash picks out the eyelids, external ear canals, hands and feet, the skin around stasis ulcers, and peri-anal skin.

Investigations

Each eczema pattern needs a different enquiry line.

Exogenous eczema

Here the main decision is whether or not to undertake patch testing (p. 32). This is of no value in irritant eczema but may be helpful in allergic contact eczema. The technique is not easy: its problems include separating irritant from allergic patch test reactions, and picking the right allergens to test. If legal issues depend on the results, the testing should be done by a dermatologist who will have the standard equipment and suitably selected allergens (Fig. 4.5). Patch testing can be used to confirm a suspected allergy, or, by the use of a battery of common sensitizers, to uncover allergies which then have to be assessed in the light of the history and the clinical picture. Photopatch-testing is more specialized and facilities are only available in a few centres. A visit to the home or work-place may be invaluable in investigating contact eczema.

Endogenous eczema

The only indication for patch testing here is when an added contact allergic element is suspected. This is most common in stasis eczema where neomycin, soframycin, lanolin or preservative allergy may perpetuate the condition or trigger dissemination. Ironically rubber gloves, so often used to protect eczematous hands, can themselves sensitize.

The role of prick testing in atopic eczema is discussed on p. 78.

Specimens should be cultured for bacterial pathogens or *Candida* if superinfection is suspected or if eczema is worsening despite treatment. Scrapings for fungal culture can be used to rule out tinea if there is clinical doubt — as in some cases of discoid/nummular eczema.

Finally, malabsorption should be considered and looked for in otherwise unexplained, widespread pigmented atypical patterns of endogenous eczema.

Treatment

Acute weeping eczema

This does best with liquid applications. Non-steroidal preparations are helpful at this stage and the technique used will vary with the facilities available and the site of the lesions. In general practice a simple and convenient way of dealing with weeping eczema of the hands or feet is to use thrice daily 10 minute soaks in a cool 1:8000 solution of potassium permanganate or 1:40 dilution of Burrow's solution (Formulary, p. 246), each soaking being followed by a smear of a corticosteroid cream or lotion and the application of a non-stick dressing or cotton gloves. One disadvantage is that permanganate stains the skin and nails brown — patients should be told about this.

Wider areas on the trunk respond well to corticosteroid creams and lotions. However, traditional remedies such as exposure and frequent applications of calamine lotion, and the use of half-strength magenta paint for the flexures, are also very effective.

An experienced doctor or nurse can supervise or teach the patient how to use wet dressings. The dilute potassium permanganate solution, Burrow's solution, saline, 0.5% silver nitrate, or even tap water, can be applied on cotton gauze, under a polythene covering, and changed twice daily. Rest at home will help too.

Subacute eczema

Steroid lotions or creams form the mainstay of treatment; their strength is determined by the severity of the attack. Neomycin or vioform can be incorporated into the application if an infective element is present, but preferably should not be used on stasis eczema as sensitization is so often induced.

Chronic eczema

This responds best to steroids in an ointment base, but is also often helped by non-steroid applications such as ichthammol and zinc cream.

The strength of the steroid is important (Fig. 9.7). Nothing stronger than 0.5 or 1% hydrocortisone ointment should be used on the face or in infancy. Even in adults one should be reluctant to prescribe more than 200 g of a mildly potent steroid, 50 g of a moderately potent or 30 g of a potent one, per week. Very potent topical steroids should not be used long term.

Bacterial superinfection may need systemic antibiotics but can often be controlled by the incorporation of antibiotics, e.g. neomycin or chlortetracycline, or antiseptics, e.g. vioform, into the steroid formulation. Many proprietary mixtures of this type are available in the U.K. Chronic localized hyperkeratotic eczema of the palms or soles can be helped by salicylic acid (1–6% in emulsifying ointment) or stabilized urea preparations (Formulary, p. 247).

Systemic treatment

Short courses of systemic steroids may occasionally be justified in extremely acute and severe eczema but prolonged systemic steroid treatment should be avoided in chronic cases, particularly in atopic eczema. Hydroxyzine, trimeprazine and other antihistamines (Formulary, p. 258) may be helpful at night. Systemic antibiotics may be needed in widespread bacterial superinfection.

Common patterns of eczema

Irritant contact eczema

This accounts for the majority of industrial cases.

Cause

Strong irritants elicit an acute reaction after brief contact and the diagnosis is then usually obvious. Prolonged exposure, sometimes over a period of years, is needed for weak irritants to cause eczema, usually of the hands and forearms (Fig. 9.8). Detergents, alkalis, solvents, cutting oils and abrasive dusts are common culprits. There is a wide range of susceptibility, those with dry skins or atopy being especially vulnerable.

Course

The need to continue at work, or with housework, seldom allows the skin to regain its normal barrier function. This may take several months. All too often, therefore, this condition, potentially reversible in the early stages, becomes chronic.

Complications

The condition may lead to loss of work.

Differential diagnosis

It is often hard to differentiate from allergic contact

Fig. 9.7 Stretch marks following the use of too potent topical steroids to the groin.

Fig. 9.8 Chronic irritant 'housewife's' hand eczema.

dermatitis and from atopic eczema of the hands. Atopic patients are especially prone to develop irritant eczema.

Investigations

Patch testing with irritants is not helpful and indeed may be misleading: patch testing to a battery of common allergens (p. 32) may be worthwhile if an allergic element is suspected.

Treatment

Management is based upon avoidance of the irritants responsible but often this is not possible and the best that can be achieved is reduced exposure and the use of protective gloves and clothing. The factory doctor or nurse can often advise here. Barrier creams seldom help established cases. Moderately potent topical corticosteroids are valuable but are secondary to the avoidance of irritants and protective measures. A wiser choice of career might have prevented the trouble arising in the first place in those with vulnerable skins.

Allergic contact dermatitis

Cause

The mechanism is that of delayed (type IV) hypersensitivity (Chapter 3). It has the following features:
- Previous contact is needed to induce allergy.
- Specificity to one chemical or its close relatives.
- All areas of skin react to the allergen.
- Sensitization persists indefinitely.
- Desensitization is seldom possible.

Fig. 9.9 Contact eczema due to allergy to nickel in a jean stud.

Presentation and clinical course

The original site of the eruption gives a clue to the likely allergen which secondary spread may later obscure. The lax skin of the eyelids and genitalia is especially likely to become oedematous.

Easily recognizable patterns exist. Nickel allergy, for example, gives rise to eczema under jewellery, bra clips and jean studs (Fig. 9.9). Possible allergens are numerous and to spot the less common ones in the environment needs specialist knowledge. Table 9.2 lists some common allergens and their distribution.

Investigations

Questioning should cover both occupational and domestic exposure to allergens. The indications for patch testing have already been discussed on p. 74. The techniques are constantly improving: dermatologists will have access to a battery of common allergens, commercially available, suitably diluted in a bland vehicle. They are applied in aluminium cups held in position on the skin for two or three days (Fig. 4.5) by tape.

Treatment

Simply to reduce exposure to the offending allergen is usually not enough and active steps have to be

Table 9.2 Some common allergens.

Allergen	Present in
Dichromate	Cement, leather, matches
Nickel	Jewellery, jean studs, bra clips
Paraphenylenediamine	Hair dye, clothing
Balsam of Peru	Perfumes, citrus fruits
Rubber chemicals	Clothing, shoes, tyres
Colophony	Sticking plaster, collodion
Neomycin Benzocaine	Topical applications
Parabens	Preservative in cosmetics and creams
Epoxy resin	Resin adhesives
Wool alcohols	Lanolin, cosmetics, creams

taken to avoid it completely. Job changes are sometimes necessary to achieve this. Some believe that reactions to nickel may be kept going by nickel in the diet, released from cans or steel saucepans — changes in diet and cooking utensils may occasionally be helpful.

Atopic eczema

Cause

Atopy is a genetic predisposition to form excessive IgE antibodies and to develop one or more of a group of disorders which includes asthma, hay fever, urticaria, food and other allergies, and a particular type of eczema. Some 15% of the population have at least one atopic manifestation.

Presentation and course

Atopic eczema usually begins before the age of six months. It affects at least 3% of infants, but the onset may be delayed until childhood or adult life. The distribution and character of the lesions vary with age (Fig. 9.10); but a general dryness of the skin may persist throughout life.

- In infancy, atopic eczema tends to be vesicular and weeping. It often starts on the face (Fig. 9.11) with a non-specific distribution elsewhere, commonly sparing the napkin (nappy/diaper) area.
- In childhood, the eczema becomes leathery, dry and excoriated, affecting mainly the elbow and knee flexures (Fig. 9.12), wrists and ankles. A stubborn 'reverse' pattern affecting the extensor aspects of the limbs is also recognized.

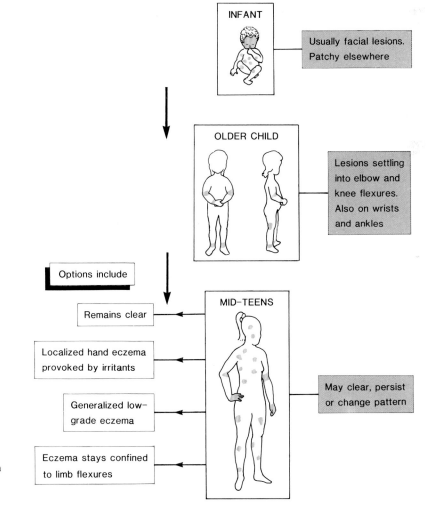

Fig. 9.10 The pattern of atopic eczema varies with age. It may clear at any stage.

- In adults, the distribution is as in childhood with a marked tendency towards lichenification and a more widespread but low-grade involvement of the trunk, face (Fig. 9.13) and hands.

The cardinal feature of atopic eczema is itching; and scratching may account for most of the clinical picture. Affected children may sleep poorly, and be hyperactive, and sometimes manipulative, using the state of their eczema to get what they want from their parents. Luckily the condition remits spontaneously before the age of 10 in at least two-thirds of affected children, though it may come back at times of stress. Eczema and asthma may see-saw so that while one is improving the other may be getting worse.

Complications

Overt bacterial infection is troublesome in many patients with atopic eczema (Fig. 9.14). They are also expecially prone to viral infections, most dangerously with widespread herpes simplex, but also with molluscum contagiosum and warts.

Investigation

Prick testing demonstrates immediate-type hypersensitivity and is helpful in the investigation of asthma and hay fever. The value of prick testing in atopic eczema, however, remains controversial; often the finding of multiple positive reactions, and a high IgE level, does little more than support a doubtful clinical diagnosis without leading to fruitful lines of treatment.

Treatment

Management here is complex and should include:
- Explanation, reassurance and encouragement.
- The avoidance of irritants, e.g. woollen clothing, and later of careers, such as hairdressing and engineering, which would inevitably lead to much exposure to irritants.
- The judicious use of topical steroids and other applications as for other types of chronic eczema (p. 75).
- The regular use of bland emollients, either directly to the skin or in the form of oils to be used in the

Fig. 9.11 Acute crusted infantile atopic eczema.

Fig. 9.12 Chronic excoriated atopic eczema behind the knees.

Fig. 9.13 Widespread excoriated adult atopic eczema.

Fig. 9.14   Bacterial superinfection of facial atopic eczema.

bath. Some of these can also be used as soap substitutes. A list of suitable preparations is given in the Formulary (p. 245).
- Those with an associated ichthyosis generally should use ointments rather than creams.
- The scratch/itch cycle can often be interrupted by occlusive bandaging, e.g. with 1% ichthammol paste.
- Sedative antihistamines, e.g. trimeprazine or hydroxyzine (Formulary, p. 258), are of value if sleep is interrupted. The newer non-sedative antihistamines do not help so much with pruritus.

- Those with active herpes simplex infections should be avoided to cut the risk of developing eczema herpeticum.
- Cow's milk and eggs possibly should be avoided for the first six months of life by children with a risk of developing atopic eczema. After this the role of diet is debatable and often minimal.
- Routine inoculations are permissible during quiet phases of the eczema. However, children who are allergic to eggs should not be inoculated against measles, influenza and yellow fever.

Seborrhoeic eczema

Cause
This condition is unrelated to seborrhoea. It may run in some families and often affects those with a tendency to dandruff. Some believe that the overgrowth of pityrosporum yeasts plays an important part in the development of seborrhoeic eczema.

Presentation and course
The term covers at least three common patterns of endogenous eczema which may merge together (Fig. 9.15):
1 A red, scaly or exudative eruption of the scalp, ears (Fig. 9.16), face (Fig. 9.17) and eyebrows. May be

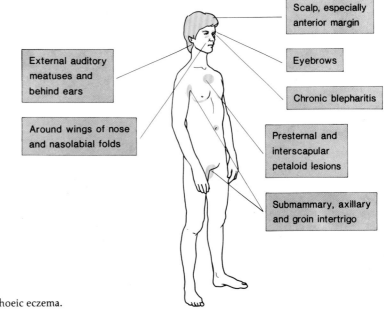

Scalp, especially anterior margin

Eyebrows

Chronic blepharitis

External auditory meatuses and behind ears

Around wings of nose and nasolabial folds

Presternal and interscapular petaloid lesions

Submammary, axillary and groin intertrigo

Fig. 9.15   Areas most often affected by seborrhoeic eczema.

associated with chronic blepharitis and otitis externa.

2 Dry, scaly, 'petaloid' lesions of the presternal (Fig. 9.18) and interscalpular areas. There may also be extensive follicular papules or pustules on the trunk (seborrhoeic folliculitis or pityrosporum folliculitis).

3 Intertriginous lesions of the armpits, umbilicus or groins, or under spectacles or hearing aids.

Seborrhoeic eczema may affect infants (Fig. 9.19) but is most common in adult males. In infants it clears quickly but in adults its course is unpredictable and may be chronic or recurrent. Some particularly severe cases have occurred in patients with AIDS.

Complications
May be associated with furunculosis. In the intertriginous type superadded *Candida* infection is common.

Investigations
None are usually needed.

Treatment
Therapy is suppressive rather than curative and patients should be told this. Topical imidazoles (Formulary, p. 250) are perhaps the first line of treatment. Two per cent sulphur and 2% salicylic acid in aqueous cream is often helpful and avoids the problem of topical steroids. It may be used to the scalp overnight and removed by a medicated shampoo which may contain tar, salicylic acid, sulphur, zinc or selenium sulphide (Formulary, p. 245). For intertriginous lesions a weak steroid–antiseptic or steroid–antifungal combination (Formulary, p. 249) is often effective.

Discoid (nummular) eczema

Cause
No cause has been established but chronic stress is often present. A reaction to bacterial antigens has been suspected as the lesions often yield staphylococci on culture, and as steroid–antiseptic or antibiotic mixtures do better than either separately.

Presentation and course
This common pattern of endogenous eczema classi-

Fig. 9.16 Dry scaly seborrhoeic eczema of the ear.

Fig. 9.17 Active seborrhoeic eczema of the face.

Fig. 9.18 Typical presternal patch of seborrhoeic eczema.

Fig. 9.19   Infantile seborrhoeic eczema.

Fig. 9.20   Vesicular and weeping patch of discoid eczema.

Fig. 9.21   Pompholyx of the palm with early secondary infection.

Fig. 9.22   Pompholyx vesicles along the side of a finger.

cally affects the limbs of middle-aged males. The lesions are multiple, coin-shaped, vesicular or crusted, highly itchy plaques (Fig. 9.20), usually less than 5 cm across. The condition tends to persist for many months.

Investigations
None are usually needed.

Treatment
With topical steroid antiseptic or antibiotic combinations (*see above*).

Pompholyx

Cause
Usually unknown but sometimes provoked by heat or emotional upsets. In allergic subjects the ingestion of small amounts of nickel in food may trigger pompholyx.

Presentation and course
In this tiresome and sometimes very unpleasant form of eczema, recurrent bouts of vesicles or larger blisters appear on the palms (Fig. 9.21), fingers (Fig. 9.22) and/or the soles of adults. Bouts lasting a few weeks recur at irregular intervals.

Investigations
None are usually needed: sometimes a pompholyx-like eruption of the hands can follow acute tinea pedis. If this is suspected, scrapings or blister roofs from the feet should be sent for mycological examination.

Treatment
As for acute eczema of the hands and feet (p. 74).

Gravitational (stasis) eczema

Cause
Often, but not always, accompanied by obvious venous insufficiency.

Presentation and course
A chronic patchy eczematous condition of the lower legs, sometimes accompanied by varicose veins, oedema, and haemosiderin deposition (Fig. 9.23). When severe it may spread to the other leg or even become generalized.

Complications
Patients often become sensitized to local antibiotic applications or to the preservatives in medicated bandages. Excoriations may lead to ulcer formation.

Treatment
This should include the elimination of oedema by elevation, pressure bandages or diuretics. One per cent hydrocortisone may be helpful but stronger topical steroids are best avoided. Bland applications, e.g. Lassar's paste or zinc cream BNF, or medicated bandages (Formulary, p. 253), are often helpful but stasis eczema is liable to persist, despite surgery to the underlying veins.

Asteatotic eczema

Cause
The low humidity of winter and central heating, diuretics, and overwashing are contributory factors.

Presentation and course
Often unrecognized, this common and itchy pattern of eczema occurs on the legs of elderly patients. Against a background of dry skin, a network of fine red superficial fissures causes a 'crazy paving' appearance (Fig. 9.24).

Investigations
None are usually needed. Very extensive cases may be part of malabsorption syndromes.

Fig. 9.23   Chronic gravitational eczema.

Fig 9.24   Asteatotic eczema with network of fine fissures in the stratum corneum.

Treatment
Can be cleared by the use of a mild or moderately potent topical steroid in a greasy base, and aqueous cream as a soap substitute for the area. Once clear, daily use of unmedicated emollients (Formulary, p. 245) usually prevents recurrence.

Localized neurodermatitis (lichen simplex)

Cause
The skin is damaged as a result of repeated rubbing or scratching, as a habit or in response to stress.

Presentation and course
Usually occurs as a single, fixed, lichenified plaque. Favourite areas are the nape of the neck in women, the legs in men, and the anogenital area in both sexes. Lesions may resolve with treatment but tend to recur either in the same place or elsewhere.

Investigations
None are usually needed.

Treatment
Potent topical steroids or occlusive bandaging, where feasible, help to break the scratch/itch cycle. Tranquillizers are often disappointing.

Juvenile plantar dermatosis

Cause
This condition is thought to be related to the impermeability of modern socks and shoe linings with subsequent sweat gland blockage and so has been called the 'toxic sock syndrome'! Some feel the condition is a manifestation of atopy.

Presentation and course
The skin of the weight-bearing areas of the feet, particularly the forefeet and undersides of the toes, be-

Fig. 9.25 The shiny skin and fissures of juvenile plantar dermatosis.

comes dry and shiny with deep painful fissures which make walking difficult (Fig. 9.25). The toe webs are spared. Onset can be at any time after shoes are first worn, and even if untreated the condition clears in the early teens.

Investigations
Much time has been wasted in patch testing and scraping for fungus.

Treatment
The child should use a commercially available cork insole in all shoes, and stick to cotton or wool socks. An emollient such as emulsifying ointment or 1% ichthammol paste, or an emollient containing lactic acid, is as good as a topical steroid.

Napkin (diaper) dermatitis

Cause
The commonest type of napkin eruption is irritant in origin, and is aggravated by the use of waterproof plastic pants. The mixture of faeces and ammonia produced by urea-splitting bacteria, if allowed to remain in prolonged contact with the skin, leads to a severe reaction.

Presentation
The moist, often glazed and sore erythema affects the napkin area generally, with the exception of the skin folds which tend to be spared (Fig. 9.26).

Complications
Superinfection with *Candida albicans* is common, and this may lead to small erythematous papules or vesicopustules appearing around the periphery of the main eruption.

Differential diagnosis
The sparing of the folds helps to separate this condition from infantile seborrhoeic eczema and candidiasis.

Treatment
It is never easy to keep the area clean and dry, but to do so remains the basis of all treatment. Theoretical-

Fig. 9.26   Irritant napkin erythema with some sparing of skin folds.

ly, the child should be allowed to be free of napkins as much as possible but this may become a messy nightmare. On both sides of the Atlantic disposable nappies (diapers) have largely replaced washable ones. The super absorbent type is best and should be changed regularly, especially in the middle of the night. When towelling napkins are used they should be washed thoroughly and changed frequently. The area should be cleaned at each nappy change with aqueous cream and water. Protective ointments, e.g. zinc and castor oil ointment, or silicone protective ointments, are often useful (Formulary, p. 246). Potent steroids should be avoided but combinations of hydrocortisone with antifungals or antiseptic (Formulary, p. 249) are often useful.

LEARNING POINTS

1 Do not accept 'eczema' as an adequate diagnosis: treatment hinges on establishing its cause and type.
2 Keep fluorinated steroids off the face and off the skin of infants.
3 Monitor repeat prescriptions of topical steroids, keeping an eye on the amount used and their potency.
4 Do not promise that atopic eczema will be clear by any particular age: guesses are always wrong and the patients lose faith.

CHAPTER 10

REACTIVE ERYTHEMAS AND VASCULITIS

As their name implies, the reactive erythemas are red or pink transient rashes arising in response to a variety of insults, both exogenous and endogenous. They and the vasculitides are diseases of blood vessels in the dermis; the epidermis is usually normal.

Urticaria (hives)

Cause

The characteristic wheals of this common condition are due to vasodilatation and leakage of fluid into the surrounding tissues. Urticaria is sometimes caused by an allergy, but is often mediated by non-allergic mechanisms. The various types of urticaria are listed in Table 10.1.

Physical urticarias

Cold urticaria
Patients develop wheals in areas exposed to cold, for example when cycling in the face of a cold wind.

A useful test in the clinic is to reproduce the reaction by immersing an extremity in cold water. A few cases are associated with the presence of cryoglobulins, cold agglutinins, or cryofibrinogens.

Solar urticaria
Wheals occur within minutes of sun exposure. Some patients with solar urticaria have erythropoietic protoporphyria (p. 217); most have an IgE-mediated urticarial reaction to sunlight.

Table 10.1 The main types of urticaria.

Physical
cold
solar
heat
cholinergic
dermographism
delayed pressure
Inherited
hereditary angioedema
Hypersensitivity
Pharmacological
Contact

Heat urticaria
In this condition wheals arise in areas in contact with hot objects or solutions.

Cholinergic urticaria
Anxiety or strenuous exercise elicits this characteristic response. The itchy, transient, 2–5 mm follicular macules or papules resemble a blush or viral exanthem. The condition is mediated by acetyl choline released from sympathetic nerves in the skin. In patients with cholinergic urticaria, vessels overdilate in response to this neuromediator, and the overlying skin becomes pink.

Dermographism
This is a physical urticaria in which skin mast cells release extra histamine after rubbing or scratching. The linear wheals are therefore an exaggerated triple response of Lewis (Fig. 10.1).

Fig. 10.1 Dermographism: linear wheals on the legs after scratching.

Table 10.2 The eight I's of antigen encounter in hypersensitive urticaria.

Ingestion
Inhalation
Instillation
Injection
Insertion
Insect bites
Infestations
Infections

Delayed pressure urticaria

Sustained pressure causes oedema of the underlying skin and subcutaneous tissue 3–6 hours later. The swelling may last up to 48 hours and it is probably mediated by kinins or prostaglandins rather than histamine. It occurs particularly on the feet after walking, on the hands after clapping and on the buttocks after sitting.

Other types of urticaria

Hereditary angioedema

This autosomal dominant condition is characterized by recurrent attacks of abdominal pain and vomiting, or massive oedema of soft tissues which may involve the larynx. Tooth extraction, cheek biting, and other forms of trauma may precipitate an attack. A deficiency of an inhibitor to C1 esterase allows complement consumption to go unchecked so that vasoactive mediators are generated. To confirm the diagnosis, a serum C1 esterase inhibitor level and a C4 level should both be checked as the level of C1 esterase inhibitor is not always depressed (there is a type where the inhibitor is present but does not work).

Hypersensitivity urticaria

This most common form of urticaria is due to hypersensitivity, often an IgE-mediated (type I) allergic reaction (Chapter 3). Allergens may be encountered in eight different ways (the eight I's listed in Table 10.2).

Pharmacological urticaria

This occurs when drugs cause mast cells to release histamine in a non-allergic manner (e.g. aspirin and morphine).

Contact urticaria

This type of urticaria may be IgE mediated or a pharmacological effect. Wheals occur most often around the mouth. Foods and food additives are the most common culprits but the reaction may be caused by drugs, animal saliva, caterpillars, and plants.

Fig. 10.2 Severe and acute urticaria due to penicillin allergy.

Fig. 10.3 Giant wheals in chronic urticaria.

Fig. 10.4 Angioedema of the face: note lack of erythema and marked swelling of the eyelids.

Fig. 10.5 Urticarial lesions simulating the target lesions of erythema multiforme.

Presentation

Most of these urticarial types share the sudden appearance of pink, itchy wheals, which may come up anywhere on the skin surface (Fig. 10.2). Each lasts less than a day, and most disappear within a few hours. Lesions may enlarge rapidly and some resolve centrally to take up an annular shape (Fig. 10.3). In an acute anaphylactic reaction, wheals may cover most of the skin surface. In contrast, in chronic urticaria, only a few wheals may develop each day.

Angioedema describes a variant of urticaria which primarily affects the subcutaneous tissues so that the swelling is less demarcated and less red than an urticarial wheal. Angioedema most commonly occurs at junctions between skin and mucous membranes (e.g. peri-orbital, peri-oral and genital) (Fig. 10.4). It may be associated with swelling of the tongue and laryngeal mucosa. It frequently accompanies chronic urticaria and its causes are the same.

Course

The course of an urticarial reaction depends on its cause. If the urticaria is allergic, it will continue until the allergen is removed, tolerated or metabolized. Most such patients clear up within a day or two, even if the allergen is not identified. Urticaria may recur if the allergen is met again. At the other end of the scale, some patients have chronic urticaria for years without any discernible cause.

Complications

Urticaria normally is uncomplicated, although its itch may be enough to interfere with sleep or daily activities. In acute anaphylactic reactions, oedema of the larynx may lead to asphyxiation and oedema of the tracheobronchial tree to asthma.

Differential diagnosis

There are two aspects to the differential diagnosis of urticaria. The first is to tell urticaria from other eruptions which are not urticaria at all. The second is to define the type of urticaria, according to Table 10.1. Insect bites and infestations commonly elicit urticarial papules, but these may have a central punctum. Erythema multiforme can also look like an annular urticaria (Fig. 10.5). A form of vasculitis (urticarial vasculitis) may resemble urticaria, but individual lesions last for longer than 24 hours and may leave bruising in their wake. Some bullous diseases, such as dermatitis herpetiformis, pemphigoid and herpes gestationis begin as urticarial areas, but later bullae make the diagnosis obvious. On the face, erysipelas can be distinguished from angioedema by its sharp margin and accompanying pyrexia (Fig. 10.6).

Investigations

The investigations will depend upon the presentation and type of urticaria. As noted above, many of the physical urticarias can be reproduced by appropriate tests.

Almost invariably, more is learned from the history than from the laboratory. It should include details of the events surrounding the onset of the eruption. A review of systems may uncover evidence of an underlying disease. Careful attention should be paid to drugs, remembering that self-prescribed ones can also cause urticaria. Over-the-counter medications (such as aspirin) and medications given by other routes (Table 10.2) can produced wheals. If a patient has acute urticaria, and its cause is not obvious, investigations are often deferred until it has persisted for a few weeks; then a physical examination (if it has not already been done) and screening tests such as a complete blood count, erythrocyte sedimentation rate, routine biochemical screen, chest X-ray, and urine analysis are worthwhile. If the urticaria continues for 2–3 months, the patient should probably be referred to a dermatologist for further evaluation. In general the focus of such investigations will be on internal disorders associated with urticaria (Table 10.3) and on external allergens (Table 10.4). Even after extensive evaluation and environmental change, the cause cannot always be found.

Fig. 10.6   Urticaria on the face simulating erysipelas: note the ill-defined margin and lack of surface change.

Table 10.3   Some endogenous causes of urticaria.

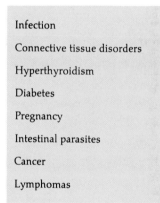

Infection
Connective tissue disorders
Hyperthyroidism
Diabetes
Pregnancy
Intestinal parasites
Cancer
Lymphomas

Table 10.4   Some exogenous causes of urticaria.

Drugs, both topical and systemic
Foods and food additives
Bites
Inhalants
Pollens
Insect venoms
Animal dander

Table 10.5 Some types of urticaria and their management.

Type	Treatment
Cold urticaria	Avoid cold Protective clothing Antihistamines
Solar urticaria	Avoid sun exposure Protective clothing Sunscreens and sunblocks β-carotene Antihistamines
Cholinergic urticaria	Avoid heat Minimize anxiety Avoid exessive exercise Anticholinergics Antihistamines Tranquillizers
Dermographism	Avoid trauma Antihistamines
Hereditary angioedema	Avoid trauma Attenuated androgenic steroids as prophylaxis Tracheostomy may be necessary
Hypersensitivity urticarias	Remove cause Antihistamines (H1 + H2) Sympathomimetics Systemic steroids (rarely justified) Avoid drugs containing aspirin

Treatment

The ideal is to find a cause and then to eliminate it. Aspirin, in any form, should be banned. The treatment for each type of urticaria is outlined in Table 10.5. In general, antihistamines are the mainstay of symptomatic treatment. Terfenidine 60 mg twice daily, or hydroxyzine, 10–25 mg up to every four hours, are useful treatments. Sometimes they can be combined with a longer acting antihistamine (such as chlorpheniramine maleate 12 mg sustained release tablets every 12 hours) so that peaks and troughs are blunted, and histamine activity is blocked throughout the night. If the eruption is not controlled, the dose can often be increased and still tolerated. H2-blocking antihistamines (e.g. cimetidine) may add a slight benefit if used in conjunction with an H1 histamine antagonist. Sympathomimetic agents can help urticaria, although the effects of adrenaline (epinephrine) are short lived. Pseudoephedrine, 30 or 60 mg every four hours, or terbutaline, 2.5 mg every eight hours, can sometimes be useful adjuncts. A tapering course of systemic corticosteroids may be used, but only when the cause is known and there are no contra-indications, and certainly not as a panacea to control chronic urticaria or urticaria of unknown cause. For treatment of anaphylaxis see p. 235.

LEARNING POINTS

1 Avoid aspirins and systemic steroids in chronic urticaria.
2 Do not promise patients that all will be solved by allergy tests.
3 Alert those with cold urticaria to the dangers of swimming and ice cream.
4 Take respiratory tract blockage seriously.

Erythema multiforme

Cause

In erythema multiforme, the victim has usually reacted to an infection, often herpes simplex, or to a drug, but other factors have occasionally been implicated (Table 10.6).

Presentation

The symptoms of an upper respiratory tract infection may precede the eruption. Typically, annular non-scaling plaques appear on the palms, soles, forearms, and legs. They may be slightly more purple than the wheals of ordinary urticaria. Individual lesions enlarge but clear centrally. A new lesion may begin at the same site as the original one, so that the two concentric plaques look like a target (Figs. 10.7 and 10.8). Occasionally lesions may blister. The Stevens–Johnson syndrome is a severe var-

Table 10.6   Some causes of erythema multiforme.

Viral infections, especially:
  herpes simplex
  hepatitis A and B
  mycoplasma
  orf

Bacterial infections

Fungal infections
  coccidioidomycosis

Parasitic infections

Drugs

Pregnancy

Malignancy, or its treatment with radiotherapy

Idiopathic

Fig. 10.7   Erythema multiforme: close-up of typical target lesions, tending to become bullous around their edges.

iant of erythema multiforme associated with fever and mucous membrane lesions. The oral mucosa, lip and bulbar conjunctivae are most commonly affected, but the nares, penis, vagina, pharynx, larynx, and tracheobronchial tree may also be involved (Fig. 10.9).

Course

Crops of new lesions appear for one or two weeks, or until the responsible drug or other factor has been eliminated. Individual lesions last several days, and this differentiates them from the more fleeting lesions of an annular urticaria. The site of resolved lesions is marked transiently by hyperpigmentation, particularly in pigmented individuals.

Complications

There are usually no complications. However, severe lesions in the tracheobronchial tree of patients with Stevens–Johnson syndrome may lead to asphyxia, and ulcers of the bulbar conjunctiva to blindness. Corneal ulcers, anterior uveitis, and panophthalmitis may also occur. Genital ulcers may cause urinary retention and phimosis or vaginal stricture after they heal.

Fig. 10.8   Bullous target lesions occurring in a favourite site. In this patient recurrent attacks of erythema multiforme followed episodes of herpes simplex.

Fig. 10.9   Stevens–Johnson type of erythema multiforme. The eyes were also severely involved.

Differential diagnosis

Erythema multiforme can mimic the annular variant of urticaria as described above. However, target lesions are pathognomonic of erythema multiforme. Its acral distribution, the way individual lesions last for more than 24 hours, their purple colour, and the involvement of mucous membranes, all help to identify erythema multiforme. Other bullous disorders may enter the differential diagnosis (Chapter 11).

Investigations

The histology of erythema multiforme is distinctive. Epidermal necrosis and dermal changes, consisting of endothelial swelling, a mixed lymphohistiocytic perivascular infiltrate and papillary dermal oedema are seen. The abnormalities may be predominantly epidermal or dermal or a combination of both; they probably depend on the stage of the lesion biopsied.

Most investigations are directed towards identifying a cause. Tzanck smears (p. 32) or culture for a precipitating herpes simplex infection are worthwhile if the disorder is recurrent. A chest X-ray and serological tests should identify mycoplasmal pneumonia. A search for other infectious agents, neoplasia, endocrine causes, or collagen disease is sometimes necessary, especially when the course is prolonged or recurrent. About 50% of cases have no demonstrable provoking factor.

Treatment

The best treatment for erythema multiforme is to identify and remove its cause. In mild cases, only symptomatic treatment is needed and this includes the use of antihistamines.

The Stevens–Johnson syndrome, on the other hand, may demand immediate consultation between dermatologists and specialists in other fields such as ophthalmology, urology, and infectious diseases, depending on the particular case. The use of systemic steroids to abort Stevens–Johnson syndrome is debatable, but many believe that a short course (e.g. prednisolone 80 mg/day in divided doses in an adult)

helps. However, the dose should be tapered rapidly or stopped because prolonged treatment in the Stevens–Johnson syndrome has been linked, controversially, with a high complication rate. Good nursing care with attention to the mouth and eyes is essential. The prevention of secondary infection, maintenance of a patent airway, good nutrition, and proper fluid and electrolyte balance, are important.

Herpes simplex infections should be suspected in recurrent erythema multiforme of otherwise unknown cause. Treatment with oral acyclovir 200 mg four times daily may prevent attacks, both of herpes simplex and of the recurrent erythema multiforme which follows it.

LEARNING POINTS

1 Look for target lesions and involvement of the palms.
2 Herpes simplex infection is the commonest provoking factor, but do not forget drugs.

Erythema nodosum

Erythema nodosum is an inflammation of the subcutaneous fat (a panniculitis). It is an immunological reaction, elicited by various bacterial, viral, and fungal infections, malignant disorders, drugs, and by a variety of other causes (Table 10.7).

Presentation

The characteristic lesion is a tender, red nodule developing alone or in groups on the legs and forearms or, rarely, on other areas such as the thighs, face, breasts, or other areas where there is fat (Fig. 10.10). Some patients also have painful joints and fever.

Course

Lesions usually resolve in 6–8 weeks. In the interim, lesions may enlarge and new lesions may occur at

Table 10.7   Some causes of erythema multiforme.

Infections
    bacteria (e.g. streptococci, tuberculosis,
    brucellosis, leprosy)
    viruses
    Mycoplasma
    Rickettsia
    Chlamydia
    fungi (especially coccidioidomycosis)

Drugs (e.g. sulphonamides, oral contraceptive
    agents)

Systemic disease (e.g. sarcoidosis, ulcerative
    colitis, Crohn's disease, Behçet's disease)

Fig. 10.10   Erythema nodosum: large painful dusky plaques on the shins. Always investigate this important reaction pattern *(see text)*.

other sites. Like other reactive erythemas, erythema nodosum may persist if its cause is not removed.

Complications

The nodules may be so tender that walking is difficult. Erythema nodosum leprosum occurs when lepromatous leprosy patients establish cell-mediated immunity to *Mycobacterium leprae*. These patients have severe malaise, arthralgia, and fever.

Differential diagnosis

The differential diagnosis of a single, tender, red nodule is extensive and includes trauma, infection (early cellulitis or abscess), and phlebitis.

When lesions are multiple, infection becomes less likely unless the lesions are developing in a sporotrichoid manner (p. 164). Other causes of a nodular panniculitis which may appear like erythema nodosum include panniculitis from pancreatitis, cold, trauma, injection of drugs or other foreign substances, withdrawal from systemic steroids, lupus erythematosus, superficial migratory thrombophlebitis, and polyarteritis nodosa. Some people use the term nodular vasculitis to describe a condition like erythema nodosum which lasts for more than six months (Fig. 10.11).

Investigations

Erythema nodosum demands a careful history, physical examination, a chest X-ray, throat culture for streptococcus, a Mantoux test, and an antistreptolysin-O (ASO) titre. If the results are normal, and there are no symptoms or physical findings to suggest other causes, extensive investigations can be deferred because the disease will resolve in most such patients.

Fig. 10.11   The smaller lesions of nodular vasculitis, the causes of which overlap with erythema nodosum.

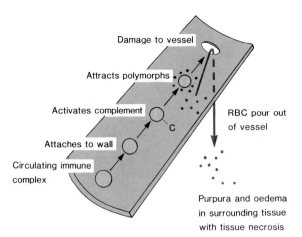

Fig. 10.12   Pathogenesis of vasculitis.

endothelial cell swelling, necrosis or fibrinoid change. The clinical manifestations depend upon the size of the blood vessel affected.

Leucocytoclastic (small vessel) vasculitis
(Syn: allergic or hypersensitivity vasculitis, anaphylactoid purpura)

Cause

Immune complexes may lodge in the walls of blood vessels, activate complement, and attract polymorphonuclear leucocytes (Fig. 10.12). Enzymes released from these can degrade the vessel wall. Antigens in these immune complexes include drugs, auto-antigens, and infectious agents such as bacteria.

Treatment

The ideal treatment for erythema nodosum is to identify and eliminate its cause if possible. For example, if a streptococcal infection is confirmed by culture or an ASO test, a suitable antibiotic will be recommended. Bed rest is also an important part of treatment. Non-steroidal anti-inflammatory agents such as aspirin, indomethacin, or ibuprofen may be helpful. Systemic steroids are usually not needed. For reasons which are not clear, potassium iodide in a dose of 400–900 mg/day can help, but should not be used for longer than six months.

Presentation

The most common presentation of vaculitis is painful, palpable, purpura (Fig. 10.13). Crops of lesions arise in dependent areas (the forearms and legs) (Fig. 10.14). Some have a small, livid or black centre, due to necrosis of the tissue overlying the affected blood vessel. The purpura is palpable because the damaged vessel has leaked fluid.

Henoch–Schönlein purpura is a small vessel vasculitis associated with palpable purpura, arthritis,

Vasculitis

Whereas the reactive erythemas are associated with some inflammation around superficial or deep blood vessels, the term vasculitis is reserved for those showing inflammation within the vessel wall, with

The three P's of cutaneous vasculitis

Fig. 10.13   The 3 P's of small vessel vasculitis.

Fig. 10.14   Palpable purpuric lesions on both legs indicate small vessel vasculitis.

and abdominal pain, often preceded by an upper respiratory tract infection.

Course

The course of the vasculitis varies with its cause, its extent, the size of blood vessel affected, and the involvement of other organs.

Complications

Vasculitis may simply be cutaneous; alternatively it may be systemic, and then other organs will be damaged, including the kidney, central nervous system, gastro-intestinal tract, and lungs.

Differential diagnosis

Small vessel vasculitis has to be separated from other causes of purpura (p. 123) such as abnormalities of the clotting system and sepsis (with or without vasculitis). Occasionally the vasculitis may look like urticaria if its purpuric element is not marked.

Investigations

Investigations should be directed toward detecting internal involvement. A physical examination, chest X-ray, erythrocyte sedimentation rate, and biochemical tests monitoring the function of various organs are indicated. The most important test, however, is urine analysis, checking for proteinuria and haematuria, because vasculitis can affect the kidney subtly and so lead to renal insufficiency.

Skin biopsy will confirm the diagnosis of small vessel vasculitis. The finding of circulating immune complexes, or a lowered level of total complement (CH50) or C4, will implicate immune complexes as its cause. Tests for cryoglobulins, rheumatoid factor, and antinuclear antibodies may also be needed.

Direct immunofluorescence can be used to identify immune complexes in blood vessel walls, but is seldom performed because of false positive and false negative results as inflammation may destroy the complexes in a true vasculitis, and induce non-specific deposition in other diseases. Henoch–Schönlein vasculitis is confirmed if IgA deposits are found in the blood vessels of a patient with the clinical triad of palpable purpura, arthritis, and abdominal pain.

Treatment

The treatment of choice is to identify the cause and eliminate it. In addition, antihistamines and bed rest are sometimes helpful. Colchicine 0.6 mg twice daily or dapsone 100 mg daily may be worth a trial, but require monitoring for side effects (Formulary, p. 262). Patients whose vasculitis is damaging the kidneys or other internal organs may require systemic corticosteroids or immunosuppressive agents such as cyclophosphamide.

LEARNING POINT

Clinical features of leucocytoclastic vasculitis are often so typical that biopsy is unnecessary.

Polyarteritis nodosa

Cause

This necrotizing vasculitis of large arteries causes skin nodules, infarctive ulcers, and peripheral gangrene. Immune complexes may initiate this vasculitis, and sometimes contain hepatitis B antigen. Other known causes are adulterated drugs, B cell lymphomas, and immunotherapy.

Presentation

Tender subcutaneous nodules appear along the line of arteries. The skin over them may ulcerate or develop stellate patches of purpura and necrosis. Splinter haemorrhages and a peculiar, net-like vascular pattern (livedo reticularis) aid the clinical diagnosis. The disorder may be of the skin only (cutaneous polyarteritis nodosa), or also affect the kidneys, heart muscle, nerves, and joints (Fig. 10.15). Patients may be febrile, lose weight, and feel pain in the muscles, joints, or abdomen. Some develop peripheral neuropathy, hypertension, and ischaemic heart disease. Renal involvement, with or without hypertension, is common.

Course

Untreated, systemic polyarteritis nodosa becomes chronic. Death, often from renal disease, is common, even in treated patients.

Differential diagnosis

Embolism, panniculitis, and infarctions can cause a similar clinical picture. Wegener's granulomatosis, allergic granulomatosis, temporal arteritis, and vasculitis which accompanies systemic lupus erythematosus and rheumatoid arthritis should be considered.

Investigations

The laboratory findings are non-specific. An elevated ESR, neutrophil count, and gamma-globulin level are common. Investigations for cryoglobulins, rheumatoid factor, antinuclear antibody, and hepatitis B sur-

face antigen are worthwhile, as are checks for disease in the kidney, heart, liver, and gut. Low levels of complement suggest active disease. The use of biopsy to confirm the diagnosis of large vessel vasculitis is not always easy as the arterial involvement may be segmental, and surgery itself difficult. Histological confirmation is most likely when biopsies are from a fresh lesion. Affected vessels show aneurysmal dilatation, necrosis, and fibrinoid changes in their walls, and an intense neutrophilic infiltrate.

Treatment

Systemic steroids and cyclophosphamide improve chances of survival. Low-dose systemic steroids alone are usually sufficient for the purely cutaneous form.

Wegener's granulomatosis

In this granulomatous vasculitis of unknown cause, fever, weight loss, and fatigue accompany nasorespiratory symptoms such as rhinitis, hearing loss, or sinusitis. Only half of the patients have skin lesions, usually symmetrical ulcers or papules on the extremities. Other organs can be affected, including the eye, joints, heart, nerves, lung, and kidney. Antineutrophil antibodies are present in most cases and are a useful diagnostic marker. Cyclophosphamide is treatment of choice, used alone or with systemic steroids.

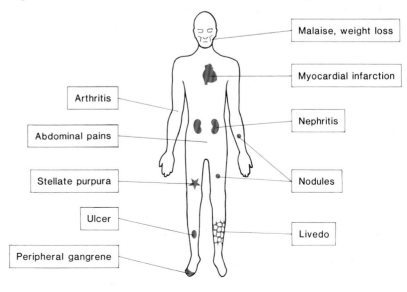

Fig. 10.15   Signs of polyarteritis nodosa.

CHAPTER 11
BULLOUS DISEASES

Blisters are accumulations of fluid lying within the epidermis, or immediately under it. They have many causes. Sometimes the morphology or distribution makes the diagnosis obvious, as in herpes simplex or zoster. Sometimes the history aids the diagnosis, as in cold or thermal injury, or in acute contact dermatitis. When the cause is not obvious, a biopsy can help by showing the level in the skin at which the blister has arisen (Fig. 11.1).

Subepidermal blisters occur between the dermis and the epidermis. Clinically these are thick-walled and may contain blood. Intra-epidermal bullae occur within the prickle cell layer of the epidermis: subcorneal blisters form just beneath the stratum corneum, at the outermost edge of the viable epidermis, and therefore have a particularly thin roof.

A list of differential diagnoses, based on histology, is given in Figure 11.1 and some clinical and patho-logical distinguishing features are listed in Table 11.1. Only the most common conditions will be discussed here.

Subcorneal blisters

Bullous impetigo (p. 136)
This is a common cause of blistering in children. The bullae are flaccid, often contain pus, and are frequently grouped or located in body folds. Bullous impetigo is caused by *Staphylococcus aureus*.

Staphylococcal scalded skin syndrome (p. 139)
A toxin elaborated by some strains of *S. aureus* makes the skin painful and red; later it peels like a scald. The staphylococcus is usually hidden (e.g. conjunctiva, throat, wound, furuncle).

Table 11.1. Distinguishing features of some bullous diseases.

	Age	Site	General health	Mouth ulcers	Nature of blisters	Circulating antibodies	Fixed antibodies	Treatment
Pemphigus	Middle age	Trunk and flexures	Poor	Common	Superficial and flaccid	IgG to inter-cellular substance	IgG in inter-cellular substance	Steroids Immunosup-pressives
Pemphigoid	Old	Often flexural	Good	Rare	Tense and blood-filled	IgG to basement membrane region	IgG at basement membrane	Steroids Immunosup-pressives
Dermatitis herpe-tiformis	Primarily adults	Elbows, knees, upper back, buttocks	Itchy	Rare	Small, excoriated and grouped	None	IgA granular deposits in papillary dermis	Gluten-free diet Dapsone Sulphapyri-dine

LOCATION OF BULLAE   DISEASES

Subcorneal bulla

Bullous impetigo
Miliaria crystallina
Staphylococcal
scalded skin syndrome

Intra–epidermal bulla

Acute eczema
Viral vesicles
Pemphigus
Miliaria rubra
Incontinentia pigmenti

Subepidermal bulla

Bullous pemphigoid
Cicatricial pemphigoid
Herpes gestationis
Dermatitis herpetiformis
Linear IgA disease
Bullous erythema multiforme
Bullous lichen planus
Bullous lupus erythematosus
Porphyria cutanea tarda
Toxic epidermal necrolysis
Cold or thermal injury
Epidermolysis bullosa

Fig. 11.1 The differential diagnosis of bullous diseases based on the histological location of the blister.

Miliaria crystallina (p. 134)

Here sweat accumulates under the stratum corneum leading to the development of thousands of uniformly spaced vesicles without underlying redness. Often this occurs after a fever or heavy exertion. The vesicles look like water droplets on the surface, but the skin is dry to the touch. The disorder is self-limiting and needs no treatment.

Subcorneal pustular dermatosis

As its name implies, the lesions are small groups of pustules rather than vesicles. However, the pustules pout out of the skin in a way that suggests they were once vesicles (like the vesico-pustules of chickenpox). The cause of this rare disease is unknown, but oral dapsone (Formulary, p. 262) usually suppresses it.

Intra-epidermal vesicles or bullae

Acute dermatitis (Chapter 9)

Severe, acute eczema, especially the contact allergic type, can produce bullae (the name eczema suggests the bubbling of boiling water). Plants such as poison ivy, poison oak, or primula are common causes. The varying size of the vesicles, their close grouping, their asymmetry, their odd configurations (e.g. linear, square, rectilinear) and a history of contact with plants are helpful guides to the diagnosis.

Pompholyx (p. 81)

In pompholyx, highly itchy, small, eczematous vesicles occur along the sides of the fingers.

Viral infections (Chapter 15)

Some viruses create blisters in the skin by destroying epithelial cells.

Pemphigus

Pemphigus is a severe, and often life-threatening blistering condition.

Cause

It is an auto-immune disease. IgG antibodies bind to the intercellular areas of the epidermis and induce the keratinocytes to release a proteolytic enzyme which dissolves the intercellular cement so that the keratinocytes fall apart.

Presentation

The disease is characterized by flaccid blisters of the

Fig. 11.2 Pemphigus vulgaris: widespread superficial blisters and erosions.

Fig. 11.3   Pemphigus vulgaris: thin-roofed blisters rupture easily leaving unhealing painful erosions.

Fig. 11.4   Painful sloughy mouth ulcers in pemphigus vulgaris.

skin (Figs. 11.2 and 11.3), and mouth (Fig. 11.4) and, after the blisters rupture, by widespread erosions. Most patients develop lesions in the mouth first. The skin lesions are flaccid blisters from the outset. Shearing stresses on normal skin may cause a new lesion to form (positive Nikolsky sign).

There are several forms of pemphigus. The common type, pemphigus vulgaris, is a blistering and erosive disease. Pemphigus vegetans leads to the formation of heaped up, cauliflower-like, weeping areas, particularly in the groin and body folds. The blisters in pemphigus foliaceus are so superficial, and rupture so easily, that there are more weeping and crusting erosions than blisters.

Course

The course is prolonged, even with treatment. The huge areas of denudation may become infected and smelly. However, with modern treatment, most patients can live relatively normal lives, with occasional exacerbations.

Complications

Infections are common. Complications are inevitable with the high doses of steroids and immunosuppressive drugs which are needed. Indeed, side effects of treatment are now the leading cause of death. Severe oral ulcers make eating painful.

Differential diagnosis

Widespread erosions may suggest a pyoderma, impetigo, epidermolysis bullosa, or ecthyma. Mouth ulcers may be mistaken for aphthae, Behçet's disease, or herpes simplex infection.

Investigations

Biopsy shows that the vesicles are intra-epidermal, with rounded keratinocytes floating free within the blister cavity (acantholysis). Direct immunofluorescence (p. 34) of adjacent normal skin shows intercellular epidermal deposits of IgG and C3 (Fig. 11.5). The serum from a patient with pemphigus contains antibodies which bind to the intercellular areas of normal epidermis, so that indirect immunofluorescence (p. 34) can also be used to confirm the diagnosis. The titre of these antibodies correlates loosely with clinical activity and may guide changes in the dose of systemic steroids.

Treatment

Because of the severity of this disease, and the difficulty in controlling it, patients should be treated by a dermatologist. Huge doses of systemic steroids, such as prednisolone (Formulary, p. 260) 80–320 mg/day, may be needed at first, and the dose is dropped only when new blisters stop appearing. Immunosuppressive agents, such as azathioprine and cyclophosphamide, are often used as steroid-sparing agents. Intramuscular or oral gold can also help. Treatment and regular follow-up is usually prolonged.

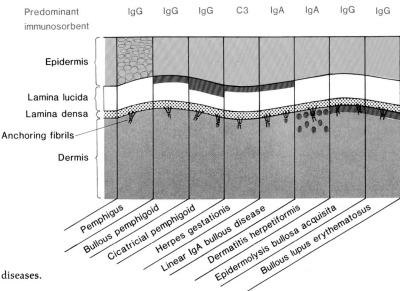

| Predominant immunosorbent | IgG | IgG | IgG | C3 | IgA | IgA | IgG | IgG |

Fig. 11.5   Immunofluorescence in bullous diseases.

Subepidermal bullous diseases

Pemphigoid (bullous pemphigoid)

Cause
Pemphigoid is also an auto-immune disease. IgG antibodies bind to the junction between the dermis and epidermis (Fig. 11.5). Serum from about 70% of patients contains antibodies which bind *in vitro* to normal skin at the basement membrane zone. The titre does not correlate with clinical disease activity. The blister is formed by enzymes released from inflammatory cells drawn to the area by chemotactic complement components.

Presentation
Pemphigoid is a chronic, sometimes itchy, blistering disease of elderly patients. Many tense bullae arise from normal skin or from large urticarial plaques (Fig. 11.6). The flexures are often affected; the mu-cous membranes usually are not. The Nikolsky test is negative.

Course
Pemphigoid is usually self-limiting and treatment can often be stopped after 1–2 years.

Complications
Untreated, the disease causes much discomfort and the loss of fluid from ruptured bullae. Systemic steroids and immunosuppressive agents carry their usual complications if used for long (Formulary, p. 260 and p. 259).

Fig. 11.6   Numerous large tense blisters in an elderly person suggest pemphigoid.

Differential diagnosis

It may look like other bullous diseases, especially bullous lupus erythematosus, dermatitis herpetiformis, herpes gestationis, bullous erythema multiforme, and linear IgA bullous disease. Immunofluorescence helps to separate it from these disorders (Fig. 11.5).

Investigations

The histology is that of a subepidermal blister, often filled with eosinophils. Direct immunofluorescence demonstrates a linear band of IgG and C3 along the basement membrane zone. Indirect immunofluorescence, using serum from the patient, identifies IgG antibodies which react with the basement membrane zone in 70% of patients (Fig. 11.7).

Treatment

In the acute phase, prednisolone (Formulary, p. 260) at the dose of 40–60 mg/day is needed to control the eruption. Immunosuppressive agents may also be required. The doses are reduced as soon as possible, with the aim of ending up with a low maintenance dose of systemic steroids, taken on alternate days until treatment is stopped.

LEARNING POINTS

1 Death is not uncommon though the disease is self-limiting.
2 Some old people get fatal side effects from their systemic steroids.

Fig. 11.7   Indirect immunofluorescence using serum from a patient with pemphigoid.

Herpes gestations

This is like pemphigoid occurring in pregnancy. As in pemphigoid, most patients have linear deposits of C3 along the basement membrane zone (Fig. 11.5), although IgG is detected less often. The condition usually remits after the birth but may return in future pregnancies. It is not caused by a herpes virus, so herpes gestationis should not be confused with herpes genitalis. Treatment is with systemic steroids.

Cicatricial pemphigoid

Like pemphigoid itself, cicatricial pemphigoid is an auto-immune skin disease characterized by deposition of IgG and C3 at the basement membrane zone (Fig. 11.5). It differs from pemphigoid as its blisters and ulcers occur mainly on mucous membranes such as the conjunctivae, the mouth and genital tract. Bullae on the skin itself are uncommon. Lesions heal with scarring; around the eyes this may cause blindness. Treatment is rather ineffective, but systemic steroids and immunosuppressive agents have been used. Good eye hygiene and the removal of ingrowing eyelashes are important.

Linear IgA bullous disease

This is similar to pemphigoid too, but affects children as well as adults. Blisters arise on urticarial plaques, and are more often grouped on extensor surfaces than in pemphigoid. Children have the most problems near the groin. Linear IgA bullous disease is, as its name implies, associated with linear deposits of IgA and C3 at the basement membrane zone (Fig. 11.5). IgG is sometimes also found. It responds well to oral dapsone (Formulary, p. 262).

Dermatitis herpetiformis

Dermatitis herpetiformis is a chronic, subepidermal, vesicular disease in which the vesicles erupt in groups as in herpes simplex.

Cause

Gluten-sensitive enteropathy, demonstrable by small bowel biopsy, is always present, but most patients do not suffer from diarrhoea, constipation, or malnutrition as this enteropathy is mild, patchy, and involves only the proximal small intestine. Absorption of gluten, or another dietary antigen, may form circulating immune complexes which lodge in the skin. Granular deposits of IgA and C3, in the superficial dermis underneath the basement membrane zone (Fig. 11.5), induce inflammation and separation of epidermis from dermis.

Presentation

The extremely itchy, grouped vesicles develop particularly over the elbows and knees, buttocks, and shoulders (Fig. 11.8). Often, before a vesicle reaches any size, it is broken by scratching. A typical patient, therefore, shows only grouped excoriations, sometimes with added eczematous changes (Fig. 11.9).

Course

The condition typically lasts for decades.

Complications

Treatment may cause side effects. The complications of gluten-sensitive enteropathy include diarrhoea, abdominal pain, and malabsorption; rarely, small bowel lymphomas have been reported.

Differential diagnosis

The disorder masquerades as scabies, an excoriated eczema, insect bites or neurodermatitis.

Investigations

If a vesicle can be biopsied before it is scratched away, its histology will be that of a subepidermal blister, with neutrophils packing the adjacent dermal papillae. Direct immunofluorescence of uninvolved skin shows granular deposits of IgA, and usually C3, in the dermal papillae and superficial dermis (Fig. 11.5). Small bowel biopsy is recommended as a routine by some centres but not by others unless bowel symptoms are present. The level of antibodies to the endomysium of muscle can be used to monitor severity of enteropathy as it heals with gluten restriction.

Treatment

The disorder responds to a gluten-free diet: the bowel reverts quickly to normal but the IgA deposits remain in the skin, and the skin disease drags on for many months. Because of this, and because a gluten-free diet is hard to follow and enjoy, many patients prefer to take dapsone (Formulary, p. 262) or sulphapyridine. Both can cause severe rashes, haemolytic anaemia, leucopenia, thrombocytopenia, methaemoglobinaemia, and peripheral neuropathy. Regular blood checks are therefore necessary.

LEARNING POINTS

1 Biopsy *non*-involved skin to demonstrate the diagnostic granular deposits of IgA in the dermal papillae.
2 Gluten enteropathy of dermatitis herpetiformis seldom causes frank malabsorption.
3 Dapsone works quickly and a gluten-free diet only very slowly. Combine the two at the start and slowly reduce the dapsone.

Fig. 11.8 The small, tense, itchy, blisters of dermatitis herpetiformis.

Fig. 11.9 The itchy blisters of dermatitis herpetiformis are quickly destroyed by scratching.

Bullous erythema multiforme

Bullous erythema multiforme in the form of Stevens–Johnson syndrome is discussed in Chapter 10.

Toxic epidermal necrolysis

(Lyell's disease, the scalded skin syndrome)

Cause

Toxic epidermal necrolysis is usually due to drug hypersensitivity or toxicity (Chapter 23), but can also be a manifestation of graft-versus-host disease. Sometimes it is unexplained.

Presentation

The skin becomes red and intensely painful, and then begins to come off in sheets like a scald. This leaves an eroded, painful, glistening surface. Nikolsky's sign is positive. The mucous membranes may be affected, including the mouth, eyes, and even the bronchial tree.

Course

The condition usually clears if the offending drug is stopped. New epidermis grows out from hair follicles so that skin grafts are not needed. The disorder may come back if the drug is taken again.

Complications

Toxic epidermal necrolysis is a skin emergency and may be fatal. Infection, and the loss of fluids and electrolytes, are life-threatening, and the painful denuded skin surfaces make life a misery.

Differential diagnosis

The staphylococcal scalded skin syndrome (p. 139) looks like toxic epidermal necrolysis, but in it only the stratum corneum comes off. Whereas toxic epidermal necrolysis affects adults, the staphylococcal scalded skin syndrome is seen in infancy or early childhood. Histology differentiates the two. Pemphigus may also look similar, but starts more slowly and is more localized.

Investigations

Biopsy helps to confirm the diagnosis. The split is subepidermal, and the entire epidermis may be necrotic. There are no tests to tell which drug, if any, caused the disease.

Treatment

If toxic epidermal necrolysis is caused by a drug, this must be stopped (Chapter 23). Intensive nursing care and medical support are necessary, including the use of central venous lines, intravenous fluids, and electrolytes. Many patients are treated in units designed to deal with extensive thermal burns. Air suspension beds may increase comfort. The decision to use systemic steroids is becoming controversial, but they are often given, for short periods, at the start.

Porphyria cutanea tarda (p. 217)

The bullae and erosions occur on the backs of the hands and on other areas exposed to sunlight.

Epidermolysis bullosa (Chapter 22)

The group of conditions known as epidermolysis bullosa are inherited diseases, present from birth. There are many forms, but the most severe are due to abnormalities of the structures anchoring the epidermis to the dermis. Poor anchoring allows blisters to develop too easily at sites of trauma.

Epidermolysis bullosa acquisita

In contrast to inherited epidermolysis bullosa, this affects adults. As in pemphigoid, linear deposits of IgG are found at the basement membrane zone, but, unlike those of pemphigoid, bullae tend to occur at the site of trauma (Fig. 11.5). The IgG in these patients binds to the anchoring fibrils attached to the lamina densa (see Fig. 2.13). Treatment is unsatisfactory.

Bullous lupus erythematosus

Vesicles and bullae may be seen in severe active systemic lupus erythematosus (p. 103). This disorder is uncommon and carries a high risk of kidney disease. Non-cutaneous manifestations of systemic lupus erythematosus do not respond to dapsone; the bullae, however, do.

CHAPTER 12

CONNECTIVE TISSUE DISORDERS

The main feature of these conditions is inflammation in the connective tissue which leads to dermal atrophy or sclerosis, to arthritis, and sometimes to abnormalities in other organs. In addition, antibodies form against normal tissues and cellular components; these disorders are therefore classed as auto-immune.

Lupus erythematosus

Lupus erythematosus (LE) is a spectrum ranging from the purely cutaneous type (discoid LE), through patterns associated with some internal problems (disseminated discoid LE and subacute cutaneous LE), to a severe, multisystem disease (systemic LE) (Table 12.1).

Acute systemic lupus erythematosus

Cause
This is unknown, but hereditary factors, for example complement deficiency, increase susceptibility. Particles looking like viruses have been seen in endothelial cells, and in other tissues, but their role is not clear. Patients with LE have auto-antibodies to DNA, nuclear proteins, and to other normal antigens, and this points to an auto-immune cause.

Presentation
The classic rash of acute systemic LE is an erythema of the cheeks and nose in the rough shape of a butterfly (Figs. 12.1 and 12.2). Typically this appears suddenly, with facial swelling. Skin lesions may also be seen in other areas. Some patients develop widespread discoid papulosquamous plaques very like those of discoid LE; others have no skin disease at all.

Other features include peri-ungual telangiectasia (see Fig. 12.7), erythema over the digits, hair fall (especially at the frontal margin of the scalp), and photosensitivity. Severe sunburn may trigger the skin disease and worsen the systemic disease. Mouth ulcers may occur.

Table 12.1 Classification of connective tissue disease.

Localized disease	Intermedial type	Aggressive multisystem disease
Discoid lupus erythematosus	Subacute lupus erythematosus	Systemic lupus erythematosus
	Juvenile dermatomyositis	Adult dermatomyositis
Morphoea	CREST syndrome	Systemic sclerosis
Cutaneous polyarteritis nodosa		Polyarteritis nodosa

SYSTEMIC LE   DISCOID LE

Fig. 12.1 In systemic LE, the eruption is often just an erythema, sometimes transient, but occupying most of the 'butterfly' area. In discoid LE, the fixed scaling and scarring plaques may occur in the butterfly area (dotted line), but can occur outside it too.

Course

The skin changes may be transient, continuous, or recurrent; they correlate well with the activity of the systemic disease. Acute systemic LE may be associated with fever, nephritis, polyarteritis, leucopenia, pleurisy, pneumonitis, pericarditis, myocarditis, and involvement of the central nervous system. Internal involvement may be fatal.

Complications

The skin disease may cause scarring or hyperpigmentation, but the main dangers lie with damage to other organs and the side effects of treatment, especially systemic steroids.

Differential diagnosis

Systemic LE is a great imitator. Its malar rash can be confused with sunburn, polymorphic light eruption, (p. 177), and rosacea (p. 131). The discoid lesions are distinctive, but are also seen in discoid LE and in subacute cutaneous LE. Occasionally they look like psoriasis (p. 42). The hair fall suggests telogen effluvium (p. 64). Plaques on the scalp may cause a scarring alopecia. Systemic LE should be suspected when a characteristic rash is combined with fever, malaise, and internal disease (Table 12.2).

Investigations

Conduct a full physical examination, looking for in-

Fig. 12.2 Ill-defined erythema in the butterfly area is suggestive of systemic LE.

Table 12.2 Criteria for the diagnosis of systemic LE (must have at least four).

Malar rash
Discoid plaques
Photosensitivity
Mouth ulcers
Arthritis
Serositis
Renal disorder
Neurological disorder
Haematological disorder
Immunological disorder
Antinuclear antibodies (ANA)

ternal disease. Biopsy of skin lesions is worthwhile because the pathology and immunopathology are distinctive. There is usually some thinning of the epidermis, a vacuolar degeneration of epidermal basal cells, and a mild perivascular mononuclear cell infiltrate. Direct immunofluorescence is helpful: IgG, IgM, IgA, and C3 are found individually or together in a band-like pattern at the dermo-epidermal junction of involved skin and often uninvolved skin as well. Relevant laboratory tests are listed in Table 12.3.

Treatment
Systemic steroids are the mainstay of treatment. Large doses of prednisolone (Formulary, p. 260) are needed to achieve control, as assessed by symptoms, signs, ESR, total complement level, and tests of organ function. The dose is then reduced to the smallest which suppresses the disease. Immunosuppressive agents, like azathioprine (Formulary, p. 259) and cyclophosphamide, and other drugs, may also be needed (e.g. antihypertensive therapy or anticonvulsants). Long-term and regular follow-up is necessary.

LEARNING POINTS

1 Do not wait for the laboratory to confirm that your patient has systemic LE: use systemic steroids quickly if indicated on clinical grounds.
2 Once committed to systemic steroids adjust their dose on clinical rather than laboratory grounds.

Subacute cutaneous lupus erythematosus
This is less severe than acute systemic LE, but is also often associated with systemic disease. Its cause is unknown.

Presentation
The skin lesions are sharply marginated, scaling, psoriasiform plaques, sometimes annular, lying on the forehead, nose, cheeks, chest, hands, and extensor surfaces of the arms. They tend to be symmetrical and are hard to tell from discoid LE, or systemic LE with widespread discoid lesions. Patients with subacute cutaneous LE are often photosensitive.

Course
As in systemic LE, the course is prolonged. The skin lesions are slow to clear but, in contrast to discoid LE, do so with little or no scarring.

Complications
Systemic disease is frequent. Children born to mothers who have, or have had, this condition are liable to neonatal LE with transient, annular skin lesions and permanent heart block.

Table 12.3 Investigations in systemic LE.

Test	Usual findings
Skin biopsy	Degeneration of basal cells, cutaneous atrophy, inflammation around appendages
Skin immunofluorescence	Fibrillar or granular deposits of IgG, IgM, IgA and/or C3 alone in basement membrane zone
Haematology	Anaemia, raised ESR, thrombocytopenia, decreased white cell count
Immunology	Antinuclear antibody, antibodies to double-stranded DNA, false positive tests for syphilis, low total complement level, lupus anticoagulant factor
Urine analysis	Proteinuria or haematuria, often with casts if kidneys involved
Tests for function of other organs	As indicated by history, always test kidney and liver function

Fig. 12.3 Red, scaly, fixed plaques of discoid LE. This degree of scaling is not uncommon in the active stage.

Differential diagnosis

The morphology is characteristic, but lesions can be mistaken for psoriasis or widespread discoid LE. Annular lesions may resemble tinea corporis (p. 157) or figurate erythemas (p. 113).

Investigations

Patients with subacute cutaneous LE should be evaluated in the same way as those with acute systemic LE, although deposits of immunoglobulins in the skin and antinuclear antibodies in serum are present less often. Many have antibodies to a cytoplasmic antigen (SSA [Ro]).

Treatment

Subacute cutaneous LE does better with antimalarials, such as hydroxychloroquine (Formulary, p. 263), than acute systemic LE. Systemic steroids may be needed too.

Discoid lupus erythematosus

Patients with discoid LE may have one or two plaques only, or many in several areas. The cause is also unknown but UVR is one factor.

Presentation

Plaques show erythema, scaling, follicular plugging (like a nutmeg grater), scarring and atrophy, telangiectasia, hypopigmentation, and a peripheral zone of hyperpigmentation. They are well demarcated and lie mostly on sun-exposed skin, of the scalp, face and ears (Figs. 12.1 and 12.3).

Course

The disease may spread relentlessly. Scarring is common and hair may be lost permanently if there is scarring in the scalp (Fig. 12.4). Whiteness remains after the inflammation has cleared. It rarely progresses to systemic LE.

Differential diagnosis

Psoriasis is hard to tell from discoid LE when plaques first arise but has larger, thicker scales, and later it is usually symmetrical (elbows, knees, scalp, and sacrum). Discoid LE is more common on the face and ears, and in sun-exposed areas.

Investigations

Most patients with discoid LE remain well. However, screening for systemic LE and internal disease is still worthwhile. A skin biopsy for pathological examination is most helpful if taken from an untreated plaque where appendages are still present (Fig. 12.5). Direct immunofluorescence shows deposits of IgG, IgM, IgA, and C3 at the basement membrane zone of skin. Biopsies for direct immunofluorescence are best taken from older, untreated plaques. Blood tests

Fig. 12.4 Discoid LE of the scalp leading to permanent hair loss. Note the marked follicular plugging.

Thin epidermis

Follicular plug of keratin

Destruction of
basal cells

Perivascular and
peri-appendageal
T lymphocyte infiltrate

Destruction of
hair follicle

Fig. 12.5 The histology of discoid LE.

are usually normal but occasionally serum contains antinuclear antibodies (Table 12.4).

Treatment

Discoid LE needs potent or very potent topical corticosteroids (Formulary, p. 248). In discoid LE, these can even be used on the face, because the risk of scarring is worse than that of atrophy. Topical steroids should be applied twice daily until the lesions disappear or side effects, such as atrophy, develop; weaker preparations can then be used for maintenance. If discoid LE does not respond to this, intralesional injections of triamcinolone (2.5 – 5 mg/ml) may help. Stubborn and widespread lesions often do well with oral antimalarials such as hydroxychloroquine (Formulary, p. 263), but rarely these cause irreversible eye damage. The eyes should therefore be tested before and at intervals during treatment. Sun avoidance and screens are also important.

Table 12.4 Some factors distinguishing the different types of LE.

	Antinuclear antibodies	Sun sensitivity	Internal organ involvement
Systemic LE	+++	+++	++
Subacute LE	+	++++	+
Discoid LE	+	+	−

Dermatomyositis

Dermatomyositis is a subset of polymyositis with distinctive skin changes. When starting after the age of 40, it may signal an internal malignancy.

Presentation

Typical patients have a faint, heliotrope discoloration around their eyes. The lilac colour of the heliotrope flower is unique. Some also develop lilac, slightly atrophic papules over the knuckles of their fingers (Gottron's papules), and streaks of erythema over the extensor tendons of the hand. Malar erythema and oedema (Fig. 12.6), peri-ungual telangiectasia (Fig.

Fig. 12.6 Acute dermatomyositis: oedematous, purple face with erythematous streaks on the backs of the fingers. Severe progressive muscle weakness, but no underlying tumour was found.

Fig. 12.7 Erythema and telangiectasia of the nail folds are important clues to systemic connective tissue disorders. This patient has dermatomyositis.

12.7), a peculiar mixture of hypo- and hyperpigmentation on light-exposed areas, and the signs of mixed connective tissue disease (*see below*) may complete the picture.

Course

Many patients have weakness of proximal muscles. Climbing stairs and combing the hair become difficult. In children the disorder is often self-limiting, but in adults it may be prolonged and progressive. Raynaud's phenomenon, arthralgia, dysphagia, and calcinosis may follow.

Complications

Myositis may lead to permanent weakness, and immobility and inflammation to contractures or cutaneous calcinosis. Some die from their severe myopathy.

Differential diagnosis

Other connective tissue disorders may look similar, particularly mixed connective tissue disease and systemic LE. In LE, finger lesions favour the skin between the knuckles whereas in dermatomyositis the knuckles are preferred. Toxoplasmosis may cause a dermatomyositis-like syndrome. Myopathy may be a side effect of systemic steroids so weakness is not always due to the disease itself.

Investigations

About 40% of adults with dermatomyositis also have an underlying malignancy. Their dermatomyositis coincides with the onset of the tumour and may improve if it is removed. Adult dermatomyositis or polymyositis therefore requires a search for such an underlying malignancy. Suprisingly, the ESR is often normal and antinuclear antibodies are usually not detected. The levels of muscle enzymes such as aldolase and creatinine phosphokinase (CPK) are often elevated. Electromyography (EMG) detects muscle abnormalities, and biopsy of an affected muscle shows inflammation and destruction.

Treatment

Systemic steroids, often in high doses (e.g. prednisolone (Formulary, p. 260) 60 mg/day for an average adult), are the cornerstone of treatment and protect the muscles from destruction. Immunosuppressive agents, such as azathioprine (Formulary, p. 259), also help to control the condition and to reduce the high steroid dose. The rash usually responds too. Maintenance treatment is adjusted according to clinical response and CPK level. Long-term and regular follow-up is necessary.

LEARNING POINT

Hunt for internal malignancy in the middle aged and elderly, but not in juvenile cases.

Systemic sclerosis

In this disorder the skin becomes hard as connective tissues thicken. Its cause is unknown. Changes like those of progressive systemic sclerosis affect workers exposed to polyvinyl chloride monomers or to severe chronic vibration, and are also seen in chronic graft-versus-host reactions after bone marrow transplants.

Presentation

Most patients suffer from Raynaud's phenomenon (p. 115) and sclerodactyly. Their fingers become immobile, hard, and shiny (Fig. 12.8). Some become hyperpigmented and itchy early in their disease. Peri-ungual telangiectasia is common (Fig. 12.7).

Course
As the disease progresses, sclerosis spreads to the face, scalp, and trunk. The nose becomes beak-like, and wrinkles radiate around the mouth (Figs. 12.9 and 12.10). Most have abnormalities of the gut including dysphagia, oesophagitis, constipation, diarrhoea, and malabsorption. Fibrosis of the lungs leads to dyspnoea, and fibrosis of the heart to congestive failure. The kidneys are involved late, but this has a grave prognosis from malignant hypertension.

Complications
Most are due to the involvement of organs other than the skin, but ulcers of the fingertips and calcinosis are distressing. Hard skin immobilizes the joints and leads to contractures (Fig. 12.8).

Differential diagnosis
Other causes of Raynaud's phenomenon are given in

Fig. 12.8 Systemic sclerosis: note the claw deformity due to sclerodactyly.

Fig. 12.9 Systemic sclerosis: radial furrowing around the mouth.

Accentuated creases on forehead

Pinched beak-like nose

Loss of pulp substance and sclerotic skin (Flecks of calcium extruding)

Diffuse hyperpigmentation

Mat-like telangiectasia

Small mouth with radial furrowing around

Shiny, indurated, tethered skin

Claw-like deformity of sclerotic hand

Fig. 12.10 Features of systemic sclerosis.

Table 13.5. The differential includes chilblains (p. 113) and erythromelalgia (p. 113). The sclerosis should be distinguished from that of porphyria cutanea tarda, mixed connective tissue disease, the results of exposure to polyvinyl chloride monomers, eosinophilic fasciitis, diabetic sclerodactyly, and an acute arthritis with swollen fingers.

Investigations
The diagnosis is made clinically as laboratory abnormalities are seldom present until the physical signs are well established. Laboratory tests should include a fluorescent antinuclear antibody test and the evaluation of the heart, kidney, lungs, joints, and muscles. Barium studies are best avoided as obstruction may follow poor evacuation. Other contrast media are available. X-rays of the hands, the measurement of muscle enzymes and immunoglobulin levels, and a blood count and ESR are also worthwhile.

Treatment
This is unsatisfactory. The calcium antagonist nifedipine may help Raynaud's phenomenon. Systemic steroids, salicylates, and antimalarials are often used, but are not of proven value. D-penicillamine has many side effects, especially on renal function. Physiotherapy is helpful.

C R E S T syndrome
This is a variant of systemic sclerosis with a relatively good prognosis associated often with serum antibodies to nuclear centromeres. The mnemonic stands for *C*alcinosis, *R*aynaud's phenomenon, *E*sophageal dysmotility, *S*clerodactyly, and *T*elangiectasia. Telangiectasia is peri-ungual on the fingers and flat, mat-like, or rectangular on the face. Many patients with this syndrome develop a diffuse, progressive, systemic sclerosis after months or years.

Eosinophilic fasciitis
Localized areas of skin become indurated, sometimes after an upper respiratory tract infection or prolonged, severe, exercise. Hypergammaglobulinaemia and eosinophilia are present, and a deep skin biopsy, which includes muscle, shows that the fascia overlying the muscle is thickened. Despite its name, and despite a profound eosinophilia in the peripheral

Fig. 12.11   Morphoea. Pale, indurated plaque on the chest; the scalloped lower margin is unusual.

blood, the fascia is not eosinophilic or permeated by eosinophils. The disease responds promptly to systemic steroids; the prognosis is good.

Morphoea
Morphoea is a localized form of scleroderma with pale indurated plaques on the skin but no internal sclerosis (Fig. 12.11). Its prognosis is usually good and the fibrosis slowly clears leaving slight depression and hyperpigmentation. A rare type may lead to arrest of growth of the underlying bones causing, for example, facial hemi-atrophy or shortening of a limb.

Lichen sclerosus
Many think that this condition is related to morphoea with which it may co-exist. However, its patches are non-indurated, white shiny macules, sometimes with obvious plugging in the sweat gland openings. Women are affected far more often than men and, though any area of skin may be involved, the classical ivory-coloured lesions often surround the vulva and anus. Intractable itching is common in these areas and the development of vulval carcinoma is a risk. In men the condition may cause stenosis of the urethral meatus and adhesions between the foreskin and glans of the penis.

Mixed connective tissue disease
This is an overlap between systemic LE and either scleroderma or polymyositis.

Presentation

As in LE, women are affected more often than men. Many develop swollen hands and sclerodactyly, and skin lesions like those of cutaneous LE may also be present. Alopecia is mild and the hair fall mimics telogen effluvium. Peri-ungual telangiectasia and pigmentary disturbances are common. About 25% of patients have a small vessel vasculitis with palpable purpura, leg ulcers, and painful dermal nodules on the hands or elbows. Many show Raynaud's phenomenon, arthritis, serositis, and myositis. Headaches, weakness, fatigue, lymph node enlargement, or hoarseness occur in about one in three patients; renal and CNS disease are less common.

Course

The disorder is chronic, and usually turns into either systemic LE or systemic sclerosis.

Differential diagnosis

The disorder can be confused with systemic LE, dermatomyositis, polymyositis, systemic sclerosis, and other sclerosing processes such as porphyria cutanea tarda (p. 217).

Investigations

Patients with mixed connective tissue disease have antibodies in high titre directed against one or more extractable nuclear antigens. These give a speckled pattern when serum is reacted against nuclei and detected by indirect immunofluorescence. Direct immunofluorescence of involved and uninvolved skin shows IgG within the epidermal nuclei, also in a speckled pattern. Only a third of patients have sub-epidermal immunoglobulin deposits in involved skin. Most have hypergammaglobulinaemia, a high ESR, oesophageal dysmotility, abnormal pulmonary function tests, and a positive rheumatoid factor. Hypocomplementaemia, leucopenia, anaemia, cryo-globulinaemia, and false positive biological tests for syphilis occur in a few patients.

Treatment

Treatment depends upon which organs are involved, but systemic steroids are usually needed, in the same dosages as for systemic LE. Immunosuppressive agents reduce the dose of systemic steroids, and non-steroidal anti-inflammatory agents help with arthralgia, myalgia, and swelling of the hands.

Other connective tissue diseases

Rheumatoid arthritis

Most patients with rheumatoid arthritis have no skin disease, but some have tiny fingertip infarcts, purpura, ulcers, palmar or peri-ungual erythema, or pyoderma gangrenosum. The commonest skin manifestations are marble-like nodules near joints. These are always associated with the presence of rheumatoid factor. Some patients with rheumatoid arthritis have a vasculitis of larger blood vessels with deep ulcers on the legs (Fig. 13.8).

Reiter's syndrome

Reiter's syndrome, precipitated by non-specific urethritis or dysentery, combines skin lesions, arthropathy, conjunctivitis, balanitis, mucositis, and spondylitis. Arthritis is the most severe element. The skin lesions (keratoderma blenorrhagicum) are psoriasis-like, red, scaling plaques, often studded with vesicles and pustules, seen most often on the feet. The toes are red and swollen, and the nails thicken. Psoriasiform plaques may also occur on the penis and scrotum, with redness near the penile meatus. Topical steroids and systemic non-steroidal anti-inflammatory drugs help, but many patients need methotrexate (Formulary, p. 259) or systemic steroids too.

Relapsing polychondritis

This process can affect any cartilage as the disorder is apparently caused by auto-immunity to collagen. The ears are the usual target. The overlying skin becomes red, swollen, and tender. The cartilage in joints, the nose, and the tracheobronchial tree may be involved, so that patients develop floppy ears, a saddle nose, hoarseness, stridor, and respiratory insufficiency. Aortic aneurysms are also seen. Treatment is with systemic steroids and non-steroidal anti-inflammatory drugs. Tracheostomy may be necessary.

Behçet's syndrome

Behçet's syndrome is uncommon and its cause is not known.

Presentation

The two main components are mouth ulcers, often multiple and large, and genital ulcers, but extracutaneous manifestations are also important. In the eye, hypopyon is characteristic, with anterior and posterior uveitis. Arthritis, meningo-encephalitis, vasculitis, and intestinal ulceration may also be features. Other skin lesions include erythema nodosum, superficial thrombophlebitis, and pustules or ulcers at sites of trauma, such as venepuncture (pathergy).

Course

The course is long but the mucocutaneous lesions have a good prognosis.

Complications

Death, blindness, and neurological damage may occur.

Differential diagnosis

The disorder is difficult to diagnose when the full syndrome is not present. Mouth ulcers must be distinguished from aphthae, the ulcers of bullous diseases and nutritional deficiency.

Treatment

It may be treated symptomatically or with systemic steroids or oral colchicine. Immunosuppressive agents including cyclophosphamide, azathioprine, and chlorambucil have also been tried.

Polyarteritis nodosa

This is discussed in Chapter 10 but is considered by some to be a connective tissue disorder.

Panniculitis

Panniculitis is an inflammation of the subcutaneous fat: it includes a number of diseases with different causes but a similar appearance. Some are listed in Table 12.5.

Presentation

Most patients have tender, ill-defined, red, nodules on the lower legs, thighs, and buttocks.

Table 12.5   Causes of panniculitis.

Erythema nodosum (p. 91)
Erythema nodosum leprosum (leprosy)
Nodular vasculitis (p. 92)
Weber–Christian type (unknown cause)
Polyarteritis nodosa (p. 94)
Associated with pancreatitis
Associated with systemic LE (lupus profundus)
Cold-induced
Withdrawal of systemic steroids
Superficial thrombophlebitis
Deficiency of α_1-antitrypsin
Factitial (e.g. from injection of milk)

Course

This depends upon the cause. Migratory thrombophlebitis may be associated with underlying malignancy. In lupus profundus, a panniculitis is associated with discoid or systemic LE. Causes of erythema nodosum are discussed in Chapter 10. Erythema induratum may be caused by tuberculosis. Erythema nodosum leprosum is a reactional state in leprosy. Patients with pancreatitis may liberate enough lipase into the systemic circulation to cause fat in the skin to liquefy and discharge through the overlying skin. The Weber–Christian variant is associated with fever, but its cause is unknown.

Investigations

The type of panniculitis can sometimes be identified by skin biopsy, which must include subcutaneous fat. A complete blood count, ESR, chest X-ray, serum lipase, serum α_1-antitrypsin and tests for antinuclear antibodies are needed.

Treatment

This depends upon the cause. Rest, elevation of affected extremities, and local heat often help symptoms. Non-steroidal anti-inflammatory agents may also bring help in the absence of specific therapy.

CHAPTER 13

DISORDERS OF BLOOD VESSELS AND LYMPHATICS

This chapter includes only those diseases in which the primary abnormality is in a blood or lymphatic vessel. In functional disease, abnormalities of flow are reversible, and there is no vessel wall damage, e.g. in urticaria (discussed in Chapter 10). The diseases of structure include the many types of vasculitis, some of which, with an immunological basis, are also covered in Chapter 10. For convenience, disorders of the blood vessels are grouped according to the size and type of the vessels affected.

Disorders involving small blood vessels

Acrocyanosis

This type of 'poor circulation', often familial, is more common in females than males. The hands, feet, nose, ears, and cheeks become blue-red and cold. The palms are often cold and clammy. The condition is due to arteriolar constriction and to cold-induced increases in blood viscosity. The best answer is warm clothes and the avoidance of cold.

Erythrocyanosis

This occurs in fat, often young, women. Purple-red mottled discoloration is seen over the buttocks, thighs, and lower legs. Cold provokes it and causes an unpleasant burning sensation. An area of acrocyanosis or erythrocyanosis may be the site where other disorders will settle in the future, e.g. perniosis, erythema induratum, lupus erythematosus, sarcoidosis, cutaneous tuberculosis, and leprosy.

Perniosis (chilblains)

In this common, sometimes familial, condition, inflamed purple-pink swellings appear on the fingers, toes, and rarely ears. They arrive with winter and are induced by cold. They are painful, and itchy or burning on rewarming. Occasionally they ulcerate. Chilblains are due to a combination of arteriolar and venular constriction. Topical remedies rarely work, but oral nifedipidine may be useful. Warm housing and clothing help; sympathectomy may be advised in severe cases.

Erythromelalgia

This is a rare condition in which the hands become red, hot, and painful when they or their owner are exposed to heat. The condition may be idiopathic, or due to a myeloproliferative disease (e.g. polycythaemia rubra vera or thrombocythaemia), lupus erythematosus, rheumatoid arthritis, diabetes, or hypertension. Small doses of aspirin give symptomatic relief.

Erythema

Erythema accompanies all inflammatory skin conditions. Discrete areas of erythema without scaling are seen in some bacterial and viral infections, and when erythema is associated with oedema ('urticated erythema') it becomes palpable. Drugs (Chapter 23) are another common cause. If no cause is obvious, the rash is often called a 'toxic' or 'reactive' erythema (Table 13.1).

Figurate erythemas

These are chronic eruptions, made up of bizarre serpiginous and erythematous rings. In the past most carried Latin labels; happily, the eruptions are now grouped under the general term of 'figurate erythe-

Table 13.1 Classification of erythemas.

Widespread
Due to infection (bacterial or viral)
Drug reactions
Connective tissue diseases
Underlying malignancy (e.g. figurate erythema)
Idiopathic

Localized
Pregnancy, liver disease, rheumatoid arthritis
  (causing palmar erythema)
Drug reaction (fixed drug eruption)
Infection (e.g. erythema chronicum migrans due to
  Borrelia burgdorferi)

mas'. Underlying malignancy, a connective tissue disorder, a bacterial, fungal, or yeast infection, worm infestation, drug sensitivity, and rheumatic heart disease should be excluded, but usually the cause remains obscure.

Palmar erythema

This may be an isolated finding in a normal person or be familial. Sometimes it is seen in pregnancy, liver disease or rheumatoid arthritis. Often associated with spider telangiectases (*see below*), it may be due to increased circulating oestrogens.

Erythema chronicum migrans

These annular lesions are usually solitary, and occur most often on exposed skin after a tick bite. They expand slowly and may become very large. The condition is due to infection with the spirochaete, *Borrelia burgdorferi*, which inhabits ticks of the family Ixodes, commonly harboured by deer. A tetracycline is the drug of choice for adults, but the condition also responds well to penicillin. The skin changes are not serious but may be part of 'Lyme disease', which includes arthritis, myocarditis and meningitis. These conditions, and a secondary rash of numerous annular plaques, occur most often when the initial lesion has gone undetected.

Telangiectases

This term refers to permanently dilated and visible small vessels in the skin. They appear as linear, punctate or stellate, crimson-purple markings. The common causes are given in Table 13.2.

Spider naevi

These stellate telangiectases do look rather like spiders, with legs radiating from a central, often palpable, feeding vessel. They are seen frequently on the faces of normal children, and may erupt in pregnancy or be the presenting sign of liver disease, with many lesions on the upper trunk. Liver function should be checked in those with many spider naevi. The central vessel can be destroyed by electrodesiccation without local anaesthesia.

Table 13.2 Causes of telangiectasia.

Primary telangiectasia	
Hereditary haemorrhagic telangiectasia	Autosomal dominant Nose and GI bleeds Lesions on face
Ataxia telangiectasia	Autosomal recessive Telangiectases develop between the ages of three and five years Cerebellar ataxia Recurrent respiratory infections Immunological abnormalities
Generalized essential telangiectasia	Runs benign course No other associations
Unilateral naevoid telangiectasia	May occur in pregnancy or in females on oral contraceptive
Secondary telangiectasia	
Atrophy	Seen on exposed skin of elderly, after topical steroid applications, after X-irradiation and with poikiloderma
Connective tissue disorders	Always worth inspecting nail folds. Mat-like on the face in systemic sclerosis
Prolonged vasodilatation	For example, with rosacea and with venous hypertension
Mastocytosis	Accompanying a rare and diffuse variant
Liver disease	Spider telangiectases are common

Livedo reticularis

This cyanosis of the skin is net-like or marbled, and due to stasis in the capillaries furthest from their arterial supply, i.e. at the periphery of the inverted cone supplied by a dermal arteriole (Fig. 2.14). 'Cutis marmorata' is the name given to the mottled skin seen in many normal chldren. It is physiological and disappears on warming, whereas true livedo reticularis remains.

The causes of livedo reticularis are listed in Table 13.3. Livedo vasculitis and cutaneous polyarteritis are forms of vasculitis associated with livedo reticularis (Chapter 10). Some patients with an apparently idiopathic livedo reticularis develop progressive disease in peripheral, cerebral, coronary and renal arteries. The presence of an anticardiolipin antibody helps to identify this group.

Erythema ab igne

The appearance of this disorder is also determined by the underlying vascular network. Its reticulate, pigmented erythema, with variable scaling, is due to damage from long-term exposure to local heat — usually from an open fire, hot water bottle, or heating pad. If on one side of the leg it gives a clue to the side of the fire on which granny likes to sit. The condition is common in northern Europe ('tinker's tartan'), but rare in the U.S.A., where central heating is the rule.

Flushing

This transient vasodilatation of the face may spread to the neck, upper chest and, more rarely, other parts of the body. The mechanism varies with the many causes which are listed in Table 13.4. There is no sharp distinction between flushing and blushing apart from the emotional provocation of the latter.

Arterial disease

Raynaud's phenomenon

This is a paroxysmal pallor of the digits provoked by cold or, rarely, emotional stress. At first the top of one or more fingers becomes white. A few minutes later a painful cyanosis appears and the area turns red before the hands return to their normal colour. In severe disease the fingers lose pulp substance, ulcerate, or become gangrenous. Some causes are listed in Table 13.5. Raynaud's disease, often familial, is the name given when no cause can be found. However, some patients with what seems to be Raynaud's disease will later develop a connective tissue disease.

The main treatment is to protect the vulnerable digits from cold. Smoking should be banned. Vasodilators such as naftidrofuryl oxalate, griseofulvin, and nifedipine have their advocates. Infusions with reserpine or prostacyclin help some severe cases. Occasionally sympathectomy is needed.

Table 13.3 Causes of livedo reticularis.

Physiological	Cutis marmorata
Vessel wall disease	Atherosclerosis
	Connective tissue disorders (especially polyarteritis and systemic LE)
	Syphilis
	Tuberculosis
Hyperviscosity states	Polycythaemia/thrombocythaemia
	Macroglobulinaemia
Cryopathies	Cryoglobulinaemia
	Cold agglutininaemia
Congenital	
Idiopathic	

Table 13.4 Causes of flushing.

Physiological	Emotional
	Menopausal
Foods	Hot drinks
	Spicy foods
	Additives (monosodium glutamate)
	Alcohol
Drugs	Vasodilators
	Bromocriptine
	Nifedipine
	Chlorpropamide + alcohol (diabetics)
	Nicotinic acid
Pathological	Rosacea
	Carcinoid tumours
	Phaeochromocytoma (type producing adrenaline)

Table 13.5 Causes of Raynaud's phenomenon.

Familial	Raynaud's disease
Connective tissue diseases	Systemic sclerosis Lupus erythematosus Mixed connective tissue disease
Arterial occlusion	Thoracic outlet syndrome Atherosclerosis Endarteritis obliterans
Repeated trauma	Pneumatic hammer/drill operators
Hyperviscosity	Polycythaemia Macroglobulinaemia
Cryopathies	Cryoglobulinaemia Cryofibrinogenaemia Cold agglutinaemia
Neurological disease	Peripheral neuropathy Syringomyelia
Toxins	Ergot Vinyl-chloride

Polyarteritis nodosa

This is discussed in Chapter 10.

Temporal arteritis

Here the brunt is borne by the larger vessels of the head and neck. The condition affects elderly people and may be associated with polymyalgia rheumatica. The classical site is the temporal arteries which become tender and pulseless, in association with severe headaches. Rarely necrotic ulcers appear on the scalp. Blindness may follow if the ophthalmic arteries are involved, and to reduce this risk systemic steroids should be given as soon as the diagnosis has been made. In active phases the ESR is high and its level can be used to guide treatment, which is often prolonged.

Atherosclerosis

This occlusive disease, most common in the developed countries, will not be discussed in detail here but involvement of the large arteries of the legs is of concern to dermatologists. It may cause intermittent claudication, nocturnal cramp, ulcers or gangrene.

These may develop slowly over the years, or within minutes if a thrombus forms on an atheromatous plaque. The feet are cold and pale, the skin is often atrophic, with little hair, and peripheral pulses are diminished or absent.

Investigations should include urine testing to exclude diabetes mellitus. Fasting plasma lipids (cholesterol, triglycerides and lipoproteins) should be checked in the young, especially if there is a family history of vascular disease. Doppler ultrasound measurements help to distinguish atherosclerotic from venous leg ulcers in the elderly (p. 121). Complete assessment is best carried out by a specialist in peripheral vascular disease or a vascular surgeon.

Arterial emboli

Emboli may lodge in arteries supplying the skin and cause gangrene, ulcers or necrotic papules, depending on the size of the vessel obstructed. Causes include dislodged thrombi (usually from areas of atherosclerosis), fat emboli (after major trauma), infected emboli (e.g. gonococcal septicaemia, or subacute bacterial endocarditis) and tumour emboli.

Venous disease

Deep vein thrombosis

The common causes are listed in Table 13.6.

The onset may be 'silent' or heralded by pain in the calf, often about 10 days after immobilization for surgery, parturition or an infection. The leg becomes swollen and cyanotic distal to the thrombus. The calf may hurt when handled or if the foot is dorsiflexed (Homan's sign). Sometimes a pulmonary embolus is the first sign of a silent deep vein thrombosis.

Suitable investigations include Doppler ultrasonography, ^{125}I-fibrinogen isotope leg-scanning, and, rarely, venography.

Treatment is anticoagulation with heparin and later with a coumarin. The value of thrombolytic regimens has yet to be assessed properly. Prevention is important. Deep vein thrombosis after a surgical operation is less frequent now with early post-operative mobilization, regular leg exercises, the use of elastic stockings over the operative period, and prophylaxis with low dose heparin.

Table 13.6 Some causes of deep vein thrombosis.

Abnormalities of the vein wall	Trauma (operations and injuries)
	Chemicals (intravenous infusions)
	Neighbouring infection (e.g. in leg ulcer)
	Tumour (local invasion)
Abnormalities of blood flow	Stasis (immobility, pressure, pregnancy, heart failure, incompetent valves)
	Impaired venous return
Abnormalities of clotting	Platelets increased or sticky (thrombocythaemia, polycythaemia vera, leukaemia, trauma, splenectomy)
	Decreased fibrinolysis (post-operative)
	Alteration in clotting factors (infection, leukaemia, pregnancy, shock and haemorrhage)
Unknown mechanisms	Malignancy (thrombophlebitis migrans)
	Smoking
	Behçet's syndrome

Thrombophlebitis

This is thrombosis in an inflamed vein. If the affected vein is varicose or superficial it will be red and feel like a tender cord. The leg may be diffusely inflamed, making a distinction from cellulitis (p. 140) difficult. There may be fever, leucocytosis, and a high ESR. *Migratory superficial thrombophlebitis* should arouse suspicion of an underlying malignancy or pancreatic disease.

Treatment is based on rest, local heat, and nonsteroidal anti-inflammatory drugs. Antibiotics or anticoagulants rarely help.

The gravitational syndrome, lipodermatosclerosis and venous leg ulceration

Ulcers of the lower leg, secondary to venous insufficiency, are commoner in women than in men and account for some 85% of all leg ulcers seen in the U.K. and U.S.A.

Cause

The proper venous drainage of a leg requires three sets of veins: the deep veins surrounded by muscles; the superficial veins; and the veins connecting these two — the perforating or communicating veins (Fig. 13.1). When the leg muscles contract, blood in the deep veins is squeezed back, against gravity, to the heart (the calf muscle pump); reflux is prevented by valves. When the muscles relax, with the help of gravity blood from the superficial veins passes into the deep veins via the communicating vessels. If the valves in the deep and communicating veins are incompetent, hypertension develops in the deep veins. The calf muscle pump now pushes blood into the superficial veins, where the pressure remains high ('venous hypertension') instead of dropping during exercise. This persisting venous hypertension enlarges the capillary bed, and forces fibrinogen out through the capillary walls. Patients with these changes develop 'lipodermatosclerosis' (*see below*) and have a high serum fibrinogen and reduced blood fibrinolytic activity. The pericapillary fibrin cuff blocks the diffusion of oxygen and nutrients, and the overlying skin becomes hypoxic. As a result, minor trauma leads to ulcers which are slow to heal. Figure 13.2 shows the factors causing venous ulceration.

Clinical features

Venous incompetence is heralded by a feeling of

Fig. 13.1 The direction of blood flow in normal leg veins.

Femoral vein

Popliteal vein

Long saphenous vein

Short saphenous vein

Medial malleolus

Communicating veins

Fig. 13.2 Factors causing venous leg ulceration.

heaviness in the legs and by oedema. Other signs include a red or bluish discoloration, loss of hair, induration, pigmentation (mainly haemosiderin from the breakdown of extravasated red blood cells), and atrophie blanche (ivory white scarring with dilated capillary loops) (Fig. 13.3). This combination of signs is sometimes called lipodermatosclerosis. Ulceration is most common near the medial malleolus (Fig. 13.4). Venous ulcers are often large, vary in depth, are sharply demarcated, and are frequently indolent. Incompetent perforating branches (blow-outs) between the superficial and deep veins are best felt with the patient standing.

Under favourable conditions the exudative phase gives way to a granulating and healing phase, signalled by a blurring of the ulcer margin, ingrowth of skin from it, and the appearance of scattered small grey epithelial islands over the base. Prolonged ulceration, with lipodermatosclerosis, gives the leg the look of an inverted champagne bottle.

Complications

Bacterial superinfection is inevitable in a long-standing ulcer, but needs systemic antibiotics only if there is a purulent discharge, rapid extension, cellulitis, lymphangitis, or septicaemia.

Eczema (p. 82) is common around venous ulcers (Fig. 13.5). Allergic contact dermatitis (p. 76) is a possibility if the rash worsens or fails to improve with local treatment. Lanolin, parabens (a preservative) and neomycin are the most common sensitizers.

Malignant change can occur. If an ulcer has a hyperplastic base or rolled edge, biopsy may be needed to rule out a squamous cell carcinoma (Fig. 13.6).

Fig. 13.3 Irregular areas of whitish scarring and dilated capillary loops — the changes of atrophie blanche.

Fig. 13.4 Large venous ulcer overlying the medial malleolus.

Fig. 13.6 Chronic ulcer failing to respond to treatment. Biopsy, taken from rolled edge, excluded malignant change.

Fig. 13.5 Eczema surrounding a small crusted venous ulcer.

Table 13.7   Causes of leg ulceration.

Venous hypertension	
Arterial disease	Atherosclerosis
	Buerger's disease
	Giant cell arteritis
	Polyarteritis nodosa
	Systemic sclerosis
Small vessel disease	Diabetes mellitus
	Systemic LE
	Rheumatoid arthritis
	Systemic sclerosis
	Allergic vasculitis
	Immune complex disease
	Sickle cell anaemia
	Cryoglobulinaemia
Neuropathy	Diabetes mellitus
	Leprosy
	Syphilis
	Syringomyelia
	Peripheral neuropathy
Infection	'Tropical ulcer'
	Tuberculosis
	Deep fungal infections
Neoplasia	Squamous cell carcinoma
	Malignant melanoma
	Kaposi's sarcoma
	Basal cell carcinoma
Trauma	Injury
	Artefact
	Iatrogenic

Differential diagnosis

The main causes of leg ulceration are given in Table 13.7. The most important differences between venous and other leg ulcers are:

Atherosclerotic

These ulcers are more common on the toes, dorsum of foot, heel, calf, and shin, and are unrelated to perforating veins. Their edges are often sharply defined, their outline may be polycyclic and the ulcers may be deep and gangrenous. Islands of intact skin are characteristically seen within the ulcer. Claudication may be present and peripheral pulses absent.

Vasculitic

These ulcers start as painful palpable purpuric lesions turning into small punched-out ulcers (Fig. 13.7). The involvement of larger vessels is heralded by painful nodules which may ulcerate. The intractable, deep, sharply demarcated ulcers of rheumatoid arthritis are due to an underlying vasculitis (Fig 13.8).

Thrombotic ulcers

Skin infarction, leading to ulceration, may be due to embolism or to the increased coagulability of polycythaemia or cryoglobulinaemia.

Infective ulcers

Infection is now a rare cause of leg ulcers in the U.K. but ulcers due to tuberculosis, leprosy, atypical mycobacteria, diphtheria, and deep fungal infections, such as sporotrichosis or chromoblastomycosis, are still seen in the tropics.

Malignant ulcers

Squamous cell carcinoma (p. 200) (Fig. 13.9) is the most common, but malignant melanoma (p. 201) and basal cell carcinoma (p. 197) can both present as flat lesions which expand, crust and ulcerate.

Fig. 13.7 Not all leg ulcers are due to venous hypertension. Surrounding palpable purpura indicates vasculitic cause of this ulcer.

Fig. 13.8 Large, shallow and recalcitrant ulcer complicating rheumatoid arthritis.

Fig. 13.9 Patient referred with a 'venous ulcer' but biopsy of hyperplastic granulating base confirmed diagnosis of poorly differentiated squamous cell carcinoma.

Pyoderma gangrenosum

This is characterized by large and rapidly spreading ulcers which may be circular or polycyclic and have a blue, indurated, undermined, or pustular margin. Pyoderma gangrenosum may complicate rheumatoid arthritis, ulcerative colitis, or blood dyscrasias.

Investigations

Most chronic leg ulcers are venous, but other causes should be considered, if the signs are atypical. A search for contributory factors, such as obesity, peripheral artery disease, cardiac failure or arthritis, is always worthwhile. Investigations should include:

- Urine test for sugar.
- Haematocrit to detect anaemia, which will delay healing.
- Swabbing for pathogens — *see* Bacterial superinfection *above*.
- Venography helps to detect surgically remediable causes of venous incompetence.
- Döppler ultrasound may help to assess arterial circulation when atherosclerosis is likely. It seldom helps if the peripheral pulses can easily be felt.

Treatment

Venous ulcers will not heal if the leg remains swollen and the patient chair-bound. Pressure bandages take priority over other measures but not for atherosclerotic ulcers with an already precarious arterial supply. A common error is to use local treatment which is too elaborate. As a last resort, admission to hospital, for elevation and intensive treatment, may be needed, but the results are not encouraging; patients may stay in the ward for many months but their apparently well-healed ulcers may break down rapidly when they go home.

The list of therapies is extensive. They can be divided into the following categories: physical, local, oral, and surgical.

Physical measures

Compression bandages and stockings. Compression bandaging is vital for most venous ulcers; it reduces oedema and aids venous return. The bandages are applied over the ulcer dressing, from the forefoot to just below the knee. Self-adhesive bandages (Formulary, p. 253) are convenient and have largely replaced elasticated bandages. Bandages stay on for 2–7 days at a time and are left on at night. Once an ulcer has healed, a graduated compression stocking (e.g. single or double Tubigrip or Venosan 2502/2003 [U.K.] or Jobst or Teds [U.S.A.]) from toes to knee (or preferably thigh), should be prescribed. A foam or felt pad may be worn under the stockings to protect vulnerable areas against minor trauma. The stocking should be put on *before* rising from bed.

Elevation of the affected limb, preferably above the hips, aids venous drainage, decreases oedema, and raises oxygen tension in the limb. Patients should rest with their legs up for at least two hours every afternoon. The foot of the bed should be raised by at least six inches; it is not enough just to put a pillow under the feet.

Walking, in moderation, is beneficial, but prolonged standing or sitting with dependent legs is not.

Physiotherapy. Some physiotherapists are good at persuading venous ulcers to heal. Their secret lies in a combination of the following: leg exercises, elevation, gentle massage, ultrasound treatment to the skin around the ulcers, and graduated compression bandaging.

Diet. Many patients are obese and should lose weight.

Local therapy

There are many preparations to choose from; those we have found most useful are listed in the Formulary (p. 253).

Clean ulcers (Fig. 13.10). Dressings need be changed only once or twice a week. Paraffin tulle dressings, plain or impregnated with 0.5% chorhexidine, 0.25%

Fig. 13.10   Clean-healing ulcer. Weekly dressing would be suitable.

silver proteinate in compound calamine cream spread on a non-stick dressing, 0.5% brilliant green, 1% silver sulphadiazine cream, and simple zinc and castor oil ointment, are all helpful and easy to apply. The area should be gently cleaned with arachis oil, 5% hydrogen peroxide or saline, before the next dressing is applied. Sometimes immersing the whole ulcer in a tub of warm water is best, and will loosen or dissolve adherent crusts.

Many dressings have absorbent and protective properties (Formulary, p. 253). These include Granuflex (which has the advantage of sticking to the surrounding skin), Geliperm and Sorbsan in the U.K. and Duoderm, Opsite and Tegaderm in the U.S.A. Actisorb (U.K.) is a useful charcoal dressing which absorbs exudate and minimizes odour.

Medicated bandages, based on zinc paste, with ichthammol, or with calamine and clioquinol, are useful when there is much surrounding eczema, and can be used for all types of ulcers, even infected, exuding ones. The bandage is applied in strips from the foot to below the knee. Worsening of eczema under a medicated bandage may signal the development of allergic contact dermatitis to a component of the paste, most often parabens (a preservative).

Infected ulcers (Fig. 13.11). These have to be cleaned and dressed more often than clean ulcers, sometimes even twice daily. Useful preparations include 0.5% silver nitrate, 0.25% sodium hypochlorite, 0.25% acetic acid, potassium permanganate (1 in 10 000 dilution) and 5% hydrogen peroxide, all made up in aqueous solution, and applied as compresses with or without occlusion. Helpful creams and lotions include 1.5% hydrogen peroxide, 20% benzoyl peroxide, 1% silver sulphadiazine, 10% povidone-iodine and 0.5% brilliant green (Formulary, p. 253). Dextran polymer beads, and starch polymer beads within cadexomer iodine, are recent expensive preparations whose main function is to absorb exudate. Although antibiotic tulles are easy to apply and are well tolerated, they should not be used for long periods as they may induce bacterial resistance or sensitize. Resistance is not such a problem with povidone-iodine, and a readily applied non-adherent dressing impregnated with this antiseptic may be useful. Surrounding eczema is helped by weak or moderate strength

Fig. 13.11 Infected ulcer with sloughing. Tendon visible at bottom of photograph. Hospital admission and frequent dressings needed to save leg.

local steroids, which must never be put on the ulcer itself. Lassar's paste, zinc cream or paste bandages (*see above*) are suitable alternatives.

Oral treatment
The following may be helpful.
- *Diuretics*. Pressure bandaging is more important as the oedema associated with venous ulceration is largely mechanical. Diuretics will combat the oedema of cardiac failure.
- *Analgesics*. Adequate analgesia is important. Aspirin may not be well tolerated by the elderly. Paracetamol (not available in the U.S.A.), or acetaminophen is often adequate but dihydrocodeine may be required. Analgesia may be needed only when the dressing is changed.
- *Antibiotics*. Ulcers need not be 'sterilized' by local or systemic antibiotics. Short courses of systemic antibiotics should be reserved for spreading infection (*see under* Complications *above*) but are sometimes tried for pain or even odour. Bacteriological guidance is needed and the drugs used include erythromycin and flucloxacillin (streptococcal or staphylococcal cellulitis), metronidazole (*Bacteroides* infection) and, recently, ciprofloxacin (*Pseudomonas aeruginosa* infection).

- *Ferrous sulphate* and *folic acid*. For anaemia.
- *Zinc sulphate*. May help to promote healing, especially if the plasma zinc level is low.
- *Stanozolol*. This anabolic steroid may not heal an existing ulcer more quickly, but may prevent ulceration in lipodermatosclerosis and may protect against recurrences. The manufacturer's advice on contra-indications, e.g. prostatic cancer and abnormal liver function, and on monitoring treatment, must not be overlooked.
- *Oxerutins*. These may help the oedema and symptoms of venous insufficiency and are said to reduce leakage from capillaries by acting on the endothelial cells.

Surgery

Autologous pinch or split-thickness grafts have a place. Lyophilized pig dermis, and synthetic films similar to skin, may also be tried. The day may soon come when more patients can be treated with sheets of epidermis grown in tissue culture. In general these work best on clean ulcers.

Venous surgery on younger patients with varicose veins may prevent recurrences, those with atherosclerotic ulcers should see a vascular surgeon for assessment. Some blockages are surgically remediable.

LEARNING POINTS

1 Whatever you put on an ulcer it will never heal if the ankle is oedematous.
2 Watch out for allergy to local applications.
3 Never put topical steroids on ulcers.
4 Most ulcers, despite positive bacteriology, are not much helped by systemic antibiotics.

Purpura

Purpura, petechiae and ecchymoses may be due to a coagulation or platelet disorder, or to an abnormal vessel wall or surrounding dermis. Some common causes are listed in Table 13.8. In general, coagulation defects give rise to ecchymoses and external bleeding. Platelet defects present more often as purpura, though bleeding and ecchymoses may still occur. Vasculitis of small vessels causes purpura, often palpable and painful, but not bleeding; this is dis-

Table 13.8 Causes of intracutaneous bleeding.

1 *Coagulation defects*
   Inherited defects, e.g. haemophilia, Christmas disease
   Connective tissue disorders
   Disseminated intravascular coagulation
   Paraproteinaemias (e.g. macroglobulinaemia)
   Acquired defects (e.g. liver disease, anticoagulant
      therapy, vitamin K deficiency, drugs)

2 *Platelet defects*
   Thrombocytopenia
      idiopathic
      connective tissue disorders, especially LE
      disseminated intravascular coagulation
      haemolytic anaemia
      hypersplenism
      giant haemangiomas (Kasabach–Merritt syndrome)
      bone marrow damage (cytostatic drugs, leukaemia,
         carcinoma)
      drugs (quinine, aspirin, thiazides and sulphonamides)
   Abnormal function
      von Willebrand's disease

3 *Vascular defect*
   Raised intravascular pressure (coughing, vomiting,
      venous hypertension, gravitational)
   Vasculitis (including Henoch–Schönlein purpura)
   Infections (e.g. meningococcal septicaemia, Rocky
      Mountain spotted fever)
   Paraproteinaemia (e.g. macroglobulinaemia,
      cryoglobulinaemia)
   Drugs (carbromal, aspirin, sulphonamides, quinine,
      phenylbutazone and gold salts)
   Painful bruising syndrome
   Idiopathic (progressive pigmented dermatoses)

4 *Lack of support from surrounding dermis*
   Senile purpura
   Corticosteroid therapy
   Scurvy (perifollicular purpura)
   Lichen sclerosus et atrophicus
   Systemic amyloidosis

cussed in Chapter 10. Purpura from vasodilatation and gravity is seen in many diseases of the legs, especially in the elderly (defective dermis around the blood vessels), and seldom requires investigation.

Cryoglobulinaemia is a rare cause of purpura, which is most prominent on exposed parts. It may also cause cold urticaria (p. 85) and livedo reticularis (p. 115). The condition may be idiopathic, or secondary to myeloma, leukaemia or an auto-immune disease.

Investigations
These must include a platelet count, prothrombin time, and a full blood count and biochemical screen. Electrophoresis is needed to exclude hypergammaglobulinaemia and paraproteinaemia. Cryoglobulinaemia should also be excluded. A coagulation screen, including measurement of fibrin degradation products, is often necessary. The bleeding time, and a Hess tourniquet test for capillary fragility, help less often. Skin biopsy will confirm a small vessel vasculitis.

Treatment
Treat the underlying condition. Replacement of relevant blood fractions may be needed initially. Systemic steroids are usually effective in vasculitis (Chapter 10).

Disorders of the lymphatics

Lymphoedema
Lymphoedema is firm and pits poorly. Long-standing lymphoedema may lead to gross hyperkeratosis, as in the so-called 'mossy foot'.

Cause
Lymphoedema may be primary or secondary. The

Table 13.9 Causes of secondary lymphoedema.

Recurrent lymphangitis	Erysipelas, infected pompholyx
Lymphatic obstruction	Filariasis, granuloma inguinale, tuberculosis, tumour
Lymphatic destruction	Surgery, radiation therapy, tumour
Uncertain aetiology	Rosacea, Melkersson–Rosenthal syndrome (facial nerve palsy, fissuring of tongue and lymphoedema of lip) Yellow nail syndrome

primary forms are developmental defects though signs may only appear in early puberty, or even in adulthood. Sometimes lymphoedema involves only one leg. Secondary causes are listed in Table 13.9.

Treatment
Elevation, compression bandages, diuretics and the early treatment of lymphangitis or erysipelas are the cornerstones of treatment. If erysipelas recurs, long-term penicillin should be given. Surgery occasionally helps to remove an obstruction or restore drainage.

Lymphangitis
This streptococcal infection of the lymphatics may occur without any lymphoedema. A tender red line extends proximally. Flucloxacillin or erythromycin is usually effective.

CHAPTER 14

SEBACEOUS AND SWEAT GLAND DISORDERS

Disorders of sebaceous glands

Acne vulgaris

Acne is a disorder of the pilosebaceous apparatus, peaking in adolescence, and characterized by comedones, papules, pustules, cysts, and scars.

Prevalence

Nearly all teenagers have some acne. Most try at some time anti-acne preparations which they buy straight from their pharmacist.

Acne affects the sexes equally. Its age of onset is usually between 12 and 14 years, tending to be earlier in females. The peak age and severity in females is 16–17 years and in males 17–19.

Cause

Many factors combine to cause acne (Fig. 14.1):

● *Sebum*. Sebum excretion is increased. However, this alone need not cause acne; patients with acromegaly, or with Parkinson's disease, have high sebum excretion rates but no acne. Furthermore, sebum excretion often remains high long after acne has gone away. The sebum of patients with acne contains an excess of free fatty acids.

● *Hormonal*. Androgens (from the testes, ovaries

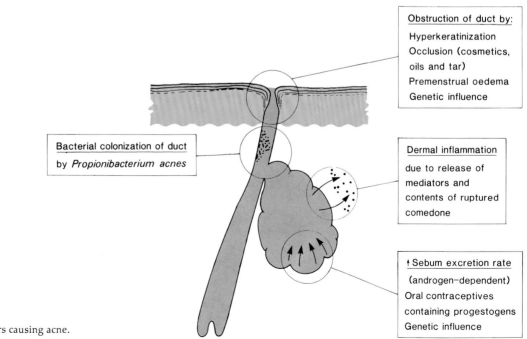

Obstruction of duct by:

Hyperkeratinization
Occlusion (cosmetics, oils and tar)
Premenstrual oedema
Genetic influence

Bacterial colonization of duct by *Propionibacterium acnes*

Dermal inflammation

due to release of mediators and contents of ruptured comedone

↑Sebum excretion rate

(androgen–dependent)
Oral contraceptives containing progestogens
Genetic influence

Fig. 14.1 Factors causing acne.

and adrenals) are the main hormones to stimulate sebum excretion, though other hormones have minor effects too (e.g. thyroid hormones and growth hormone). Those castrated before puberty never develop acne. In acne the sebaceous glands respond excessively to what are usually normal levels of these hormones (increased sensitivity of the target organ). Infantile acne may follow transplacental stimulation of a child's adrenals.

- *Mechanical.* Increased and abnormal keratinization within the follicle can obstruct the pilosebaceous ducts. Fluid retention swells keratin and accounts for premenstrual flares.
- *Bacterial. Propionobacterium acnes*, a normal skin commensal, plays a pathogenic role. It colonizes the pilosebaceous ducts, breaks down triglycerides and sparks off the inflammatory reaction.
- *Genetic.* The condition is familial but its mode of inheritance is debatable.

Fig. 14.2 The seborrhoea, comedones and scattered inflammatory papules of teenage acne.

Presentation

Common type
Lesions are confined to the face, shoulders, upper chest and back. Seborrhoea (greasy skin) (Fig. 14.2), is often present. Open comedones (blackheads), due to the plugging by keratin and sebum of the pilosebaceous orifice, or closed comedones (whiteheads), due to accretions of keratin and sebum deeper in the pilosebaceous duct, are always seen. Inflammatory papules, nodules and cysts occur, with one or two types of lesion predominating. Depressed or hypertrophic scarring may follow.

Variants

Conglobate. Conglobate means gathered into balls (Latin: *globus*, ball). This severe form of acne consists of abscesses or cysts, with intercommunicating sinuses, which contain thick serosanguinous fluid or pus. On resolution, it leaves deeply pitted or hypertrophic scars, sometimes joined by keloidal bridges (Fig. 14.3).

Fulminans. Acne fulminans is a rare variant in which conglobate acne is accompanied by fever, joint pains and a high ESR.

Fig. 14.3 Conglobate acne with inflammatory nodules, pustulocystic lesions and depressed scars.

Exogenous. Tars, chlorinated hydrocarbons, oils, and oily cosmetics may cause or exacerbate acne. Suspicion should be raised if the distribution is odd or if comedones predominate (Figs. 14.4, 14.5 and 14.6).

Excoriated. This is seen most often in young girls. Obsessional picking or rubbing leaves discrete denuded areas (Fig. 14.7).

Fig. 14.4   A group of open comedones (blackheads) following the use of a greasy cosmetic.

Fig. 14.5   Acne with numerous closed comedones. Caused by frequent use of a sunscreen oil.

Fig. 14.6   Papulopustular lesions in an odd distribution. The patient played the violin ('fiddler's neck').

Fig. 14.7   Excoriated acne with typical lesions.

Late onset. This type too occurs mainly in women and is often limited to the chin (Fig. 14.8). Nodular and cystic lesions predominate. It is stubborn and persistent.

Infantile. This rare type is more common in males, and may last for up to three years. Its morphology is like that of common acne (Fig. 14.9). Unfortunately it may be the forerunner of severe acne in adolescence.

Drug-induced. Corticosteroids, androgenic steroids, lithium, oral contraceptives, iodides, bromides, anti-tuberculosis and anticonvulsant therapy may cause an acneiform rash (Fig. 14.10).

Tropical. This affects Caucasoids in hot, humid cli-

Fig. 14.8 Late onset acne in a woman. Often localized to the chin.

Fig. 14.10 Steroid-induced acne in a seriously ill patient.

Fig. 14.9 Infantile acne. Pustulocystic lesions on the cheeks.

mates. It occurs mainly on the trunk, and responds poorly to any treatment other than return to a temperate climate.

Course
Although acne clears by the age of 23–25 years in 90% of patients, some 5% of women and 1% of men still need treatment in their thirties or even forties.

Investigations
None are usually necessary. Cultures are occasionally needed to exclude a pyogenic infection, an anaer-obic infection, or Gram-negative folliculitis. Any acne, including infantile acne, which is associated with virilization needs investigation to exclude an androgen-secreting tumour of the adrenals, ovaries or testes. Tests should then include the measurement of plasma testosterone, sex hormone binding globulin, dehydroepiandrosterone sulphate, androstenedione and, depending on the results, ultrasound examination of the ovaries and adrenals.

Differential diagnosis
Rosacea affects older individuals: comedones are absent, lesions occur only on the face, and the rash has an erythematous background. Pyogenic folliculitis can be excluded by culture. Hidradenitis suppurativa (p. 134) is associated with acne conglobata, but attacks the axillae and groin.

Treatment
Local treatment is enough for most patients with comedo-papular acne. Both local and systemic treatment are needed for pustular–cystic–scarring acne (Fig. 14.11).

Local treatment (Formulary, p. 251)
1 *Regular cleansing* with soap and water should be

Fig. 14.11 Therapeutic approaches to acne.

encouraged, to remove surface sebum. Antibacterial cleansers are also useful — e.g. chlorhexidine.

2 *Benzoyl peroxide.* This is applied only at night initially, but can be used twice daily in the absence of excessive dryness and irritation. It is wise to start with a 2.5% or 5% preparation, moving up to 10% if necessary. Benzoyl peroxide bleaches coloured sheets and towels.

3 *Retinoic acid* (tretinoin). This vitamin A analogue normalizes follicular keratinization, and is especially effective against comedones. Patients should be warned about skin irritation and photosensitivity. It can be prescribed as a lotion, cream or gel. The weakest preparation should be used first, and applied overnight on alternate nights. Sometimes, after a week or two, it has to be stopped temporarily because of irritation. As with benzoyl peroxide it may be worth increasing the strength of tretinoin after six weeks if it is tolerated well. The combination of benzoyl peroxide in the morning and tretinoin at night has many advocates.

4 *Abrasive pastes* containing aluminium oxide may also help with comedones, but aggressive scrubbing should be discouraged.

5 *Sulphur.* A number of time-honoured preparations containing sulphur are available on both sides of the Atlantic. Some are included in the Formulary (p. 251).

6 *Local antibiotics.* These are used more often in the U.S.A. than in Britain. They include topical tetracycline, clindamycin, and erythromycin (Formulary, p. 251) and are alternatives to benzoyl peroxide or tretinoin.

7 *Aluminium chloride.* Alcoholic solutions of aluminium chloride act as antiperspirants, and may help tropical acne.

8 *Cosmetic camouflage.* Cover-ups are useful is some patients, especially females, whose scarring is unsightly. They also help to obscure post-inflammatory pigmentation. A range of make-ups is available in the U.K. and U.S.A. (Formulary, p. 247).

Systemic treatment

Antibiotics:

● *Tetracycline.* An average dose for an adult is 250 mg up to four times daily, but up to 1.5 g/day may be needed in resistant cases. It should not be used for less than four months and may be needed for a year or two, or even longer. It should be taken on an empty stomach, one hour before meals or four hours after food, including milk. The dose should be tapered in line with clinical improvement, an average maintenance dose being 250–500 mg/day. Even with long courses serious side effects are rare, though candidal vulvovaginitis may force a change to a narrower spectrum antibiotic such as erythromycin. Minocycline, 50 mg twice daily, is a useful alternative if the response has been poor; it may be taken with meals. Neither antibiotic should be taken in pregnancy. Tetracyclines should not be given to children under 12 who deposit them in growing bone and developing teeth, causing stained teeth and dental hypoplasia. The absorption of tetracyclines is decreased by milk, antacids and calcium, iron and magnesium salts. Tetracyclines may cause photosensitivity.

- Erythromycin (dosage as for oxytetracycline) is the antibiotic of second choice, but may be preferred by teenagers who nibble continuously and whose stomachs are never empty.
- Trimethoprim is used by some as a third-line antibiotic for acne, when a tetracycline and erythromycin have not helped.

Hormonal. A combined antiandrogen/oestrogen treatment (Dianette: 2 mg cyproterone acetate and 0.035 mg ethinyloestradiol) is available in many countries and may help with persistent acne in women. Monitoring is as for any patient on an oral contraceptive and further contraceptive measures are unnecessary. Courses last for 8–12 months. These drugs must not be used for males.

For women with acne who also require oral contraception, a relatively high oestrogen/low progestogen preparation or a triphasic pill is best. Women taking antibiotics should be warned of their possible interaction with oral contraceptives; they should use other contraceptive precautions, especially if the antibiotics induce diarrhoea.

13-cis-retinoic acid (isotretinoin). Ro-Accutane (U.K.) (Accutane, U.S.A.) is an oral retinoid which inhibits sebum excretion, the growth of *P. acnes*, and acute inflammatory processes. The drug is reserved for se-

vere acne, unresponsive to the measures outlined above. It is given for 4–6 months only, in a dose of 0.5–1 mg/kg body weight per day; young men with truncal acne usually require the higher dose. Liver function and fasting lipid levels should be checked before the start of a course, and monitored for at least six weeks thereafter, though the drug seldom has to be stopped because of abnormalities. Isotretinoin is highly teratogenic; women should sign a form confirming that they have been warned about this, and should take an oral contraceptive throughout treatment, and for three months thereafter. A test for pregnancy should usually be done before starting treatment. Other side effects of isotretinoin include dry skin, dry and inflamed lips and eyes, nosebleeds, muscle aches and hair loss; these are often tolerated, especially if the acne is doing well. Occasionally isotretinoin flares acne at first, but this effect is usually short-lived and the drug may be continued.

Diet. It is sensible for patients to avoid foods (e.g. nuts, chocolates and wine) which they think make their acne worse, but there is little evidence that any dietary constituent, except iodine, causes acne.

Physical

Ultraviolet B radiation therapy often helps with exacerbations. Two-month courses, during which the patient attends twice weekly, are usually adequate.

Cysts can be incised and drained under local anaesthetic.

Intralesional injections of 0.1 ml of triamcinolone acetonide (2.5–10 mg/ml) hasten the resolution of stubborn cysts, but may leave atrophy.

Dermabrasion. This may be useful to flatten hypertrophic scars. A high-speed rotating wire brush planes down to a bleeding dermis. It should not be carried out if there are any active lesions and does not help depressed 'ice-pick' scars. Unsightly hyperpigmentation may follow in darker skins.

Collagen injections. Bovine collagen may be injected

into depressed scars to improve their appearance. Patients with a history of any auto-immune disorder are excluded from this treatment. Shallow atrophic lesions do better than discrete 'ice-pick' scars. The procedure is expensive and has to be repeated every six months as the collagen is resorbed.

LEARNING POINTS

1 Do not prescribe short courses of many different antibiotics.
2 Avoid tetracyclines in children and pregnant women.
3 Make sure that females with acne are not pregnant before you put them on isotretinoin, and that they do not become pregnant during the course and for three months after it.

Rosacea

Rosacea affects the face of adults, usually women. Although its peak incidence is in the thirties and forties, it may be seen too in the young or old. It may co-exist with acne but is distinct from it.

Cause and histopathology

The cause is still unknown. The condition is often seen in those who flush easily, in response to warmth, spicy food, alcohol or embarrassment. Any psychological abnormalities, including neuroticism and depression, are secondary to the skin condition. No pharmacological defect has been found which explains these flushing attacks. Sebum excretion rate and skin microbiology are normal. A pathogenic role for the tiny hair follicle mite, *Demodex folliculorum*, has not been proved.

Clinical course and complications

The cheeks, nose, centre of forehead, and chin are most commonly affected; the peri-orbital and peri-oral areas are spared (Fig. 14.12). Intermittent flushing is followed by a fixed erythema and telangiectases. Discrete, domed, inflamed papules, papulopustules and, rarely, nodules develop later (Fig.

Fig. 14.12   Typical rosacea of a middle-aged woman, with papules and pustules on a background of erythema.

Fig. 14.13   Severe rosacea and rhinophyma.

14.12). Rosacea, unlike acne, has no comedones or seborrhoea. It is usually symmetrical. Its course is prolonged, with exacerbations and remissions. Complications include blepharitis, conjunctivitis and, occasionally, keratitis. Rhinophyma, due to hyperplasia of the sebaceous glands and connective tissue on the nose, is a striking complication (Fig. 14.13) which is more common in males. Lymphoedema, below the eyes and on the forehead, is a tiresome feature in a few cases. Patients treated with potent topical steroids will develop a rebound flare of pustules, worse than the original rosacea, when treatment is stopped.

Differential diagnosis
Acne has already been mentioned. Rosacea can be distinguished from it by the background of erythema and telangiectases, and by the absence of comedones. The distribution of lesions is different and it develops later in life. Seborrhoeic eczema (p. 79), systemic lupus erythematosus (p. 103) and photodermatitis should be considered, but the papulopustules of rosacea are not seen. The flushing of rosacea may be confused with menopausal symptoms and, rarely, with the carcinoid syndrome. Superior vena caval obstruction may be mistaken for lymphoedematous rosacea.

Treatment
Tetracyclines, prescribed as for acne (p. 129), are usually effective. Erythromycin is the antibiotic of second choice. Courses should last for at least 10 weeks, and, after gaining control with 500–1000 mg daily, the dose may be cut to 250 mg daily. The condition recurs in about half of the patients within two years but repeated antibiotic courses, rather than prolonged maintenance, are generally recommended. Rarely metronidazole or 13-*cis*-retinoic acid (p. 130) is needed for stubborn rosacea. Rosacea and topical steroids go badly together (Fig. 14.14); if possible patients should use traditional applications such as 2% sulphur in aqueous cream or 1% ichthammol in zinc cream. Sunscreens may help if sun exposure is an aggravating factor. Changes in diet or drinking habits seldom help.

LEARNING POINT

Never put strong topical steroids on rosacea. If you do, skin addiction, rebound flares, and a cross dermatologist will all figure in your nightmares.

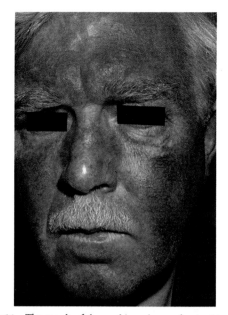

Fig. 14.14   The result of the prolonged use of potent topical steroids for rosacea. Note the extreme telangiectasia, but absence of papules and pustules.

The sweat glands

Eccrine and apocrine glands have been discussed in Chapter 2. Disorders may follow increased or decreased sweating, or blockage of their ducts.

Disorders of eccrine sweat apparatus

Generalized hyperhidrosis

Thermal hyperhidrosis
The 'thermostat' for sweating lies in the pre-optic area of the hypothalamus. Sweating follows any rise in body temperature whether it is due to exercise, environmental heat or an illness. The sweating in acute infections, and in some chronic illnesses (e.g. Hodgkin's disease), may be due to a lowering of the 'set' of this thermostat.

Other causes of general hyperhidrosis
• Emotional stimuli, hypoglycaemia, opiate withdrawal, and shock cause sweating by a direct or reflex stimulation of the sympathetic system at hy-

pothalamic or higher centres. When sweating is accompanied by a general sympathetic discharge it occurs on cold, pale skin.

- Lesions of the central nervous system (e.g. a cerebral tumour or cerebrovascular accident) may cause generalized sweating, presumably by interfering directly with the hypothalamic centre.
- Phaeochromocytoma, the carcinoid syndrome, diabetes mellitus, thyrotoxicosis, Cushing's syndrome, and the hot flushes of menopausal women, have all been associated with general sweating. The mechanisms are not clear.

Local hyperhidrosis

Local hyperhidrosis mainly plagues young adults. The commonest areas are the palms, soles and axillae. Too much sweating there is embarrassing, if not socially crippling. A sodden shirt in contact with a dripping armpit, a wet handshake, and stinking feet, are hard crosses to bear. Seldom is any cause found, but organic disease, especially thyrotoxicosis, acromegaly, tuberculosis and Hodgkin's disease, should be considered. A blatant anxiety state is occasionally present, but more often an otherwise normal person is understandably concerned about his or her antisocial condition. A vicious circle emerges in which increased anxiety drives further sweating.

The problem may be no more than one end of the normal physiological range. How many students sitting exams have to dry their hands before putting pen to paper? It is only when the sweating is gross, or continuous, that medical advice is sought. Such sweating is often precipitated by emotional stimuli and stops during sleep.

Treatment
Topical applications. The most useful preparation for axillary hyperhidrosis is 20% aluminium chloride hexahydrate in an alcohol base (Formulary, p. 247). It is applied to the dry axillae every night at first. Soon the interval can be increased, and many need to use the preparation only once or twice a week. The frequency of application may have to be cut down if the preparation irritates the skin; this is most likely if it

is applied soon after shaving. Aluminium chloride also helps hyperhidrosis of the palms and soles, but it is less effective there.

Potassium permanganate soaks (1:10 000 aqueous solution) combat the bacterial superinfection of sweaty feet which is responsible for their foul smell. The patient should soak the feet for 15 minutes twice a day until the smell has improved and be warned that potassium permanganate stains the skin and everything else brown. Occasionally glutaraldehyde solutions are used instead, but allergy and yellow-stained skin are potential complications.

Iontophoresis is the passage of a low-voltage direct current across the skin. Iontophoresis with tap water or with the anticholinergic drug glycopyrronium bromide may help palmar or plantar hyperhidrosis. Patients attend two to three times a week for treatment until the condition improves. Repeated courses or maintenance therapy may be required.

Systemic treatment. The side effects of anticholinergic therapies often limit their usefulness.

Surgery is seldom used now, as the above measures are usually effective. However, recalcitrant axillary hyperhidrosis may be treated by removing the vault of the axilla which bears most of the sweat glands; these can be identified pre-operatively by applying starch and iodine which interact with sweat to colour the starch blue. Cervical sympathectomy is the last resort in palmar hyperhidrosis; the gains seldom outweigh the drawbacks.

LEARNING POINT

20% aluminium chloride hexahydrate in an alcohol base has now taken over from anticholinergic drugs and surgery for those with sweaty armpits and hands. Iontophoresis is the second choice of therapy.

Hypohidrosis and anhidrosis

Anhidrosis due to abnormality of the sweat glands

Heat stroke

Heat stroke, due to sweat gland exhaustion, is a medical emergency seen most often in an elderly person moving to a hot climate. It may also occur in the young, during or after prolonged exercise. Patients present with hyperthermia, dry skin, weakness, headache, cramps and confusion leading to vomiting, hypotension, oliguria, metabolic acidosis, hyperkalaemia, delirium and death. They should be cooled down immediately with cold water, and fluids and electrolytes must be replaced.

Anhidrotic ectodermal dysplasia

This rare disorder is inherited as an X-linked recessive trait, in which the sweat glands are either absent or decreased. Affected boys have a characteristic facial appearance, with poor hair and poor teeth, and are intolerant of heat.

Prematurity

The sweat glands function poorly in premature babies nursed in incubators and hot nurseries.

Anhidrosis due to abnormalities of the nervous system

Anhidrosis may follow abnormalities anywhere in the sympathetic tract, from the hypothalamus to the peripheral nerves. It may therefore be a feature of multiple sclerosis, a cerebral tumour, trauma, Horner's syndrome, or peripheral neuropathy (e.g. leprosy, alcoholic neuropathy and diabetes). Patients with widespread anhidrosis are heat-intolerant, developing nausea, dizziness, tachycardia and hyperthermia in hot surroundings.

Anhidrosis or hypohidrosis due to skin disease

Local hypohidrosis has been reported in many skin diseases, especially in those which scar (e.g. lupus erythematosus and morphoea). It may be a feature of Sjogren's syndrome, ichthyosis, psoriasis and miliaria profunda (*see below*).

Interference with sweat delivery

Miliaria

This is the result of plugging or rupture of sweat ducts. It occurs in hot, humid climates, at any age, and is common in overclothed infants in hot nurseries. The physical signs depend on where the ducts are blocked.

Miliaria crystallina

Tiny clear, non-inflamed vesicles which look like dew. The most superficial type.

Miliaria rubra (prickly heat)

Tiny erythematous and very itchy papules.

Miliaria profunda

Larger erythematous papules or pustules. The deepest type.

Treatment

The best treatment is to move to a cooler climate or into air conditioning. Clothing which prevents the evaporation of sweat (e.g. nylon shirts) should be avoided; cotton is best. Claims have been made for ascorbic acid by mouth, but in our hands it rarely if ever helps. Topical steroids reduce irritation but should only be used briefly. Calamine lotion cools and soothes.

Disorders of the apocrine sweat gland

Suppurative hidradenitis (apocrine acne)

This is a severe, chronic, suppurative disease of the apocrine glands. Many papules, pustules, cysts, sinuses and scars occur in the axillae, groin and perianal areas. It may co-exist with conglobate acne. Its cause is unknown but slightly raised androgen levels are found in some affected females. It is probably not a primary infection of the apocrine glands, though *Staphylococcus aureus*, anaerobic streptococci and *Bacterioides* spp. are frequently present, and one group of workers has implicated *Streptococcus milleri* as the main pathogen. Treatment is unsatisfactory but should be as for acne vulgaris in the first instance. Systemic anti-androgens may be useful in women. Severe cases need plastic surgery to remove large areas of affected skin.

Fox–Fordyce disease

This rare disease of the apocrine ducts is comparable to miliaria rubra of the eccrine duct. It occurs in women after puberty. Itchy skin-coloured or light brown papules appear in the axillae and other areas where apocrine glands are found, such as the breasts and vulva. Treatment is not usually necessary but removal of the affected skin, or electrodesiccation of the most irritable lesions may be considered.

CHAPTER 15

INFECTIONS

Bacterial infections

Skin flora

The surface of the skin teems with harmless micro-organisms. These, the resident flora, are most numerous in moist hairy areas, rich in sebaceous glands. Organisms are found, in clusters, in irregularities in the stratum corneum and within the hair follicles. The skin bacteria are a mixture of harmless and poorly classified micrococci and diphtheroids. *Staphylococcus epidermidis* predominates on the surface and anaerobic diphtheroids deep in the hair follicles. The proportion of the different types varies from person to person; but, once established, an individual's skin flora tends to remain stable. Overgrowth of skin diphtheroids leads to three conditions:

Trichomycosis axillaris
The axillary hairs become beaded with concretions, usually yellow, made up of colonies of commensal diphtheroids. Clothing may become stained in the armpits. Topical antibiotic ointments, or shaving, clears the condition.

Pitted keratolysis
The combination of unusually sweaty feet and occlusive shoes encourages the growth of organisms which can digest keratin. The result is a cribriform pattern of fine, punched-out depressions on the soles, coupled with an unpleasant smell. Four per cent formalin soaks or 20% aluminium chloride hexahydrate in alcohol are helpful.

Erythrasma
Some diphtheroid members of the skin flora can produce porphyrins when grown in a suitable medium: as a result their colonies fluoresce coral pink under Wood's light. Overgrowth of these strains is sometimes the cause of symptom-free macular, wrinkled, slightly scaly, pink, brown or macerated white areas, most often found in the armpits or groins, or between the toes. These areas also fluoresce coral pink with Wood's light. Topical fusidic acid or miconazole will clear the condition.

Staphylococcal infections

Staphylococcus aureus is not part of the resident flora of the skin other than in a minority who carry it in their nostrils, perineum or armpits. Carriage rates vary with age. Nasal carriage is almost invariable in babies born in hospital, becomes less frequent during infancy, and rises again during the school years to the adult level of roughly 20%. Rather fewer carry the organism elsewhere (Fig. 15.1). Staphylococci can also grow, without causing obvious sepsis, on areas of diseased skin such as eczema. A minor breach in the skin's defences is probably necessary for a frank staphylococcal infection to establish itself: some strains seem particularly likely to cause skin sepsis.

Impetigo

Cause
This condition can be caused by staphylococci, streptococci, or by both together. As a useful rule of

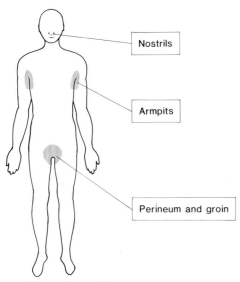

Fig. 15.1 Sites of possible staphylococcal carriage.

thumb, the bullous type is usually caused by *S. aureus*, whereas the crusted ulcer type is caused by beta-haemolytic strains of streptococci. It is highly contagious.

Presentation
A thin-walled blister forms, but ruptures rapidly, leaving an extending area of exudation and yellowish crusting (Fig. 15.2). Multiple lesions often occur, particularly around the face. The lesions may be more obviously bullous in infants. A follicular type of impetigo (superficial folliculitis) is also common.

Course
The condition may spread rapidly through a family or class. It tends to clear slowly even without treatment.

Complications
Streptococcal impetigo may trigger an acute glomerulonephritis.

Differential diagnosis
Herpes simplex may become impetiginized, as may eczema. Always think of a possible underlying cause such as this. For example, recurrent impetigo of the head and neck should prompt a search for scalp lice.

Investigation and treatment
The diagnosis is usually made on clinical grounds. Swabs should be taken and sent to the laboratory for culture, but treatment should not be held up until the results are available. Systemic antibiotics are needed for severe cases (flucloxacillin or erythromycin), or if a nephritogenic strain of streptococcus is suspected (penicillin V). For minor cases the removal of crusts and a topical antibiotic such as neomycin, mupirocin, or bacitracin will suffice (Formulary, p. 250).

Ecthyma
This is the term used to describe ulcers forming under a crusted surface infection. The site may have been that of an insect bite or of neglected minor trauma. The bacterial pathogens and their treatment are similar to those of impetigo; however, in contrast to impetigo, ecthyma heals with scarring.

Furunculosis (boils)

Cause
A boil is an acute pustular infection of a hair follicle, usually with *Staphylococcus aureus*. Adolescent boys are especially susceptible to them.

Fig. 15.2 Impetigo on a common site showing the typical honey-coloured crusting.

Fig. 15.3 A single furuncle on the forearm.

Presentation and course

A tender red nodule (Fig. 15.3) enlarges and later may discharge pus and its central 'core', before healing to leave a scar. Fever and enlarged draining nodes complete the picture. Most patients have one or two boils only and then clear; a few patients suffer from a tiresome sequence of boils (chronic furunculosis).

Complications

Cavernous sinus thrombosis is an unusual complication of boils on the central face. Septicaemia may occur but is rare.

Differential diagnosis

The diagnosis is straightforward but hidradenitis suppurativa (p. 134) should be considered if only the groin and axillae are involved.

Investigations in chronic furunculosis

- General examination: look for underlying skin disease, e.g. scabies, pediculosis, eczema.
- Test the urine for sugar. Full blood count.
- Culture swabs from lesions, and carrier sites (nostrils, perineum) of patient and immediate family.
- Immunological evaluation only if the patient has recurrent or unusual internal infections too.

Treatment

Acute episodes will respond to an appropriate antibiotic; sometimes incision speeds healing.

In chronic furunculosis (Fig. 15.4):
- Treat carrier sites such as the nose and groin twice daily for six weeks with an appropriate antiseptic or antibiotic cream (e.g. mupirocin). Treat family carriers similarly.

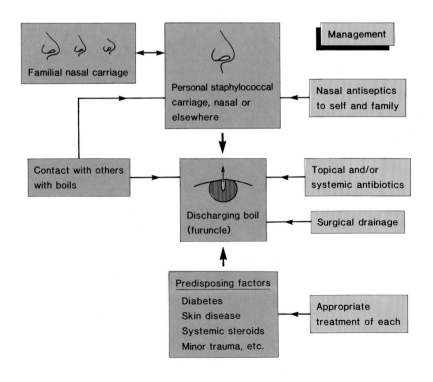

Fig. 15.4 Chronic furunculosis.

- Treat lesions with a local antibiotic cream. In stubborn cases add six weeks of a systemic antibiotic chosen to cover organism's proven sensitivities.
- Daily bath using an antiseptic soap.
- Improve hygiene and nutritional state, if faulty.

Carbuncle

A group of adjacent hair follicles becomes deeply infected with *Staphylococcus aureus*, leading to a swollen, painful, suppurating area discharging pus from several points. The pain and systemic upset are greater than those of a boil. Diabetes must be excluded; treatment needs both topical and systemic antibiotics. The multiple deep, pus-filled pockets are not easy to drain surgically. Consider the possibility of a fungal kerion (p. 158) in unresponsive carbuncles.

Toxic epidermal necrolysis

In this condition the skin changes resemble a scald. Erythema and tenderness are followed by the loosening of large areas of overlying epidermis (Fig. 15.5). In children the condition is staphylococcal in origin. Organisms in what may be only a minor local infection, such as impetigo, release a toxin (exfoliatin) which causes a split to occur high in the epidermis. With systemic antibiotics the outlook is good.

This is in contrast to the toxic epidermal necrolysis of adults which is usually drug-induced; the damage to the epidermis here is full thickness, and the mortality is high.

Streptococcal infections

Erysipelas

The first warning of an attack is often malaise, shivering and a fever. After a few hours the affected area of skin becomes red, and the eruption spreads with a well-defined advancing edge (Fig. 15.6). Untreated, the condition may even be fatal, but it responds rapidly to systemic penicillin. The causative streptococci may gain their entry through a split in the skin, for example between the toes or under an ear lobe.

Episodes may repeatedly affect the same area and lead to persistent lymphoedema. Low dosage long-term oral penicillin V will usually cut down the frequency of recurrences. The cause of the original skin split, perhaps a minor tinea pedis, should be treated too.

LEARNING POINTS

1 Unlike lightning, erysipelas often strikes in the same place twice.
2 Shivering and malaise precede the rash but that is when the penicillin should be given.
3 Recurrent bouts may need long-term prophylactic penicillin.

Fig. 15.5 Staphylococcal toxic epidermal necrolysis in a child. The overlying epidermis is loosening in the red areas.

Fig. 15.6 Erysipelas — note sharp demarcation and gross oedema. The portal of entry here was in the external ear.

Cellulitis

This refers to an inflammation of the skin occurring at a deeper level than erysipelas. The subcutaneous tissues are involved and the area is more raised and swollen; the erythema is less marginated than in erysipelas. The condition often follows an injury and favours areas of hypostatic oedema. Streptococci, staphylococci, or other organisms may be the cause. Treatment is elevation, rest and systemic antibiotics.

Necrotizing fasciitis

A mixture of pathogens, usually including streptococci and anaerobes, is responsible for this condition which, at first, resembles a dusky cellulitis, but which quickly turns into an extending necrosis of the skin and subcutaneous tissues. The prognosis is often poor despite early surgical debridement and systemic antibiotics.

Erysipeloid

The causative organism, *Erysipelothrix insidiosa*, infects a wide range of animals, birds, and fish. In man, infections are most common in butchers, fishmongers, and cooks, the organism penetrating the skin after a prick from an infected bone. Usually such infections are mild, and localized to the area around the inoculation site. The swollen purple area spreads slowly with a clear-cut advancing edge. With penicillin the condition clears quickly; without it, resolution may take several weeks.

Spirochaetal infections

Syphilis

Cause
Infection with the causative organism, *Treponema pallidum*, may be congenital, or acquired through tranfusion with contaminated blood, or by accidental inoculation. The most important route, however, is through sexual contact with an infected partner.

Presentation

Congenital syphilis
A high standard of antenatal care ensures that syphi-

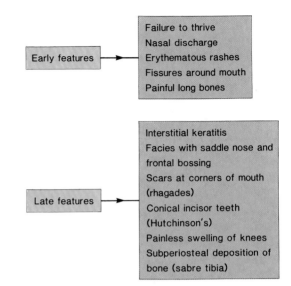

Fig. 15.7 The early and late features of congenital syphilis.

lis in the mother is detected and treated during pregnancy — congenital syphilis is then rare. Otherwise, stillbirth is a common outcome, though some children with congenital syphilis may develop the stigmata of the disease only in late childhood. Some features of early and late congenital syphilis are listed in Fig. 15.7.

Acquired syphilis
The features of the different stages are given in Fig. 15.8. After an incubation period (9–90 days), a primary chancre develops at the site of inoculation. Often this is genital, but oral and anal chancres are not uncommon. A typical chancre is an ulcerated, though not painful, button-like lesion of up to 1 cm in diameter. Untreated it lasts about six weeks and then clears leaving an inconspicuous scar.

The secondary stage may be reached while the chancre is still subsiding. Systemic symptoms and lymphadenopathy usher in eruptions which at first are macular and inconspicuous, and later papular and more obvious. Lesions are distributed symmetrically and are of a coppery, ham colour. Classically there are obvious lesions on the palms and soles. Annular lesions are also not uncommon. Condyloma lata are moist papules in the genital and anal areas. Other signs include 'moth-eaten' alopecia and mucus patches in the mouth.

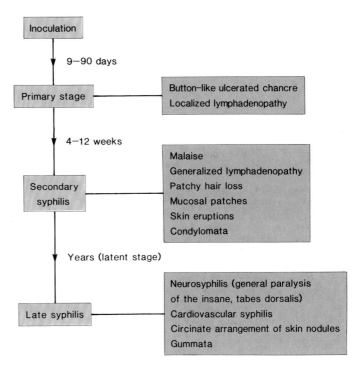

Fig. 15.8 The stages of syphilis

The skin lesions of late syphilis may be nodules which spread peripherally and clear centrally, leaving a serpiginous outline. Gummas are granulomatous areas; in the skin they quickly form punched-out ulcers which heal poorly to leave papery white scars.

Clinical course
Even if left untreated, most of those who contract syphilis have no further problems after the secondary stage has passed.

Differential diagnosis
The skin changes of syphilis may mimic many other skin diseases. Always consider the following:
- *Chancre*. Chancroid (multiple and painful), herpes simplex, anal fissure, cervical erosions.
- *Secondary syphilis:*
  Eruption — measles, german measles, drug eruptions, pityriasis rosea, lichen planus, psoriasis.
  Condylomas — genital warts, piles.
  Oral lesions — aphthous ulcers.
- *Late syphilis*. Bromide and iodide reactions, other granulomas, erythema induratum.

Investigations
The diagnosis of syphilis in its infectious (primary and secondary) stages can be confirmed using dark-field microscopy to show up spirochaetes in smears from a chancre, an oral lesion, or a moist area in a secondary eruption.

Serological tests for syphilis become positive only some 5–6 weeks after infection (usually a week or two after the appearance of the chancre). The traditional tests (WR and VDRL) have now largely been replaced by more specific ones (e.g. the *Treponema pallidum* haemagglutination test and the fluorescent treponemal antibody/absorption test). These more sensitive tests tend not to become negative after treatment if an infection has been present for more than a few months.

Treatment
Penicillin is still the treatment of choice (e.g. for early syphilis benzathine penicillin 1.2 mega units given intramuscularly into each buttock at a single session, or procaine penicillin, 600 000 units intramuscularly, daily for 10 days), with erythromycin and tetracycline effective alternatives for those with penicillin

allergy. The use of long-acting penicillin injections overcomes the ever-present danger of poor compliance with oral treatment. Every effort must be made to trace and treat infected contacts.

LEARNING POINTS

1 Syphilis is still around and today's general was yesterday's lieutenant.
2 It is still worthwhile checking for syphilis in perplexing rashes.

Yaws

Yaws is distributed widely across the poorer parts of the tropics. The spirochaete, *Treponema pertenue*, gains its entry through skin abrasions. After an incubation period of up to six months, the primary lesion, a crusting and ulcerated papule known as the 'mother yaw', develops at the site of inoculation; later it may enlarge to an exuberant raspberry-like swelling which lasts for several months before healing to leave an atrophic pale scar. In the secondary stage, other lesions may develop in any area but do so especially around the orifices. They are not unlike the primary lesion but are smaller and more numerous ('daughter yaws'). Hyperkeratotic plaques may appear on the palms and soles. The tertiary stage is characterized by ulcerated gummatous skin lesions, hyperkeratosis of the palms and soles, and a painful periostitis which distorts the long bones. Serological tests for syphilis are positive. Treatment is with penicillin.

Erythema chronicum migrans (Lyme disease)

The spirochaete *Borrelia burgdorferi* is responsible for this condition. It is transmitted to man by ticks of the genus *Ixodes*. The site of the tick bite becomes the centre of a slowly expanding erythematous ring. Later, many annular non-scaly plaques may develop. Some patients, especially in the U.S.A., have an associated arthritis. The condition clears rapidly with penicillin or doxycycline.

Other infections

Chronic gonococcal septicaemia

Skin lesions are important as a clue to the diagnosis of this condition, in which the symptoms and signs of classical gonorrhoea are usually absent. A patient with recurring fever and joint pains develops sparse crops of skin lesions, usually around the hands and feet. The grey, often haemorrhagic, vesicopustules are characteristic. Rather similar lesions may occur in chronic meningococcal septicaemia.

Mycobacterial infections

Tuberculosis

Tuberculous infections of the skin are becoming less common as the incidence of pulmonary disease falls.

Inoculation tuberculosis
Lupus vulgaris follows the inoculation of tubercle bacilli into the skin of a person with a high degree of immunity. Lesions occur most often around the head and neck. A reddish-brown scaly plaque slowly enlarges, and may damage deeper tissues such as cartilage, leading to ugly mutilation. Scarring and contractures may follow.

Diascopy (p. 31) shows up the characteristic brownish 'apple jelly' nodules and the clinical diagnosis should be confirmed by a biopsy. A warty variant exists.

Scrofuloderma
The skin overlying a tuberculous lymph node or joint may become involved in the process. The subsequent mixture of lesions (irregular puckered scars, fistulae and abscesses) is most commonly seen in the neck.

Tuberculides
A number of skin eruptions have been, in the past, attributed to a reaction to internal foci of tuberculosis. Of these the best authenticated are the 'papulonecrotic tuberculides', recurring crops of firm dusky papules, which may ulcerate, and which favour the points of the knees and elbows.

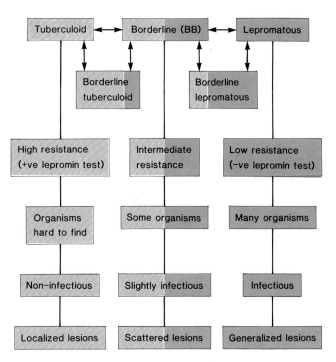

Fig. 15.9 The spectrum of leprosy: tuberculoid to lepromatous.

Erythema induratum (Bazin's disease)

Erythema induratum is the presence of deep purplish ulcerating nodules on the backs of the lower legs, usually in women with a poor, 'chilblain' type of circulation. Sometimes this is associated with a tuberculous focus elsewhere. Erythema nodosum (p. 91) may also develop as the result of tuberculosis elsewhere.

Treatment

The treatment of all types of cutaneous tuberculosis should be with a full course of a standard antituberculosis regimen. There is no longer any excuse for the use of one drug alone.

Leprosy

Cause

Mycobacterium leprae was discovered by Hansen in 1874, but has still not been cultured *in vitro*, though it can be made to grow in some animals (armadillos, mouse foot-pads, etc.). In man the route of infection is through nasal droplets from cases of lepromatous leprosy.

Epidemiology

Some 15 million people suffer from leprosy. Most live in the tropics and subtropics, but the ease of modern travel means that some cases are seen in northern Europe and the U.S.A.

Presentation

The range of clinical manifestations and complications depends upon the immune response of the patient (Fig. 15.9). Those with a high resistance tend to develop a tuberculoid type and those with low resistance a lepromatous type. Between the extremes lies a spectrum of reactions, classified as 'borderline'. Those most like the tuberculoid type are known as borderline tuberculoid (BT) and those nearest to the lepromatous type as borderline lepromatous (BL). The clinical differences between the two polar types are given in Fig. 15.10.

Differential diagnosis

Tuberculoid leprosy

Consider the following — in none of which is there any loss of sensation:

- Vitiligo (p. 182) — loss of pigment is usually complete.
- Pityriasis versicolor (p. 162) — scrapings show mycelia and spores.

Fig. 15.10 Tuberculoid versus lepromatous leprosy.

- Pityriasis alba — a common cause of fine scaly and hypopigmented areas on the cheeks of children.
- Post-inflammatory depigmentation of any cause.
- Sarcoidosis, granuloma annulare, necrobiosis lipoidica.

Lepromatous leprosy

Widespread leishmaniasis may closely simulate lepromatous leprosy. The nodules seen in neurofibromatosis and mycosis fungoides and multiple sebaceous cysts may cause confusion, as may the acral deformities seen in yaws and systemic sclerosis. Leprosy is a great imitator.

Investigations

- Biopsy of skin or sensory nerve.
- Skin or nasal smears, with Ziehl–Nielsen stain, will show up the large number of organisms seen in the lepromatous type.
- Lepromin test. This is of no use in the diagnosis of leprosy, but once the diagnosis has been made it will help in deciding on the type of disease present (positive in tuberculoid type).

Treatment

The emergence of resistant strains of *M. leprae* means that it is no longer wise to treat leprosy with dapsone alone. It should now be used in combination, usually with rifampicin, and perhaps also with clofazimine for lepromatous leprosy. A brief period of isolation is needed only for patients with infectious lepromatous leprosy; with treatment they quickly become non-infectious and can return to the community. However, their management should remain in the hands of physicians with a special interest in the disease. Special care is needed with the two types of lepra reaction which may occur during treatment.

- Type I reactions are seen in tuberculoid disease — lesions become red and angry, and pain and paralysis may follow neural inflammation.
- Type II reactions occur in lepromatous leprosy and include erythema nodosum.

Tuberculoid forms should be treated for two years after disease activity has ceased: lepromatous leprosy needs treatment for life. The household contacts of lepromatous patients are at risk of developing leprosy and should be followed up.

Other mycobacterial infections

Mycobacteria are widespread in nature, living as environmental saprophytes. Some can infect man.

Mycobacterium marinum lives in water. Human infections have occurred in epidemics centred on infected swimming pools. Another route of infection is through minor skin breaches in those who clean out tropical fish tanks. After a three-week incubation period an indolent abscess or ulcerated nodule forms at the site of inoculation; later nodules may develop along the draining lymphatics (sporotrichoid spread) (p. 164). The lesions heal spontaneously, but slowly. Resolution may be speeded by an eight-week course of trimethoprim/sulphamethoxazole or minocycline.

Mycobacterium ulcerans. Infections are confined to certain humid tropical areas where the organism lives on the vegetation, and are most common in Uganda (Buruli ulcers). The necrotic spreading ulcers, with their undermined edges, are usually found on the legs. Drug therapy is disappointing and the treatment of choice is probably surgical removal of infected tissue.

Leishmaniasis

Leishmania organisms are protozoa whose life cycle includes stages in phlebotomus flies, from which they are transmitted to man. Different species, in different geographical areas, cause different clinical pictures.

- *Leishmania tropica* is found around the Mediterranean coast and in southern Asia; it causes chronically discharging skin nodules (oriental sores).
- *Leishmania donovani* is the cause of kala-azar, a disease characterized by fever, hepatosplenomegaly and anaemia. The skin may show an irregular darkening, particularly on the face and hands.

Antimony compounds are still the treatment of choice in most types of leishmaniasis. Destructive measures, including cryotherapy, are sometimes used for localized skin lesions.

Viral infections

The viral infections dealt with here are those which commonly present at dermatology clinics. A textbook of infectious diseases should be consulted for details of systemic viral infections, many of which, like measles and german measles, have their own specific rashes.

Viral warts

Cause
The human papilloma virus (HPV) has still not been cultured *in vitro*. Nevertheless, it is now known that there are more than 50 subtypes of the virus, and that particular strains cause particular varieties of wart. Infections occur when infected skin scales come into contact with breaches in the skin or mucous membranes.

Presentation (Fig. 15.11)

Common warts (Figs. 15.12 and 15.13)
The first sign is a smooth skin-coloured papule, often more easily felt than seen. As the lesion enlarges, an irregular hyperkeratotic surface develops with the classic 'warty' appearance. Common warts usually

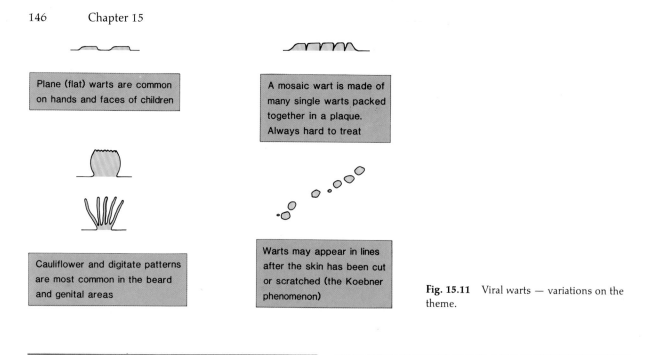

Plane (flat) warts are common on hands and faces of children

A mosaic wart is made of many single warts packed together in a plaque. Always hard to treat

Cauliflower and digitate patterns are most common in the beard and genital areas

Warts may appear in lines after the skin has been cut or scratched (the Koebner phenomenon)

Fig. 15.11 Viral warts — variations on the theme.

Fig. 15.12 Typical common warts on the fingers.

Fig. 15.13 Multiple hand warts in a fishmonger.

Fig. 15.14 Solitary plantar wart on the heel.

Fig. 15.15 Group of warts under the forefoot pared to show mosaic pattern.

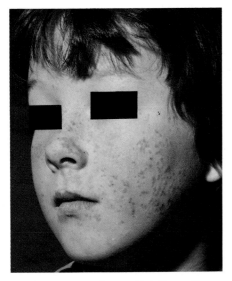

Fig. 15.16   Plane warts resolving with inflammation.

Fig. 15.17   Exuberant peri-anal warts.

occur on the hands but are also often on the face and genitals. They are more often multiple than single. Pain is rare.

Plantar warts
These are characterized by a rough surface, protruding only slightly from the skin and surrounded by a horny collar (Fig. 15.14). On paring, oozing capillary loops distinguish plantar warts from corns. Often multiple, plantar warts may be painful.

Mosaic warts (Fig. 15.15)
These plaque-like hyperkeratotic lesions, often extensive, are made up of multiple, small, tightly packed but discrete individual warts. They are most common on the soles but are also seen on palms and around finger nails. They are usually not painful.

Plane warts (Fig. 15.16)
These smooth, flat-topped papules are most commonly seen on the face and brow and on the backs of the hands. Usually skin-coloured or light brown, they become inflamed as they resolve spontaneously. Lesions are multiple, painless, and, as with common warts, sometimes arranged along a scratch line.

Facial warts
These are most common in the beard area of the

adult male and are liable to be spread by shaving. A digitate appearance is common. Lesions may be ugly but are painless.

Anogenital warts (condyloma acuminata) (Fig. 15.17)
Papillomatous cauliflower-like lesions, with a moist macerated vascular surface, may appear anywhere in this area. They may coalesce to form huge lesions causing discomfort and irritation. The vaginal and anorectal mucosae may be affected.

Course
Warts resolve spontaneously in the healthy as their immune response overcomes the infection: this happens within six months in 30% of patients. Spontaneous resolution, sometimes heralded by punctate blackening due to capillary thrombosis (Fig. 15.18), leaves no trace. Mosaic warts are notoriously slow to resolve and often resist all treatment. Warts persist and spread in immunocompromised patients, e.g. those on immunosuppressive therapy or with lymphoreticular disease. Seventy per cent of renal allograft recipients will have warts five years after transplantation.

Complications
1 Some plantar warts are very painful.
2 Epidermodysplasia verruciformis is a rare univer-

Fig. 15.18 Spontaneous resolution of a group of plantar warts. The blackness is due to capillary thrombosis.

sal wart infection, usually with HPV of unusual strains. The cause is not known but ensuing carcinomatous change frequently occurs.

3 Malignant change is otherwise rare though infections with HPV of certain genital strains may predispose to cervical carcinoma. HPV infections in immunocompromised patients (e.g. renal allograft recipients) have also been linked with skin cancer.

Differential diagnosis

Most warts are easily recognized. The following must be ruled out:

- *Molluscum contagiosum* (p. 153) — smooth dome-shaped and pearly, with central umbilication. Caused by a pox virus.
- *Plantar corns* — on pressure areas, no capillary bleeding on paring. Have a central keratotic core and are painful.
- *Granuloma annulare* (p. 213) — surface is smooth, the lesions dermal, and the outline often annular.
- *Condyloma lata* — seen in syphilis. Rare but should not be confused with condyloma acuminata (warts). Lesions are flatter, greyer and less well defined. In doubt, other signs of secondary syphilis (p. 140) should be looked for, and serological tests carried out.
- *Amelanotic melanomas and other epithelial malignancies* — verrucose nodules in patients over the age of 40 should be examined with special care. Mistakes have been made in the past.

Treatment

Palmoplantar warts

Home treatment is best and can be carried out with one of the many wart paints now available (Formulary, p. 250). Most contain salicylic acid (12–20%). The success rate is good if the patient is prepared to persist with regular treatment. Paints should be applied once daily, after moistening the warts in hot water for at least five minutes. After drying, dead tissue and old paint are removed with an emery board or pumice stone. Enough paint to cover the surface of the wart, but not the surrounding skin, is applied and allowed to dry. Warts on the plantar surface should be covered with plasters though this is not necessary elsewhere. Side effects are rare if these instructions are followed. Wart paints should not be applied to facial or anogenital skin, or used in patients with adjacent eczema.

If no progress is being made after regular and correct use of the salicylic acid wart paint for 12 weeks, then a paint containing formaldehyde or glutaraldehyde is worth trying. A useful way of dealing with multiple small plantar warts is for the area to be soaked for 10 minutes each night in a 4% formalin solution. A few patients may become allergic to this.

Cryotherapy, with carbon dioxide or liquid nitrogen, is effective. However, it is painful and should perhaps remain, after wart paints, the second line of treatment for most patients. A cotton-tipped applicator dipped into liquid nitrogen, or a CO_2 stick, is applied to the wart until a small frozen halo appears in the surrounding normal skin (Fig. 15.19). If further treatment is necessary the optimal interval is three weeks. A few minutes tuition from a dermatologist will help a practitioner wishing to start cryotherapy. Blisters should not be provoked intentionally, but occur from time to time, and should not alarm patients who have been forewarned.

Anogenital warts

Women with anogenital warts, or who are the partners of men with anogenital warts, should have regular tests of cervical cytology since the wart virus can cause cervical cancer.

Cryotherapy is suitable for treating anogenital warts. Some prefer to use podophyllin paint (Formu-

Fig. 15.19 A wart treated with cryotherapy: area includes a small frozen halo of normal surrounding skin.

Fig. 15.20 Multiple scars following the injudicious surgical treatment of warts.

lary, p. 250) which should be applied carefully to the warts and allowed to dry before powdering with talc. On the first occasion it should be washed off with soap and water after two hours but if there has been little discomfort this may be increased stepwise to six hours. Treatment is best carried out weekly by a doctor or nurse and not by the patient. Podophyllin must not be used in pregnancy.

Facial common warts
These are best treated with electrocautery or a hyfrecator but also surrender to careful cryotherapy. Shaving, if essential, should be with a brushless foam and a disposable razor.

Plane warts
On the face these are best left untreated and the patient or parent can be reasonably assured that spontaneous resolution will occur. When treatment is demanded, careful freezing is the best method.

Solitary, stubborn, or painful warts
These may be removed under local anaesthetic with a curette, though cure is not assured with this or any other method and a scar often follows. Surgical excision is never justifiable (Fig. 15.20). Bleomycin can also be injected into such warts with much success.

LEARNING POINTS

1 Do not hurt children with cryotherapy without a good trial of a wart paint first.
2 Treat most warts with a wart paint for 12 weeks before referring.
3 Do not leave scars: nature does not.
4 Avoid podophyllin during pregnancy.
5 Do not miss an amelanotic malignant melanoma.

Varicella (chickenpox)

Cause
The herpes virus varicella-zoster is spread by the respiratory route; its incubation period is about 14 days.

Presentation and course
Slight malaise is followed by the development of papules which turn rapidly into clear vesicles, the contents of which soon become pustular. Over the next few days the lesions crust and then clear, sometimes leaving white depressed scars. Lesions appear in crops, are often itchy and are most profuse on the trunk and least profuse on the periphery of the limbs (centripetal). Second attacks are rare.

Complications
• Pneumonitis, with pulmonary opacities on X-ray.
• Secondary infection of skin lesions.
• Haemorrhagic or lethal chickenpox in the immunocompromised.
• Scarring.

Differential diagnosis
Smallpox, mainly centrifugal anyway, has been universally eradicated now, and the diagnosis is seldom in doubt.

Investigations
None are usually needed.

Treatment
Acyclovir (Formulary, p. 258) should be reserved for severe attacks and for immunocompromised patients; for the latter hyperimmune globulin can also be used to prevent disease if given within a day or two of exposure. For mild attacks calamine lotion topically is all that is required.

Herpes zoster

Cause
Shingles is also caused by the herpes virus varicella-zoster. An attack is due to the reactivation, usually for no apparent reason, of virus which has remained dormant in a sensory root ganglion since an earlier episode of chickenpox (varicella). The incidence of

shingles is highest in old age, and in conditions such as Hodgkin's disease, AIDS, and leukaemia, which weaken the normal defence mechanisms. Shingles does not occur in epidemics; its clinical manifestations are due to virus acquired in the past; however, patients with zoster may transmit the virus to others in whom it will cause chickenpox (Fig. 15.21).

Presentation and course
Attacks usually start with a burning pain soon followed by erythema and grouped, sometimes blood-filled, vesicles scattered over a dermatome. The clear vesicles quickly become purulent, and over the space of a few days burst and crust. Scabs usually separate in 2–3 weeks, sometimes leaving depressed depigmented scars.

Zoster is characteristically unilateral (Figs. 15.22 and 15.23). It may affect more than one adjacent dermatome. The thoracic segments and the ophthalmic division of the trigeminal nerve are involved disproportionately often.

It is not uncommon for few pock-like lesions to be found outside the main segment of involvement, but

Fig. 15.21   Zoster/varicella relationships.

Fig. 15.22 Herpes zoster of a mid-thoracic dermatome.

Fig. 15.23 Herpes zoster of the second division of the trigeminal nerve with severe ulceration of one side of the palate.

a generalized chickenpox-like eruption accompanying segmental zoster should raise suspicions of an underlying immunocompromised state or malignancy, particularly if the lesions are unusually haemorrhagic or necrotic.

Complications
- Secondary bacterial infection is common.
- Motor nerve involvement is much less common, but has led to paralysis of ocular muscles, the facial muscles, the diaphragm, and the bladder.
- Zoster of the ophthalmic division of the trigeminal nerve may lead to corneal ulcers and scarring. A good clinical clue here is involvement of the naso-ciliary branch (vesicles grouped on the side of the nose).
- Persistent neuralgic pain, after the acute episode is over, is most common in the elderly.

Differential diagnosis
Occasionally the initial pain, before the rash has appeared, is taken for an emergency such as acute appendicitis or myocardial infarction. Otherwise the dermatomal distribution, and the pain, allow zoster to be distinguished easily from herpes simplex, eczema, and impetigo.

Investigations
Blister fluid can be sent to the laboratory for culture in the few cases when the diagnosis is in doubt. Clinical suspicions about underlying conditions, such as Hodgkin's disease, chronic lymphatic leukaemia, or AIDS, will require further investigation.

Treatment
Mild attacks need only rest, analgesics, and bland applications such as calamine. Secondary bacterial infection should be treated appropriately.

Systemic acyclovir (Formulary, p. 258) can be used with good effect in severe cases. Some recommend, if there are no contra-indications, a tapered course of prednisolone to help prevent neuralgia in the elderly. A trial of systemic carbamazepine or topical capsaicin cream is worthwhile in established post-herpetic neuralgia.

LEARNING POINTS

1 Post-herpetic neuralgia affects the old rather than the young.
2 Systemic acyclovir only works if given within 48 hours of the onset.
3 Look for an underlying cause when there is widespread involvement.

Herpes simplex

Cause

Herpes virus hominis is the cause of herpes simplex. The virus is ubiquitous and carriers may continue to shed virus particles in their saliva or tears. It has been separated into two types. The lesions caused by type II virus occur mainly on the genitals, while those of type I are usually extragenital: this distinction is not absolute however.

The route of infection may be through mucous membranes or abraded skin. After the episode associated with the primary infection, the virus may become latent, possibly within nerve ganglia, but still capable of giving rise to recurrent bouts of vesication (recrudescences).

Presentation

The primary infection

The most common recognizable manifestation of a primary type I infection in children is an acute gingivostomatitis accompanied by malaise, headache, fever, and enlarged cervical nodes. Vesicles, soon turning into ulcers, can be seen scattered over the lips and mucous membranes. The illness lasts about two weeks.

Primary type II virus infections, usually transmitted sexually, cause multiple and painful genital or peri-anal blisters which rapidly ulcerate.

The virus can also be inoculated directly into the skin, for example during wrestling. A herpetic whitlow is one example of this direct inoculation: the uncomfortable pus-filled blisters on a finger tip are seen most often in medical personnel attending patients with unsuspected herpes simplex infections.

Recurrent (recrudescent) infections

These occur in roughly the same place each time: they may be precipitated by respiratory tract infections (cold sores), UVR, menstruation or even stress. Common sites include the face and lips (type I) (Fig. 15.24) and the genitals (type II) but lesions can occur anywhere. Tingling, burning, or even pain, is followed within a few hours by the development of erythema and clusters of tense vesicles. Crusting occurs within 24–48 hours and the whole episode lasts about a week.

Fig. 15.24　The grouped vesicles of herpes simplex, here provoked by sunlight.

Complications

- Herpes encephalitis or meningitis may occur without any cutaneous clues.
- Disseminated herpes simplex: widespread vesicles may be part of a severe illness in newborns, debilitated children or immunosuppressed adults.
- Eczema herpeticum: patients with atopic eczema are particularly susceptible to widespread cutaneous herpes simplex infections. Those looking after patients with atopic eczema should stay away if they develop cold sores.
- Herpes simplex may cause recurrent dendritic ulcers leading to corneal scarring.
- Erythema multiforme (p. 89) may in some patients regularly follow recurrent herpes simplex infections.

Investigations

None are usually needed. Doubts over the diagnosis can be dispelled by culturing the virus from vesicle fluid. Antibody titres rise with primary, but not with recurrent, infections.

Treatment

'Old-fashioned' remedies will suffice for occasional mild attacks of recurrent herpes simplex. Dabbing with surgical spirit is helpful and secondary bacterial infection may be reduced with topical framycetin sulphate or sodium fusidate. For more severe and frequent attacks, a topical 5-idoxuridine lotion or acyclovir cream applied five or six times a day for the

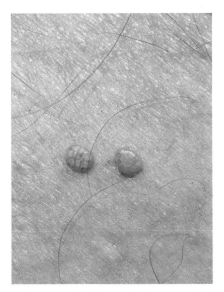

Fig. 15.25 Two typical molluscum lesions, one of which shows a mosaic appearance.

Fig. 15.26 Multiple lesions scattered over the foot of a child: some show the typical punctum.

first four days of the episode may cut down the length of attacks and perhaps increase the intervals between them.

Acyclovir tablets (Formulary, p. 258), 200 mg five times daily for five days, will also shorten an attack, and should be prescribed for those with widespread or systemic involvement. Recurrences in the immunocompromised can usually be prevented by long-term treatment at a lower dose.

Molluscum contagiosum

Cause
This common pox virus infection can be spread by direct contact, for example sexually, or by towels, clothing, etc.

Presentation and course
The incubation period varies from two to six weeks. Often several members of one family are affected. Individual lesions are shiny, white or pink, and hemispherical; they grow slowly up to 0.5 cm in diameter. A central punctum which may contain a cheesy core, gives the lesions their characteristic umbilicated look.

On close inspection a mosaic appearance may be seen (Fig. 15.25). Multiple lesions are common (Fig.

Fig. 15.27 Molluscum lesions concentrated in an area of atopic eczema in the elbow flexures.

15.26) and their distribution depends on the mode of infection. Atopic individuals and the immunocompromised are prone to especially extensive infections, spread by scratching and the use of topical steroids (Fig. 15.27).

Untreated lesions usually clear, often after a brief local inflammation, in 6–9 months. Large solitary lesions may take longer. Some leave depressed scars.

Complications
Eczematous patches often appear around mollusca. Traumatized or overtreated lesions may become secondarily infected.

Differential diagnosis
Inflamed lesions may simulate a boil. Large solitary lesions in adults may be confused with a kerato-canthoma (p. 195), an intradermal naevus (p. 191), or even a cystic basal cell carcinoma (p. 197). Confusion with warts should not arise — these have a rough surface and no central pore.

Investigations
None are usually needed, but the diagnosis can be confirmed by looking under the microscope for large swollen epidermal cells which are easily seen in unstained preparations of debris expressed from a lesion.

Treatment
Many simple destructive measures cause inflammation and then resolution. These include squeezing out the lesions with forceps, piercing them with an orange stick (preferably without phenol), and curettage. Liquid nitrogen is also effective.

These measures are fine in adults, but young children dislike them and it is reasonable to play for time using aureomycin ointment, or instructing the mother carefully how to apply a wart paint once a week to lesions well away from the eyes. Sparse eyelid lesions can be left alone but patients with numerous lesions may need to be referred to an ophthalmologist for curettage. Common sense measures will help to limit spread within the family.

LEARNING POINTS

1 If you can not tell mollusca from warts buy a lens.
2 Do not hurt young children with mollusca with radical treatment. You will not be able to get near them next time something goes wrong.

Orf

Cause
Contagious pustular dermatitis is a common condition in lambs. Its cause is a pox virus which can be transmitted to those handling infected animals. The condition is, therefore, most commonly seen on the hands of shepherds, of their wives who bottle-feed lambs, and of butchers, vets and meat porters.

Presentation and course
The incubation period is 5–6 days. Lesions, which may be single or multiple, start as small firm papules which change into flat-topped apparently pustular nodules with a violaceous and erythematous surround. The condition clears up spontaneously in about a month.

Complications
● Lymphadenitis and malaise are common.
● Erythema multiforme.
● 'Giant' lesions in the immunosuppressed.

Differential diagnosis
Diagnosis is usually simple if contact with sheep is recognized. Milker's nodules, a pox virus infection acquired from cow's udders, may look similar to orf, as may staphylococcal furuncles.

Investigations
None are usually needed. In doubt the diagnosis can be confirmed by the distinctive electron microscopic appearance of the virus obtained from crusts.

Treatment
A topical antibiotic will help prevent secondary infection; otherwise no active therapy is needed.

Acquired immune deficiency syndrome (AIDS)

Cause
The condition is caused by the human immune deficiency virus (HIV-1) which, by infecting and depleting T helper lymphocytes, reduces the effectiveness of the immunological defence system. A variety of opportunistic infections may then follow.

The virus is spread by contaminated body fluids — particularly semen and blood. Groups at high risk are male homosexuals, intravenous drug abusers, and haemophiliacs who have been given infected blood products. These populations also include many who carry the virus, sometimes with a persistent lymphadenopathy, but who have not yet developed the full-blown AIDS picture.

Presentation
Skin conditions are often the first clue to the presence of AIDS. They may be grouped into:

1 *Kaposi's sarcoma* is the initial presentation in up to one quarter of AIDS patients. The lesions of classical Kaposi's sarcoma are multiple, purplish nodules (Fig. 19.44); in AIDS the lesions may be fewer and atypical, sometimes looking like small bruises (p. 208). The diagnosis can easily be missed.
2 *Seborrhoeic eczema and folliculitis* — both are common in all groups positive for HIV, and particularly those with full-blown AIDS. The underlying cause may be an overgrowth of pityrosporum yeasts.
3 *Florid examples of common infections* — recurrent or unusually extensive infections, often atypical, may be seen with one or more of the following: herpes simplex, herpes zoster, molluscum contagiosum, candida, tinea, scabies, staphylococci.
4 *Unusual infections* — e.g. with histoplasmosis, cryptococci, atypical mycobacteria.
5 *Others* — e.g. 'hairy' oral leucoplakia, vasculitis.

Course
AIDS is associated with a very high mortality.

Treatment
No specific therapy of the underlying condition exists and so the emphasis at present must be on the avoidance of infection and on the education of the public. Treatment is symptomatic and varies according to the types of infection detected. The role of azidothymidine (AZT) has still to be assessed fully.

Cat-scratch disease
The infective agent has not yet been identified. Some two weeks after a cat bite or scratch, a reddish granulomatous papule appears at the site of inoculation. Tender regional lymphadenopathy follows some weeks later, and lasts for several weeks, often being accompanied by a mild fever. The glands may discharge before settling spontaneously. There is no specific treatment.

Mucocutaneous lymph node syndrome
(Kawasaki's disease)
The cause is thought to be a *Rickettsia*-like organism. The disease affects young children whose erythema, though often generalized, becomes most marked in a glove and stocking distribution. Peeling around the fingers and toes is one obvious feature but is not seen at the start.

The episode is accompanied by fever and usually resolves within two weeks. Despite its name, not all patients have lymphadenopathy. The danger of this condition lies in the proportion of children who develop myocarditis and coronary artery disease. The pathology is close to that of polyarteritis nodosa. Treatment with aspirin has been recommended as a way of reducing the risk of coronary artery involvement.

Gianotti–Crosti syndrome
This is a rather uncommon reaction to infection with hepatitis B virus in childhood. Small reddish papules erupt bilaterally over the limbs and face, and fade over the course of a few weeks. Jaundice is uncommon though tests of liver function give abnormal results.

Herpangina
This is an acute infectious illness, caused by group A Coxsackie viruses. The patient is usually a child with a fever, and a severe sore throat covered in many small vesicles which rapidly become superficial ulcers. Episodes resolve in about a week.

Hand, foot and mouth disease
This is usually due to Coxsackie A16. Minor epidemics occur in institutions. The oral vesicles are larger and fewer than those of herpangina. The hand and foot lesions are small greyish vesicles with a narrow rim of redness around. The condition settles within a few days.

Measles
An incubation period of 10 days is followed by fever, conjunctival injection, photophobia, and upper respiratory tract catarrh. Koplik's spots are seen at this stage on the buccal mucosa. The characteristic rash starts after a few days, on the brow and behind

the ears, and soon becomes extensive before fading with much desquamation.

German measles (rubella)

Lymphadenopathy occurs a few days before the evanescent pink macular rash which fades, first on the trunk, over the course of a few days. Rubella during the first trimester of pregnancy carries a risk of damage to the unborn child.

Erythema infectiosum (fifth disease)

This is caused by the human parvovirus and occurs in small outbreaks, often in the spring. A slapped-cheek erythema is quickly followed by a reticulate erythema of the shoulders. The affected children feel well, and the rash clears over the course of a few days. Other features, sometimes not accompanied by a rash, include transient anaemia and arthritis.

Fungal infections

Dermatophyte infections (ringworm)

Cause

Three genera of dermatophyte fungi cause tinea infections (ringworm):
- *Trichophyton* (skin, hair and nail infections).
- *Microsporum* (skin and hair).
- *Epidermophyton* (skin and nails).

Dermatophytes invade keratin only, and the inflammation they cause is due to metabolic products of the fungus or to delayed hypersensitivity. In general, zoophilic fungi (those transmitted to man by animals) cause a more severe inflammation than anthropophilic ones (spread from person to person).

Presentation and course

This depends upon the site (Fig. 15.28), and on the strain of fungus involved.

Tinea pedis (athlete's foot)

This is the commonest type of fungal infection in man. The sharing of wash places, for example in coal mines, and of swimming pools, predisposes to infection: occlusive footwear encourages relapses.

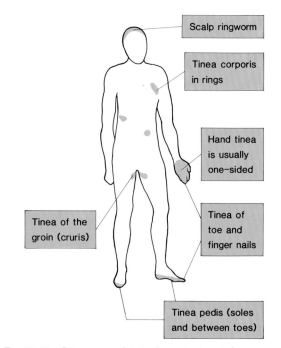

Fig. 15.28 Sites susceptible to dermatophyte infections.

Fig. 15.29 Tinea pedis. Scaly area spreading to the sole from the toe webs.

Fig. 15.30 Chronic tinea of the big toe nail. Starting distally, the thickness and discoloration are spreading proximally.

Most cases are due to one of three organisms: *Trichophyton rubrum* (the most common and the most stubborn), *T. mentagrophytes* var. *interdigitale* and *Epidermophyton floccosum*.

There are three common clinical patterns:

1 Soggy interdigital scaling, particularly in the fourth and fifth interspace (all three organisms) (Fig. 15.29).
2 A diffuse dry scaling of the soles (usually *T. rubrum*).
3 Recurrent episodes of vesication (usually *T. mentagrophytes* var. interdigitale or *E. floccosum*).

Tinea of the nails

Toe nail infection is usually associated with tinea pedis. The initial changes occur at the free edge of the nail which becomes yellow and crumbly (Fig. 15.30). Subungual hyperkeratosis, separation of the nail from its bed, and thickening may then follow. Usually a few nails only are infected but rarely all are. Finger nail lesions are similar, but less common, and are seldom seen without a chronic *T. rubrum* infection of the skin of the hands.

Tinea of the hands

This is usually asymmetrical and associated with tinea pedis. *T. rubrum* may cause a barely perceptible erythema of one palm with a characteristic powdery scale in the creases (Fig. 15.31).

Tinea of the groin

This is common and affects men more often than women. The eruption is often unilateral or asymmetrical. The upper inner thigh is involved and lesions expand slowly to form sharply demarcated plaques with peripheral scaling (Fig. 15.32). A few vesicles or pustules may be seen within the lesions. The organisms are the same as those causing tinea pedis.

Tinea of the trunk and limbs

Tinea corporis is characterized by plaques with scaling and erythema most pronounced at the periphery (Fig. 15.33). A few small vesicles and pustules may be seen within them. The lesions expand slowly and healing in the centre leaves a typical ring-like pattern.

Tinea of the scalp (tinea capitis)

This is usually a disease of children. The causative organism varies from country to country.

Fungi derived from animal sources (zoophilic fungi) induce a more intense inflammation than do

Fig. 15.31 Chronic *T. rubrum* infection of one palm. Minimal erythema, and dry powdery scaling most marked in the skin creases. Always look for similar changes on the feet.

Fig. 15.32 A very gross example of tinea of the groins. The *T. rubrum* infection has spread onto the abdomen and thighs, aided by the use of topical steroids.

Fig. 15.33 Typical tinea of the trunk showing an active red scaly edge and central clearance.

Fig. 15.34 Animal ringworm of the beard area showing boggy inflamed swellings (kerion).

Fig. 15.35 Tinea capitis of the type spread from person to person. Scaly area with broken hairs.

those spread from person to person (anthropophilic fungi). In ringworm acquired from cattle, for example, the boggy swelling, inflammation and pustulation is often so fierce that a bacterial infection may be suspected; such a lesion is called a kerion and the hair loss associated with it may be permanent. Tinea of the beard area is usually due to zoophilic species and shows the same features (Fig. 15.34).

Anthropophilic organisms cause bald rather scaly areas, with minimal inflammation, and hairs broken off 3–4 mm from the scalp (Fig. 15.35). In favus, due to *Trichophyton schoenleinii*, the picture is dominated by foul-smelling yellowish crusts surrounding many scalp hairs, and sometimes leading to scarring alopecia.

Complications
1 Fierce animal ringworm of the scalp may lead to permanent scarring alopecia.
2 A florid fungal infection anywhere may induce vesication on the sides of the fingers and palms (trichophytide).
3 Epidemics of ringworm may occur in schools.
4 The usual appearances of a fungal infection may be masked when it is mistreated with topical steroids (tinea incognito) (Fig. 15.36).

Fig. 15.36 'Tinea incognito'. Topical steroid applications have thinned the skin and altered much of the morphology. A recognizable active spreading edge is still visible.

Table 15.1 Common problems in the differential diagnosis of dermatophyte infections.

Area	Differential diagnosis
Scalp	Alopecia areata, psoriasis, seborrhoeic eczema, carbuncle, trichotillomania
Feet	Erythrasma, interdigital intertrigo, eczema
Trunk	Discoid eczema, psoriasis, candidiasis, pityriasis rosea
Nails	Psoriasis, paronychia
Hand	Chronic eczema, granuloma annulare

Differential diagnosis
This varies with the site. Some of the commoner problems are listed in Table 15.1.

Investigations

Microscopic examination of a skin scraping, nail clipping or plucked hair is a simple procedure. The scraping should be taken from the scaly margin of a lesion with a scalpel blade, and clippings from the most crumbly part of a nail. Broken hairs should be plucked with tweezers. Specimens are cleared in potassium hydroxide (p. 31). Branching hyphae are easily seen (Fig. 4.4) using a scanning (x 10) or low-power (x 25) objective lens with the iris diaphragm almost closed and the condenser racked down. Hyphae may also be seen within a cleared hair shaft, or spores may be noted around it.

Cultures should be carried out in a mycology or bacteriology laboratory. Transport medium is not necessary, and specimens should be sent in folded black paper. The report may take as long as a month; microscopy is much quicker.

Wood's light (ultraviolet light) examination of the scalp usually reveals a green fluorescence of the hairs in *Microsporum audouini* and *M. canis* infections. The technique is useful for screening children

in institutions where outbreaks of tinea capitis still sometimes occur, but some fungi (e.g. *Trichophyton tonsurans*) do not fluoresce.

Treatment

Local
This is all that is needed for minor infections of the skin. The more recent imidazole preparations, e.g. miconazole and clotrimazole (Formulary, p. 250), have largely superseded time-honoured remedies such as benzoic acid ointment (Whitfield's ointment) and tolnaftate. They should be applied twice daily. Magenta paint (Castellani's paint), although highly coloured, is helpful for exudative or macerated areas in body folds or toe webs. Occasional dusting with an antifungal powder is useful to prevent relapses.

Systemic
This is needed for tinea of the scalp and of the nails, and for widespread or chronic infections of the skin which have not responded to local measures.

Griseofulvin (Formulary, p. 257) is the drug of choice. Ultramicrosize formulations are preferred. The average duration of treatment is: scalp — three months; trunk — two months; finger nails — 12 months; toe nails — 18 months (some never clear but the addition of tioconazole nail solution may help). Griseofulvin should be taken with meals (adults 500 mg daily as a single dose; children 10 mg/kg body weight taken in two divided doses). Side effects are uncommon but treatment may have to be stopped because of persistent headache, nausea, vomiting, and skin eruptions. Griseofulvin should not be given in pregnancy, or to patients with liver failure or porphyria. The drug interacts with coumarin anticoagulants, the dose of which may have to be increased. The effectiveness of griseofulvin falls if barbiturates are being taken at the same time.

Ketoconazole (Formulary, p. 257) is now available but remains a second-line treatment for those who cannot take griseofulvin. The lack of data on the side effects of prolonged courses means that it cannot yet be recommended for the routine treatment of tinea of the nails. The drug should not be prescribed for pregnant patients, and liver functions should be checked regularly.

LEARNING POINTS

1 Do not prescribe griseofulvin for psoriasis of the nails or chronic paronychia. Always get mycological proof first.
2 Think of a dermatophyte infection in asymmetrical 'eczemas' which are worsening with local steroids.
3 Consider tinea in acute inflammatory and purulent reactions of the scalp and beard.

Candidiasis

Cause
Candida albicans is a classic opportunistic pathogen. Even in transient and trivial local infections, in the apparently fit, one or more predisposing factors such as obesity, moisture and maceration, diabetes, pregnancy, the use of broad-spectrum antibiotics, or perhaps the use of the contraceptive pill, will often be found to be playing some part. Opportunism is even more obvious in the overwhelming systemic infections of the immunocompromised (Fig. 15.37).

Presentation
This varies with the site (Fig. 15.38).

Oral candidiasis
One or more whitish adherent plaques (like bread sauce) appear on the mucous membranes. If wiped off they show an erythematous base. Under dentures candidiasis will produce sore red areas. Angular stomatitis, usually in denture wearers (Fig. 15.39), may be candidal.

Candida intertrigo
A moist glazed area of erythema and maceration appears in a body fold; the edge shows soggy scaling, and outlying satellite papulopustules. These changes

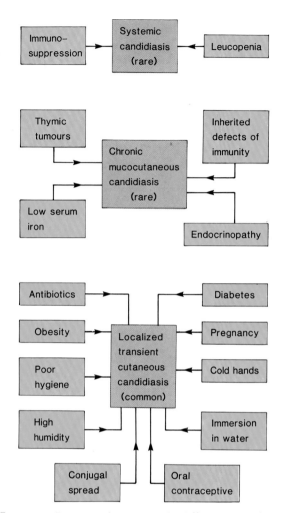

Fig. 15.37 Factors predisposing to the different types of candidiasis.

are most common under the breasts, and in the armpits and groin, but can also occur between the fingers of those whose hands are often in water (Fig. 15.40).

Genital candidiasis
Most commonly presents as a sore itchy vulvovaginitis, with white curdy plaques adherent to the inflamed mucous membranes, and a whitish discharge. The eruption may extend to the groin folds. Conjugal spread is common, and in males similar changes may occur under the foreskin. Diabetes, pregnancy, and antibiotic therapy are common predisposing factors.

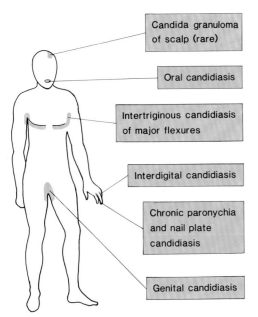

Fig. 15.38 Sites susceptible to *Candida* infection.

Fig. 15.39 Candidal angular stomatitis associated with severe candidiasis of the tongue.

Fig. 15.40 A barmaid whose hands, constantly immersed in water, have developed candidal intertrigo between the middle and index fingers.

Paronychia

Acute paronychia is usually bacterial, but in chronic paronychia *Candida* may be the sole pathogen or be found with other opportunists such as *Proteus* or *Pseudomonas*. The proximal and sometimes the lateral nail folds of one or more fingers become bolstered and red (Fig. 15.41). The cuticles are lost and small amounts of pus may be expressed. The adjacent nail plate becomes ridged and discoloured. Predisposing factors include wet work, poor peripheral circulation and vulval candidiasis.

Chronic mucocutaneous candidiasis

Persistent candidiasis, affecting most or all of the areas described above, may start in infancy. Sometimes the nail plates as well as the nail folds are involved. *Candida* granulomas may appear on the scalp. Several different forms have been described including those with autosomal recessive and dominant inheritance patterns. In the *Candida* endocrinopathy syndrome chronic candidiasis occurs with one or more endocrine defect, the most common of which are hypoparathyroidism, and Addison's disease. A few late-onset cases have underlying thymic tumours.

Fig. 15.41 Chronic paronychia with loss of the cuticle and bolstering of the proximal nail fold. Secondary ridging and discoloration of the nail plate are common.

Systemic candidiasis
This is seen against a background of severe illness, leucopenia and immunosuppression. The skin lesions are firm red nodules which can be shown by biopsy to contain yeasts and pseudohyphae.

Investigations
Swabs from suspected areas should be sent for culture. The urine should always be tested for sugar. In chronic mucocutaneous candidiasis a detailed immunological work-up will be needed, focussing on cell-mediated immunity.

Treatment
Underlying predisposing factors should be sought and eliminated. For example, denture hygiene may be important. Infected skin folds should be separated and kept dry. Those with chronic paronychia should keep their hands warm and dry.

Amphotericin, nystatin and the imidazole group of compounds are all effective topically. For the mouth, these are available as oral suspensions, lozenges and oral gels (Formulary, p. 249). False teeth should be removed at night, washed and steeped in a nystatin solution. For other areas of candidiasis, creams, ointment and pessaries are available (Formulary, p. 250). Magenta paint is also a useful but messy remedy for the skin flexures. In chronic paronychia the nail folds can be packed with an imidazole cream or drenched in an imidazole solution several times a day, particularly just before immersion in water. A course of nystatin tablets may be useful to reduce bowel carriage if this seems to be important in recurrent candidiasis. A five-day course of ketoconazole (200 mg twice daily for adults) may also be helpful. Ketoconazole will be needed long term in mucocutaneous candidiasis.

LEARNING POINTS

1 Always check the urine for diabetes.
2 Remember that griseofulvin has no action against *Candida.*

Fig. 15.42 Pityriasis versicolor: fawn areas stand out against the untanned background.

Pityriasis versicolor

Cause
The old name, tinea versicolor, should be dropped now as the disorder is caused by commensal yeasts (*Pityrosporum orbiculare*), but not by dermatophyte fungi. It is the overgrowth of these yeasts, particularly in hot humid conditions, which is responsible for the clinical lesions.

Carboxylic acids released by the organisms inhibit the normal increase in pigment production by melanocytes after exposure to sunlight. The term 'versicolor' refers to this process through which the superficial scaly patches, fawn or pink on non-tanned skin (Fig. 15.42), become pale after exposure to sunlight (Fig. 15.43). The condition should be regarded as non-infectious.

Presentation and course
The fawn or depigmented areas, with their slightly branny scaling and wrinkling (Fig. 15.44), look ugly. Otherwise they are symptom-free or only slightly itchy. Lesions are most common on the upper trunk but may become widespread. Untreated lesions persist, and depigmented areas, even after adequate treatment, are slow to regain their former colour. Recurrences are common.

Differential diagnosis
In vitiligo (p. 182), the border is clearly defined, scal-

Fig. 15.43 This patient's holiday was spoilt by pale versicolor ruining her expensive tan.

Fig. 15.44 A common site for pityriasis versicolor. The hint of scaling becomes more obvious after gentle scraping with a blade.

ing is absent, lesions are larger, the limbs and face are often affected, and depigmentation is more complete; however, it may sometimes be hard to distinguish vitiligo from the pale, non-scaly areas of treated versicolor. Seborrhoeic eczema of the trunk tends to be more erythematous, and is often confined to the presternal or interscapular areas. Pityriasis alba often affects the cheeks. Pityriasis rosea, tinea corporis, secondary syphilis, and erythrasma seldom cause real confusion.

Investigations
Scrapings, prepared and examined as for a dermatophyte infection (p. 31), show a mixture of short, branched hyphae and spores (spaghetti and meatballs). Culture is not helpful.

Treatment
A topical preparation of one of the imidazole group of antifungal drugs (Formulary, p. 250) can be applied at night to all affected areas for 2–4 weeks. Systemic ketoconazole is rarely necessary but a single dose of 400 mg is often curative. Equally effective, but messier and more irritant, is a 2.5% selenium sulphide mixture in a detergent base (Selsun shampoo).

This should be lathered onto the patches after an evening bath, and allowed to dry. Next morning it should be washed off. Three applications at weekly intervals are adequate.

LEARNING POINTS

1 This is not a dermatophyte infection, so do not try griseofulvin.
2 Patients think the treatment has not worked if their pale patches do not disappear straight away — warn them about this in advance.

Deep fungal infections

Histoplasmosis
Histoplasma capsulatum is found in soil and in the droppings of some animals, for example of bats. Airborne spores are inhaled and cause lung lesions which are in many ways like those of tuberculosis. Later, granulomatous skin lesions may appear, particularly in the immunocompromised. Amphotericin B

or ketoconazole, given systemically, is often helpful.

Coccidioidomycosis

The causative organism, *Coccidioides immitis*, is present in the soil in arid areas in the U.S.A. Its spores are inhaled, and the pulmonary infection may be accompanied by a fever. At this stage erythema nodosum (p. 91) may be seen. In a few patients the infection becomes disseminated, with ulcers or deep abscesses in the skin. Treatment is with amphotericin B or ketoconazole.

Blastomycosis

Infections with *Blastomyces dermatitidis* are virtually confined to rural areas of the U.S.A. Rarely the organism is inoculated into the skin; more often it is inhaled and then spreads systemically from the pulmonary focus to other organs including the skin. There the lesions are ulcerated discharging nodules which spread peripherally with a verrucose edge, while tending to clear and scar centrally. Treatment is with systemic amphotericin B or ketoconazole.

Sporotrichosis

The causative fungus, *Sporotrichium schenkii*, lives saprophytically in soil or on wood in warm humid countries.

Infection is through a wound, where later a lesion like an indolent boil arises. Later still nodules appear, in succession, along the draining lymphatics. Potassium iodide is still the most effective treatment.

Actinomycosis

The causative organism, *Actinomyces israelii*, is bacterial but traditionally considered with the fungi. It has long, branching hyphae and is part of the normal flora of the mouth and bowel. In actinomycosis, a lumpy induration and scarring co-exist with multiple sinuses discharging pus containing 'sulphur granules', made up of tangled filaments. Favourite sites are the jaw, and the chest and abdominal walls. Long-term penicillin is the treatment of choice.

Mycetoma (Madura foot)

Various species of fungus or actinomycetes may be involved. They gain access to the subcutaneous tissues, usually of the feet or legs, via a penetrating wound. The area becomes lumpy and distorted, later enlarging and developing multiple sinuses. Pus exuding from these shows tiny diagnostic granules. Surgery may be a valuable alternative to the often poor results of medical treatment with amphotericin B.

CHAPTER 16

INFESTATIONS

To be infested is to harbour animal parasites on or in the body. Such parasites are common in tropical countries and less so in temperate ones. Infestations fall into two main groups:
1 Those due to arthropods.
2 Those due to worms.

Arthropods

Table 16.1 lists some of the ways in which arthropods can affect the skin. Only a few can be discussed here.

Insect bites

The skin changes are due in part to the pharmacologically active substances injected and in part to a sensitization reaction to injected antigens. A wheal may appear within a few minutes, to be followed by a firm itchy persistent papule, often with a central haemorrhagic punctum. Bullous reactions are common on the legs of children. The diagnosis is usually obvious: when it is not the term papular urticaria may be used.

Papular urticaria

Cause
Papular urticaria is nothing more than an excessive, possibly allergic, reaction to insect bites. The source of the bites may be simple garden pests but more often is a parasite on a domestic pet; sometimes it cannot be traced. Human fleas are now rather uncommon. Perhaps the term 'papular urticaria', with its

Table 16.1 Arthropods and their effects on the skin.

	Manifestations
Insects	
Hymenoptera	Bee and wasp stings
	Ant bites
Lepidoptera	Caterpillar dermatitis
Coleoptera	Blisters from cantharidin
Diptera	Mosquito and midge bites
	Myiasis
Aphaniptera	Human and animal fleas
Hemiptera	Bed bugs
Anaplura	Lice infestations
Mites	
Demodex folliculorum	Normal inhabitant of facial hair follicles
Sarcoptes scabei	Human and animal scabies
Food mites	Grain itch, grocer's itch, etc.
Harvest mites	Harvest itch
House dust mite	Possible role in atopic eczema
Cheyletiella	Papular urticaria
Ticks	Tick bites
	Vector of rickettsial infections and erythema chronicum migrans (p. 142)

hint that the condition is a variant of ordinary urticaria, should now be dropped.

Presentation
Lesions are usually most marked on the arms or

Fig. 16.1 Florid insect bites on the chest. Note the tendency of the now infected lesions to lie in lines and groups.

legs. They consist of recurrent groups or lines of small itchy excoriated urticarial papules which may become bullous and infected (Fig. 16.1). Some clear to leave small scars or pigmented areas.

Course
Surprisingly often only one member of a family is affected. Lesions tend to start after infancy and a child will usually 'grow out' of the problem in a few years even if the source of the bites is not dealt with. Individual lesions last for one or two weeks and recur in distinct crops, especially in the summer — hence the lay term 'heat bumps'. The lesions will disappear with any change of environment, for example on holiday.

Complications
Itching may lead to much discomfort and loss of sleep. Impetiginization is common.

Differential diagnosis
The grouped excoriated papules of papular urticaria are quite distinct from scabies, in which burrows are the diagnostic feature. Atopic prurigo may be more difficult to distinguish but here there is usually a family history of atopy and often frankly eczematous plaques in a typical distribution.

Investigations
The parents should be encouraged to act as detectives in their own environment, but some resist the idea that the lesions are due to bites. This attitude is often supported by veterinarians who, after a superficial look at infested animals, pronounce them clear. In such cases the animal should be brushed vigorously while standing on a polythene sheet. Enough dandruff-like material can then be obtained to send to a reliable veterinary laboratory. Often the cause is a *Cheyletiella* mite infestation.

Treatment
Local treatment with Eurax HC ointment or calamine lotion, and the regular use of insect repellants, may be of some help but the ultimate solution is to trace the source of the bites.

Infested animals should be treated by a veterinarian and insecticidal powders should be used for soft furnishings in the home. Sometimes professional exterminators are needed. It has to be admitted that even these measures sometimes meet with little success.

Bed bugs (hemiptera)
During the day bed bugs hide in crevices in walls and furniture: at night they can travel considerable distances to reach a sleeping human. Burning wheals, turning into firm papules, occur in groups wherever the crawling bugs have easy access to the skin; the face, neck and hands are the most common sites. Treatment should be directed towards the application of insecticides to walls and furniture likely to be harbouring the bugs.

Myiasis
The larvae of several species of fly will develop only if deposited in living flesh: man is one of several possible hosts. The skin lesions may look like boils, but movement may be detected within. The diagnosis is proved by incising the nodule and extracting the larva.

Lice infestations (pediculosis)

Lice are flattened wingless insects which suck blood. Their eggs, attached to hairs or clothing, are known as nits. The main features of all lice infestations are severe itching, followed by scratching and secondary infection.

Two species are obligate parasites in man: *Pediculus humanus* (with its two varieties *P. humanus capitis*, the head louse, and *P. humanus corporis*, the body louse) and *Phthirus pubis* (the pubic louse).

Head lice

Cause

Head lice are still common, affecting up to 10% of children even in the smartest schools. The head louse itself measures some 3–4 mm in length and is greyish, and often rather hard to find. However, its egg cases (nits) can be seen easily enough, firmly stuck to the hair shafts (Fig. 16.2). Spread from person to person is achieved by head-to-head contact, shared combs or hats.

Presentation and course

The main symptom is itching, at first around the sides and back of the scalp and then more generally over it. Scratching and secondary infection soon follow and, in heavy infestations, the hair may become matted and smelly. Draining lymph nodes often enlarge.

Fig. 16.2 Pediculosis capitis: numerous oval eggs (nits) can be seen scattered throughout the scalp hair, but the adult lice are not seen here.

Complications

Secondary bacterial infection may be severe enough to cause the child to become generally listless and feverish.

Differential diagnosis

All patients with recurrent impetigo or crusted eczema on their scalps should be carefully examined for the presence of nits.

Investigations

None are usually required.

Treatment

Malathion lotion or pyrethrin shampoos (Formulary, p. 251) are probably the treatments of choice now. Lindane (gamma-benzene hexachloride) or carbaryl lotions can be used as reasonable alternatives. They should be applied to the scalp and left on for 12 hours. A toothcomb helps to remove nits, and occasionally matting is so severe that the hair has to be clipped short. The application should be repeated after one week, and other members of the family and schoolmates should be checked. A systemic antibiotic may be needed to deal with severe secondary infection.

Body lice

Cause

Body louse infestations are now uncommon except in the unhygienic and socially deprived. Morphologically the body louse looks just like the head louse, but lays its eggs in the seams of clothing in contact with the skin. Transmission is via infested bedding or clothing.

Presentation and course

Self-neglect is usually obvious: against this background there is severe and widespread itching, especially on the trunk. The bites themselves are soon obscured by excoriations and crusts of dried blood or serum. In chronic untreated cases ('vagabond's disease') the skin becomes generally thickened, eczematized, and pigmented; lymphadenopathy is common.

Differential diagnosis

In scabies characteristic burrows will be seen (p. 169). Other causes of chronic itchy erythroderma include eczema and lymphomas, but these are ruled out by the finding of lice and nits.

Investigations

Clothing should be examined for the presence of eggs in the inner seams.

Treatment

One per cent gamma-benzene hexachloride lotion (Formulary, p. 251) may be used on the patient's skin. Infested clothing and bedding should be destroyed or treated with gamma-benzene hexachloride powder before thorough laundering. Less competent patients will need help with this.

Pubic lice

Cause

Pubic lice (crabs) are broader than scalp and body lice, and their second and third pairs of legs are well adapted to cling on to hair. These lice are usually spread by sexual contact, and most commonly infest young adults.

Presentation

Severe itching in the pubic area is followed by eczematization and secondary infection. Among the excoriations will be seen small blue-grey macules of altered blood at the site of bites. The shiny, translucent nits are less obvious than those of head lice (Fig. 16.3). Pubic lice spread most extensively in hairy males and may affect the eyelashes.

Differential diagnosis

Eczema of the pubic area may give rise to similar symptoms but lice and nits are not seen.

Investigations

The possibility of other co-existing sexually transmitted diseases should be kept in mind.

Treatment

The pubic hair, and hair on the thighs and around the anus, should be treated with malathion lotion or

Fig. 16.3 The shiny translucent nits of the pubic louse, together with one or two shy adult lice.

Fig. 16.4 The adult female acarus (scabies mite).

with 1% gamma-benzene hexachloride lotion (Formulary, p. 251). Shaving is not necessary. Infested sexual partners should also be treated.

Scabies

Cause

Scabies is caused by the mite *Sarcoptes scabei* var. *hominis* (Fig. 16.4). Adult mites are 0.3–0.4 mm long and therefore just visible, though hard to see except through a lens. It is now well established that the mites are transferred from person to person by close bodily contact and not via inanimate objects.

Once on the skin, fertilized female mites burrow through the stratum corneum at the rate of about 2 mm per day, and produce two or three oval eggs each day. These turn into sexually mature mites in 2–3 weeks. The number of mites varies from case to case, from less than 10 in a clean adult to many more in an unwashed child.

The generalized eruption of scabies, and its itchiness, are thought to be due to a sensitization to the mites or their products.

Presentation

For the first 4–6 weeks after infestation there may be no itching; but thereafter pruritus dominates the picture, often affecting several people and being particularly bad at night.

The most dramatic part of the eruption — excoriated, eczematized or urticarial papules — is usually on the trunk, but these changes are non-specific and a burrow has to be identified to confirm the diagnosis (Figs. 16.5 and 16.6).

Most burrows lie on the sides of the fingers, finger webs, sides of the hand, and on the flexural aspects of the wrists. Other favourite sites include the elbows, ankles and feet (especially in infants; Fig. 16.7), nipples and genitals (Fig. 16.8). Only in infancy does scabies affect the face. Burrows are easily missed, grey-white, slightly scaly, tortuous lines of up to 1 cm in length. The acarus may be seen through a lens as a small dark dot at the most recent, least scaly end of the burrow. With experience it can be removed for microscopic confirmation (p. 32). On the genitals, burrows are associated with erythematous, rubbery nodules (Fig. 16.9).

Course

Scabies persists indefinitely unless treated. In the chronic stage, the number of mites may be small and diagnosis is correspondingly difficult. Relapses after apparently adequate treatment are common and can be put down to reinfestation from undetected and untreated contacts.

Complications

- Secondary infection, with pustulation, is common (Fig. 16.10). Rarely glomerulonephritis may follow this.
- Repeated applications of scabicides may cause skin irritation and eczema.

Fig. 16.5   A group of typical burrows on the side of the hand.

Fig. 16.6   Obvious burrows on the side of a foot.

Fig. 16.7   The characteristic plantar lesions of scabies in infancy.

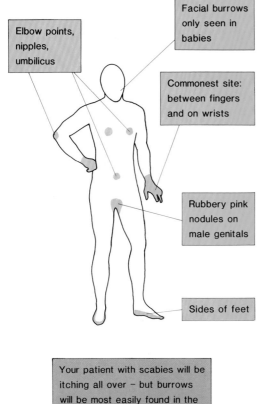

Elbow points,
nipples,
umbilicus

Facial burrows
only seen in
babies

Commonest site:
between fingers
and on wrists

Rubbery pink
nodules on
male genitals

Sides of feet

Your patient with scabies will be
itching all over – but burrows
will be most easily found in the
areas shown above

Fig. 16.8 Common sites of burrows in scabies.

Fig. 16.9 Unmistakable rubbery nodules on the penis —
diagnostic of scabies.

Fig. 16.10 Crusting due to infection of finger web burrows.

- Persistent itchy red nodules may remain on the genitals or armpits of children for some months after adequate treatment.
- Venereal disease may be acquired at the same time as scabies.
- Crusted (Norwegian) scabies, which may not be itchy, is a widespread crusted eruption in which vast numbers of mites are found. It affects mental defectives or the immunosuppressed, and may be the unsuspected source of epidemics of ordinary scabies.

Differential diagnosis

Only scabies shows the characteristic burrow. Animal scabies from pets induces an itchy rash in humans but this lacks burrows. The lesions of papular urticaria (p. 165) are excoriated papules, in groups, mainly on the legs. Late-onset atopic eczema (p. 71), cholinergic urticaria (p. 85), lichen planus (p. 55), and dermatitis herpetiformis (p. 100) have their own distinctive features. Fibreglass can also cause epidemics of itching.

Investigations

With practice an acarus can be picked neatly from the end of its burrow and identified microscopically; failing this, eggs and mites can be seen microscopically in burrow scrapings mounted in potassium hydroxide (p. 32).

Treatment

- Use an effective scabicide: there is little to choose

between benzyl benzoate, gamma-benzene hexa-chloride (Lindane) and crotamiton (Formulary, p. 251) on this score, but the last two may be less irritant. We avoid gamma-benzene hexachloride in young children and pregnant women as absorption leading to CNS toxicity is a theoretical risk, and prefer 6 % precipitated sulphur in soft white paraffin (petrolatum) applied nightly to the entire body for 3 days (Formulary, p. 251).

- Do not just treat the patient: treat all members of the family, and sexual contacts, whether they are itching or not (Fig. 16.11).
- Have a printed instruction sheet to hand to the patient — scabies victims are notoriously confused. On the first night, the scabicide is applied to all areas below the jaw-line; no baths are allowed until the end of the course. If the hands are washed the scabicide should be reapplied there. On the second night — one further application. On the third night — bath and fresh clothing and sheets.
- Ordinary laundering deals satisfactorily with clothing and sheets. Mites die in clothing unworn for one week.
- Residual itching may last for several days, or even a few weeks, but this does not need more applications of the scabicide. Rely instead on calamine lotion.

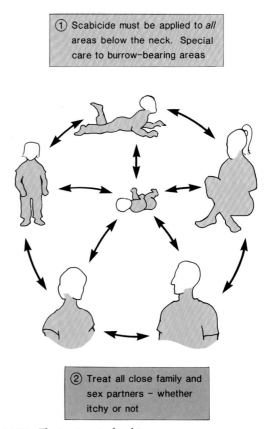

Fig. 16.11   The treatment of scabies.

LEARNING   POINTS

1 Paravenereal diseases hunt in packs: has your patient with scabies also got pubic lice, genital mollusca, or even something worse?
2 Never forget the contacts — itchy or not — as they will reinfect your patient and waste everybody's time.

Parasitic worms

A textbook of tropical medicine should be consulted for more details on this subject.

Onchocerciasis
This is endemic in much of Central America and Africa where it is an important cause of blindness. The buffalo gnat (*Simulium* species) carries the filarial worm to man. Infested humans become itchy with an excoriated papular eruption. Later the skin may thicken and become hyper- or hypopigmented. Dermal nodules are found, mainly near bony prominences, and contain both mature worms and microfilariae. It is the latter which invade the eye leading to blindness. The diagnosis is confirmed by detecting active microfilariae in skin snips teased out in saline and examined microscopically. The condition is treated with diethylcarbamazine but this may lead to a violent reaction and the drug must be given with great care if the eyes are involved.

Filariasis
This condition is endemic throughout much of the tropics. The adult filarial worms, usually *Wuchereria bancrofti*, inhabit the lymphatics where they excite

an inflammatory reaction with episodes of lymphangitis and fever, gradually leading to lymphatic obstruction and lymphoedema, usually of the legs or scrotum. Such swellings may be massive (elephantiasis). Microfilariae are found in the peripheral blood, mainly at night; their vector from man to man is the mosquito in which the larvae mature. Diethylcarbamazine is again the treatment of choice.

Larva migrans
The larvae of hookworms, which can go through their full life cycle only in cats or dogs, may penetrate human skin in contact with soil or sand contaminated by the faeces of these animals. The movement of the larvae under the skin causes tortuous red itchy lines to appear, moving forwards at the rate of a few millimetres a day. The larvae eventually die but this can be speeded up by freezing with liquid nitrogen the area just ahead of the advancing linear lesion. Local applications of thiabendazole are also effective.

Other worm manifestations
- Threadworm infestation in children can cause severe anal and vulval pruritus. The small worms are seen best at night time when the itch is worst. Treatment is with piperazine.
- Swimmer's itch, in tropical waters, may be due to the penetration through the skin of the cercariae of human and non-human schistosomes.
- Multiple firm nodules in the skin may be due to the larval stages of the pork tapeworm (cysticercosis).
- Larger fluctuant cysts may be due to hydatid disease.

CHAPTER 17
SKIN REACTIONS TO LIGHT

Exposure to the sun offers some benefits but causes some problems (Fig. 17.1).

Ultraviolet radiation (UVR) is divided into three parts (Fig. 17.2). The C spectrum does not penetrate the ozone layer of the atmosphere and so far is irrelevant to skin disease. The B wavelengths (UVB: 290–320 nm) cause sunburn and are effectively screened out by window glass. The A spectrum (UVA) is long-wave ultraviolet light, from 320 nm to the most violet colour perceptible to the eye (about 400 nm). It ages and tans the skin. UVR is non-ionizing but changes the skin chemically by reacting with endogenous light-absorbing chemicals called chromophores.

Sunburn

Cause
UVB penetrates the epidermis and superficial dermis, stimulating the production and release of prostaglandins, leukotrienes and histamine, which cause pain and redness.

Presentation and course
Areas of skin exposed to too much UVB tingle and become red several hours later. Severe sunburn is painful and may blister. Redness is maximal after one day and then settles over the next two or three days, leaving a sheet-like desquamation, pigmentation, and eventually scattered lentigines. Sunburn damages both the epidermis and the dermis, and may cause wrinkling, pigmentary changes, and cancer.

Differential diagnosis
Phototoxic reactions due to drugs are like an exaggerated sunburn.

Investigations
None are required.

BENEFITS

Attractive tan
↑ Sense of well-being
↑ Vitamin D production
Clearing of psoriasis, eczema, etc.

DRAWBACKS

Sunburn
↑ Skin ageing
↑ Skin cancer
Photosensitivity
Worsening of LE, porphyria, etc.

Fig. 17.1 The balance between the benefits and drawbacks of sun exposure.

Fig. 17.2   Skin disorders and the wavelengths which cause them.

Treatment

The treatment is symptomatic. Baths may be cooling and oily shake lotions (e.g. oily calamine lotion or oil-in-water lotions and creams) may be comforting. Potent topical corticosteroids (Formulary, p. 248) help if used early and briefly. Oral aspirin (a prostaglandin synthesis inhibitor) relieves the pain.

Phototoxicity

A basic photochemical law states that a drug must absorb UVR to cause such a reaction. Most drugs listed in Table 17.1 absorb UVA as well as UVB, and so window glass, protective against sunburn, will not protect against most phototoxic drug reactions.

Presentation and course

Tenderness and redness occur only in areas exposed to sufficient UVR (Fig. 17.3). The signs and symptoms are those of sunburn. The skin may become hyperpigmented on healing.

Cause

These reactions are not immunological. Everyone exposed to enough of the drug and to enough UVR

Fig. 17.3 Extreme photosensitivity of a patient taking a thiazide diuretic. Note sparing of the area covered by his cap.

Fig. 17.4 Severe bullous eruption in areas in contact with giant hogweed (contains psoralens) and then exposed to sunlight (phytophotodermatitis).

Table 17.1 Drugs commonly causing photosensitivity.

Amiodarone	Psoralens
Chlorpropamide	Quinidine
Nalidixic acid	Sulphonamides
Oral contraceptives	Tetracyclines
Phenothiazines	Thiazides

Table 17.2 Features which distinguish phototoxicity from photo-allergy.

Phototoxicity	Photo-allergy
Erythematous	Eczematous
Immediate	Delayed
Often drug-induced	Often drug-induced
Photopatch testing negative	Photopatch testing positive

will develop the reaction. Some drugs which can cause phototoxic reactions are listed in Table 17.1. In addition, psoralens in plants can cause phototoxicity, termed 'phytophotodermatitis' (Fig. 17.4).

Differential diagnosis
Photo-allergic reactions are difficult to distinguish, the more so as the same drugs can often cause both photo-allergic and phototoxic reactions. The main differences between phototoxicity and photo-allergy are shown in Table 17.2.

Investigations
None are usually required. Phototesting may be carried out in special centres in difficult cases. The action spectrum (those wavelengths which cause the reaction) may incriminate a particular drug.

Treatment
This is the same as for sunburn. Drugs should be stopped if further exposure to ultraviolet light is likely.

Photo-allergy
Drugs, topical or systemic, and chemicals on the skin can interact with UVR and cause immunological reactions.

Cause
UVR converts an immunologically inactive form of a

drug into an antigenic molecule, or into a hapten which reacts with a carrier protein to become a complete antigen. An immunological reaction, analogous to allergic contact dermatitis, is induced if antigen remains in the skin or is formed there on subsequent exposure to the drug and UVR. Many of the same drugs which cause toxic reactions can cause allergic ones.

Presentation
Photo-allergy is often similar to phototoxicity. The areas exposed to UVR become inflamed, but the reaction is more likely to be eczematous. The eruption will be on exposed areas such as the hands, the V of the neck, the nose, the chin, and the forehead. There is also a tendency to spare the upper lip under the nose, the eyelids, and the submental region (Fig. 17.5). Often the eruption does not occur on the first exposure to ultraviolet, but only after a second or further exposures. A lag phase of one or more weeks is necessary for induction of an immune response.

Course
The original lesions are red patches, plaques, vesicles, or bullae, which usually become eczematous. They tend to resolve when either the drug or the exposure to UVR is stopped, but this may take several weeks.

Complications
Some drugs, like the sulphonamides, may cause a persistent light reaction (*see below*).

Investigations
Photopatch testing can confirm the diagnosis. The chemical is applied for 24 hours and the skin is then irradiated with UVA. An acute photo-allergic contact dermatitis is then elicited. A control patch, not irradiated, rules out ordinary allergic contact dermatitis.

Treatment
The drug should be stopped and the patient protected from additional UV exposure (avoidance, clothing, and sunscreens). Potent topical or a short course of systemic corticosteroids hastens resolution and provides symptomatic relief.

Persistent light reaction
Some patients with a photo-allergic reaction never get over it and continue to develop eczematous areas after sun exposure long after the drug has been stopped.

Cause
This is not clear but some believe minute amounts of the drug persist in the skin indefinitely.

Presentation
This is the same as a photo-allergic reaction to a drug.

AIRBORNE ALLERGY   PHOTOSENSITIVITY

Spared areas include behind the ears

Fig. 17.5 Features distinguishing airborne allergy from photosensitivity.

Course

These patients may be exquisitely sensitive to UVR. They are usually middle-aged or elderly men who react after the slightest exposure, even through window glass or from fluorescent lights.

Complications

None, but the persistent, severe, pruritic eruption may lead to depression and even suicide.

Differential diagnosis

Airborne allergic contact dermatitis may be confusing, but does not require sunlight. Sometimes the diagnosis is difficult as exposure both to sunlight and to the airborne allergen occurs only out of doors. Airborne allergic contact dermatitis also affects sites which sunlight is less likely to reach, such as under the chin (Fig. 17.5). A continuing drug photo-allergy, a polymorphic light eruption (*see below*), or eczema due to some other cause must also be considered.

Investigations

Persistent light reaction can be confirmed experimentally by exposing uninvolved skin to UVA or UVB. Patch tests and photopatch tests help to distinguish between photo-allergy and airborne allergic contact dermatitis, and the action spectrum may point to a certain drug. Testing is difficult, and should be carried out only in specialist centres.

Treatment

Persistent light reactors need extreme measures to protect their skin from UVR. These include protective clothing, and frequent applications of combined UVA and UVB blocking agents (Formulary, p. 247). Patients must protect themselves from UVR coming through windows or from fluorescent lights. Some can only go out at night. The disorder is helped by potent topical steroids: others may need systemic therapy.

Actinic reticuloid

This may be a severe form of persistent light reaction. A chronic dermatitis, with thick plaques, occurs on sun-exposed areas. It affects elderly men who also become allergic to a range of contact allergens,

especially oleoresins in some plants (e.g. chrysanthemum). Histology shows a dense, lymphocytic infiltrate with some atypical lymphocytes suggestive of a lymphoma and the disorder must be differentiated histologically from cutaneous T cell lymphoma (mycosis fungoides). Fortunately it seldom becomes malignant. Combined UVA and UVB sunscreens and topical steroids are used initially. As even the most potent topical steroids are often ineffective, systemic steroids or immunosuppressants (e.g. azathioprine) may be needed for long periods.

Polymorphic light eruption

This is the most frequent cause of 'sun allergy'.

Cause

It is speculated that UVR causes a natural body chemical to change into an allergen or hapten. Mechanisms are similar to those in drug photo-allergy.

Presentation

Small itchy, red papulovesicles or eczematous plaques arise from two hours to five days, most commonly at 24 hours, after exposure to UVB. The eruption is itchy and usually confined to sun-exposed areas (Fig. 17.6), remembering that some UVR passes through thin clothing.

Fig. 17.6 Polymorphic light eruption: excoriated erythematous papules on the face of a young girl. Persists throughout the summer but fades in the winter.

Course

Patients may continue to erupt after UVR exposure for year after year. Tanning protects some patients so that if the initial exposures are limited, few or no symptoms occur later. Such patients can still enjoy sun exposure and outdoor activities. Others are so sensitive, or their skin pigments so little, that fresh exposures continue to induce reactions throughout the summer. They require photoprotection, and must limit their sun exposure and outdoor activities. The rash disappears during the winter.

Differential diagnosis

Phototoxic reactions, photo-allergic reactions, persistent light reaction, ordinary eczemas, and airborne allergic contact dermatitis should be considered.

Investigations

It may be possible to reproduce the dermatitis by testing non-sun-exposed skin with UVB.

Treatment

If normal tanning does not confer protection, sunscreens (Formulary, p. 247) should be used. Protective clothing, such as wide-brimmed hats, long-sleeved shirts, and long trousers are helpful. In some patients, a four-week PUVA course (p. 51) in the late spring can create enough of a tan to confer protection for the rest of the season. Moderately potent topical steroids (Formulary, p. 248) usually improve the eruption.

Actinic prurigo

This is probably distinct from polymorphic light eruption. Papules, crusts, and excoriations arise on sun-exposed areas and sometimes also on other sites: lesions may persist through the winter. It is common among North American Indians and may resemble excoriated acne, bites, eczemas, or neurotic excoriations. It may be associated with atopy.

Solar urticaria

This is discussed in Chapter 10. Wheals occur in the sun-exposed areas within minutes. Some patients have erythropoietic protoporphyria (p. 237) and this should be considered particularly when solar urticaria starts in infancy.

Actinic keratoses

These are discussed in Chapter 19.

Actinic cheilitis

This term describes the inflammation and scaling of the lower lips of those who have led an outdoor life. It can be treated by cryosurgery, excision with lip advancement, or the judicious use of 5-fluorouracil cream (Formulary, p. 253).

Lupus erythematosus

Many patients with lupus erythematosus (p. 102) notice that they get worse after exposure to UVR, especially to UVB. They should be warned about this, and protect themselves from the sun (avoidance, clothing and sunscreens).

Carcinoma

The sun can cause basal cell carcinomas, squamous cell carcinomas, and malignant melanomas. These are discussed in Chapter 19.

Exacerbated diseases

UVR is useful in the treatment of many skin diseases, but it can also make some worse (Table 17.3).

Porphyria cutanea tarda

This condition is described in Chapter 20.

Table 17.3 The effect of sunlight on some skin diseases.

Helps	Worsens
Atopic eczema	Albinism
Mycosis fungoides (plaques)	Darier's disease
Parapsoriasis	Herpes simplex
Pityriasis lichenoides	Lupus erythematosus
Pityriasis rosea	Pellagra
Psoriasis	Photo-allergy/toxicity
	Porphyrias (excluding acute intermittent)
	Vitiligo
	Xeroderma pigmentosum

Cutaneous ageing

The trouble with old skin is the way it looks rather
than the way it behaves. UVR is the main factor
speeding the ageing process in the skin. The bronzed
young skins of today will become the wrinkled
prune-like ones of tomorrow.

Wrinkles occur when the dermis loses its elastic
recoil, failing to snap back properly into shape. UVR
damages elastic tissue and hastens the process. In
skin chronically exposed to UVR, the elastic fibres
are clumped and amorphous, leading clinically to a
yellow, pebbly look called *actinic elastosis*.

Although face lifts can smooth wrinkles out, there
is no way to reverse this damage fully, although tretinoin cream (Formulary, p. 251) seems to help some
patients. Prevention, by reducing exposure to UVR,
is better than any cure.

Skin ages even in sun-protected areas, albeit much
more slowly. The dermis thins. Skin collagen falls by
about 1% per year throughout adult life, and it becomes more stable (less elastic). Fibroblasts become
sparser in the dermis, accounting for reduced collagen synthesis and slower wound healing.

CHAPTER 18

DISORDERS OF PIGMENTATION

Normal skin colour

It is a mixture of pigments, and not one alone, that gives normal skin its colour. Untanned Caucasoid skin is pink, due to oxyhaemoglobin in the blood within the papillary loops and superficial horizontal plexus (Fig. 2.14). Melanin may blend with this colour, for example after a suntan. Melanin is, of course, responsible too for the shades of brown seen in Negroid skin. Other hues are due to the addition to these pigments of yellow from carotene, found mainly in subcutaneous fat and in the horny layer of the epidermis. There is no natural blue pigment; when blue is seen it is due either to an optical effect from normal pigment (usually melanin) in the dermis or to the presence of an abnormal pigment (*see below*).

Abnormal skin colours

These may be due to an imbalance of the normal pigments mentioned above (e.g. in cyanosis, chloasma and carotenaemia) or to the presence of abnormal pigments (Table 18.1).

Sometimes it is difficult to distinguish between the colours of these pigments. For example, the gingery brown colour of haemosiderin is readily confused with melanin. Histological stains may be needed to settle the issue.

In practice, apart from tattoos, most pigmentary problems are due to too much, or too little melanin.

Table 18.1 Some abnormal pigments.

Endogenous	
Haemoglobin-derived	
methaemoglobin ⎫	cyanosis
sulphaemoglobin ⎰	
carboxyhaemoglobin	pink
bilirubin ⎫	yellow to green
biliverdin ⎰	
haemosiderin	brown
Drugs	
gold	blue-grey (chrysiasis)
silver	blue-grey (agyria)
bismuth	grey
mepacrine	yellow
clofazamine	red
phenothiazines	slate-grey
amiodarone	blue-grey
Diet	
carotene	orange

Exogenous	
Tattoo pigments	
carbon	blue-black
coal dust	blue-black
cobalt	blue
chrome	green
cadmium	yellow
mercury	red
iron	brown
Local medications	
silver nitrate	black
magenta paint	magenta
gentian violet	violet
eosin	pink
potassium permanganate	brown
dithranol	puple
tar	brown
iodine	yellow

Decreased melanin pigmentation

Some common conditions in which there is a lack of melanin are listed in Table 18.2. A few of the more important, and the mechanisms involved, are summarized in Figure 18.1.

Oculocutaneous albinism

At least six forms exist but only the two most common are described here: the tyrosinase-positive and tyrosinase-negative types. Their prevalence is estimated at 1:20 000, being highest in countries where marriages between cousins are common.

Cause

Oculocutaneous albinism is inherited as an autosomal recessive trait. Melanocytes are found in normal numbers in the epidermis but the synthesis of melanosomes within them is abnormal, due to a mutation of the gene coding for tyrosinase.

Presentation and course

The whole skin is white and pigment is also lacking in the hair, iris, and retina (Fig. 18.2). Albinos have poor sight, photophobia, and a rotatory nystagmus. As they grow older tyrosinase-positive albinos gain a little pigment in their skin, iris, and hair. Negroid skin becomes yellow-brown and the hair becomes yellow. Albinos may also develop freckles. Sunburn is common on unprotected skin. As melanocytes are present, albinos have non-pigmented melanocytic naevi and may develop amelanotic malignant melanomas.

Table 18.2 Some causes of hypopigmentation.

Genetic	Albinism
	Piebaldism
	Phenylketonuria
	Waardenburg's syndrome
	Chediak–Higashi syndrome: autosomal recessive lysosomal defect (susceptible to infections)
	Tuberous sclerosis
Endocrine	Hypopituitarism
Chemical	Substituted phenols (in rubber industry)
	Chloroquine and hydroxychloroquine
Post-inflammatory	Eczema
	Pityriasis alba
	Psoriasis
	Sarcoidosis
	Lupus erythematosus
	Lichen sclerosus et atrophicus
	Cryotherapy
Infections	Leprosy
	Pityriasis versicolor
	Syphilis, yaws and pinta
Tumours	Halo naevus
	Malignant melanoma
Miscellaneous	Vitiligo
	Idiopathic guttate hypomelanosis

Fig. 18.1 The mechanisms involved in some types of hypopigmentation.

Fig. 18.2 Oculocutaneous albinism in an Asian. The skin and hair are depigmented and the irides translucent. The patient had a rotatory nystagmus.

Complications
In the tropics these unfortunate individuals develop numerous skin tumours even when they are young, confirming the protective role of melanin.

Differential diagnosis
Piebaldism and vitiligo are described below.

Investigations
Prenatal diagnosis of albinism is now possible. A biopsy from fetal skin, taken at 20 weeks, is examined by electron microscopy for arrested melanosome development.

The hair bulb test, in which plucked hairs are incubated in dihydroxyphenylalanine, distinguishes tyrosinase-positive from tyrosinase-negative types. Those whose hair bulbs turn black (tyrosinase-positive) are less severely affected.

Treatment
Avoidance of sun exposure, and protection with opaque clothing, wide-brimmed hats, and sunscreen creams (Formulary, p. 247), are essential and allow albinos in temperate climates to live a relatively normal life. In the tropics the outlook is less good and the termination of affected pregnancies should be considered.

Piebaldism
These patients often have a white forelock of hair and patches of depigmentation lying symmetrically on the limbs, trunk and central part of the face, especially the chin. The condition is present at birth and is inherited as an autosomal dominant trait. Melanocytes are absent from the hypopigmented areas. The depigmentation, often mistaken for vitiligo, may improve with age. There is no effective treatment. The Waardenburg syndrome includes piebaldism, widening of the medial epicanthic folds, irides of different colour, and deafness.

Phenylketonuria
This rare metabolic cause of hypopigmentation has a prevalence of about 1:25 000. It is described in Chapter 20.

Hypopituitarism
The skin changes here may alert an astute physician to the diagnosis. The complexion has a pale, yellow tinge; there is thinning or loss of the sexual hair; the skin itself is atrophic. The hypopigmentation is due to a decreased production of pituitary melanotrophic hormones (see Chapter 2).

Vitiligo
The word vitiligo comes from the Latin word 'vitellus', which means veal, that is pale, pink flesh. It is an acquired circumscribed depigmentation, found in all races; its prevalence may be as high as 0.5–1%; its inheritance is polygenic.

Cause and types
There is a complete loss of melanocytes from affected areas. There are two main patterns: a common generalized one and a rare segmental type. Generalized vitiligo, including the acrofacial variant, usually starts after the second decade. There is a family history in 30% of patients and this type is most frequent in those with auto-immune diseases such as diabetes, thyroid disorders and pernicious anaemia. Segmental vitiligo is restricted to one part of the body, but not necessarily to a dermatome. It occurs earlier than generalized vitiligo, and is not associated with auto-immune diseases. Trauma and sunburn may precipitate both types.

Clinical course

Generalized type

The sharply defined, white patches are especially common on the backs of the hands (Fig. 18.3), wrists, fronts of knees, neck and around body orifices. The hair of the scalp and beard may depigment too. The surrounding skin in Caucasoids is sometimes hyperpigmented.

The course is unpredictable: lesions may remain static, or spread; occasionally they repigment spontaneously from the hair follicles (Fig. 18.4).

Segmental type

The individual areas look like the generalized type but their segmental distribution is striking (Fig. 18.5). Spontaneous repigmentation occurs more often in this type than in generalized vitiligo.

Differential diagnosis

Contact with depigmenting chemicals, such as hydroquinones and substituted phenols in the rubber industry, should be excluded. Pityriasis versicolor (p. 162) must be considered; its fine scaling and less complete pigment loss separate it from vitiligo. Post-inflammatory depigmentation (*see below*) may look very like vitiligo but is less white and improves spontaneously. The patches of piebaldism are present at birth. In the tropics, leprosy must be excluded by sensory testing and a general examination. Other tropical diseases which cause patchy hypopigmentation are leishmaniasis (p. 145), yaws (p. 142), and pinta.

Treatment

Treatment is unsatisfactory. A short course of a potent topical steroid, applied to a few recent patches, occasionally helps. Some patients improve with psoralens (trimethylpsoralen or 8-methoxypsoralen, in a dose of 0.6 mg/kg body weight), taken 1–2 hours before graduated exposure to natural sunshine or to artificial UVA (PUVA, p. 51). Therapy is needed daily for at least six months: new lesions seem to respond best. As a general rule, however, established vitiligo is best left untreated in most whites, though advice about suitable preparations (Formulary, p. 247) to

Fig. 18.3   Vitiligo: note the rough symmetry, and the coffee colour of the surrounding skin.

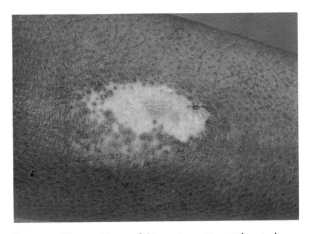

Fig. 18.4   The spottiness of this repigmenting vitiligo is due to the revival of melanocytes in and around the hair follicles.

Fig. 18.5   Segmental vitiligo in a young girl. The distribution is not dermatomal.

cover unsightly patches should be given. Sun avoidance and screening preparations are needed to avoid sunburn of the affected areas (Formulary, p. 247). Patients with extensive vitiligo can be completely and irreversibly depigmented by creams containing the monobenzyl ether of hydroquinone. Carefully considered informed consent is needed before such treatment.

LEARNING POINTS

1 Vitiligo looks ugly and burns easily in the sun: treat with cosmetic cover and efficient sunscreens or sun avoidance.
2 Do not promise a cure.

Post-inflammatory depigmentation
This may follow eczema, psoriasis, sarcoidosis, lupus erythematosus and, rarely, lichen planus. It may also result from cryotherapy or a burn. In general, the more severe the inflammation, the more likely pigment is to decrease rather than increase in its wake. These problems are most significant in Negroids or Asians. With time, repigmentation usually occurs.

White hair
Melanocytes in hair bulbs become less active with age (Chapter 2), and white hair (canities) is a universal sign of ageing. Early greying of the hair is seen in the rare premature ageing syndromes, such as Werner's syndrome, and in auto-immune conditions such as pernicious anaemia, thyroid disorders, and Addison's disease.

Disorders with increased pigmentation
(hypermelanosis)

Some of these disorders are listed in Table 18.3. The most common will be described below and the mechanisms involved are summarized in Figure 18.6.

Freckles (ephelides)
Freckles are so common that to describe them seems

Table 18.3 Some causes of hyperpigmentation.

Genetic	Freckles
	Lentigines
	Café au lait macules
	Peutz–Jeghers syndrome
	Xeroderma pigmentosum
	Albright's syndrome:
	segmental hyperpigmentation
	fibrous dysplasia of bones
	precocious puberty
Endocrine	Addison's disease
	Cushing's syndrome
	Pregnancy
	Renal failure
Metabolic	Biliary cirrhosis
	Haemochromatosis
	Porphyria
Nutritional	Malabsorption
	Carcinomatosis
	Kwashiorkor
	Pellagra
Drugs	Photosensitizing drugs
	ACTH and synthetic analogues
	Oestrogens and progestogens
	Psoralens
	Arsenic
	Busulphan
	Minocycline
Post-inflammatory	Lichen planus
	Eczema
	Secondary syphilis
	Systemic sclerosis
	Lichen and macular amyloidosis
	Cryotherapy
Poikiloderma	
Tumours	Acanthosis nigricans
	Pigmented naevi
	Malignant melanoma
	Mastocytosis

unnecessary. They are most often seen in the red-haired or blond as sharply demarcated light brown-ginger macules, of usually less than 5 mm in diameter (Fig. 18.7). They multiply and become darker with sun exposure.

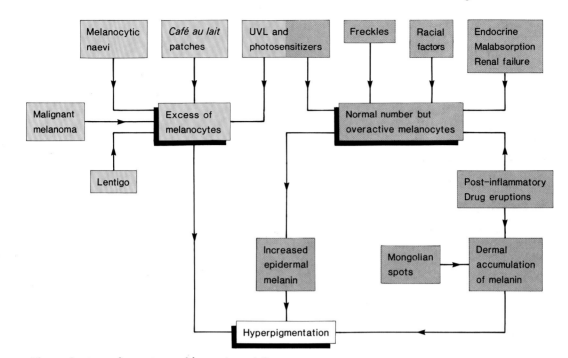

Fig. 18.6 The mechanisms of some types of hyperpigmentation.

Fig 18.7 Characteristic freckling in a red-headed boy.

Increased melanin is seen in the basal layer of the epidermis without any increase in the number of melanocytes, and without elongation of the rete ridges (Fig. 18.8). No treatment is necessary.

Lentigo
Simple and senile lentigines look alike. They are light or dark brown macules, ranging from 1 mm to 1 cm across. Although usually discrete, they may have an irregular outline. Simple lentigines arise most often in childhood as a few scattered lesions, often on areas not exposed to sun. Senile or solar lentigines are common after middle age on the backs of the hands ('liver spots') (Fig. 18.9) and on the face. In contrast to freckles, lentigines have increased numbers of melanocytes (Fig. 18.8). They should be distinguished from freckles, from junctional melanocytic naevi (p. 191), and from a lentigo maligna (p. 202). Treatment is usually unnecessary. Ugly lesions may be excised or frozen with liquid nitrogen.

Conditions associated with multiple lentigines
Three rare but striking syndromes feature multiple lentigines:

Peutz–Jeghers syndrome
Profuse lentigines are seen on and around the lips in this autosomal dominant condition (Fig. 18.10). Scattered lentigines also occur on the buccal mucosa, gums, hard palate, hands and feet. The syndrome is important because of its association with polyposis of the small intestine which may lead to recurrent intussusception and, rarely, to malignant transformation of the polyps. Ten per cent of affected women have ovarian tumours.

FRECKLE   NORMAL   LENTIGO

Fig 18.8   Histology of a freckle and a lentigo.

Fig. 18.9   Senile lentigines on the back of an elderly hand ('liver spots'). Note accompanying atrophy.

Fig. 18.10   Profuse lentigines on and around the lips in the Peutz–Jeghers syndrome.

Cronkhite–Canada syndrome
This consists of multiple lentigines on the backs of the hand and a more diffuse pigmentation of the palms and volar aspects of the fingers. It may also associate with gastro-intestinal polyposis. Alopecia and nail abnormalities complete the rare but characteristic clinical picture.

'Leopard' syndrome
This is an acronym for generalized *L*entiginosis associated with cardiac abnormalities demonstrated by *E*CG, *O*cular hypertelorism, *P*ulmonary stenosis, *A*bnormal genitalia, *R*etardation of growth and *D*eafness.

Chloasma
Chloasma is a patterned pigmentation of the face occurring in women during pregnancy or on oral contraceptives. The areas of increased pigmentation are well-defined, symmetrical, and their edge is often scalloped (the mask of pregnancy) (Fig. 18.11). The light brown colour becomes darker after exposure to the sun. The placenta may secrete hormones which stimulate melanocytes. Chloasma should be differen-

tiated from a phototoxic reaction to a scented cosmetic or to a drug. Treatment is unsatisfactory, though some find bleaching agents which contain hydroquinone helpful. A sunscreen will make the pigmentation less obvious during the summer.

Endocrine hyperpigmentation

Addison's disease
Hyperpigmentation due to the overproduction of ACTH is often striking (Fig. 18.12); it may be generalized or limited to the skin folds, creases of the palms, scars and the buccal mucosa.

Cushing's syndrome
Increased ACTH production may cause a picture like that of Addison's disease. The hyperpigmentation may become even more marked after adrenalectomy (Nelson's syndrome).

Pregnancy
There is a generalized increase in pigmentation during pregnancy, especially of the nipples and areolae,

Fig. 18.11   Chloasma which became more obvious after a holiday in the sun.

Fig. 18.12   Marked, diffuse, facial pigmentation in Addison's disease.

and of the linea alba. Chloasma (*see above*) may also occur. The nipples and areolae remain pigmented after parturition.

Chronic renal failure

The hyperpigmentation of chronic renal failure and of patients on haemodialysis is due to an increase in levels of pituitary melanotrophic peptides, normally degraded by the kidney.

Porphyria

Formed porphyrins, especially uroporphyrins, are produced in excess in cutaneous hepatic porphyria and erythropoietic porphyria (p. 217). These endogenous photosensitizers induce hyperpigmentation on exposed areas; skin fragility, blistering and hypertrichosis are equally important clues to the diagnosis.

Nutritional hyperpigmentation

Any severe wasting disease, such as malabsorption, AIDS, tuberculosis or cancer, may be accompanied by diffuse hyperpigmentation. Kwashiorkor is a cause of hyperpigmentation in the tropics, and in this condition the hair is red-brown or grey.

Drugs causing hyperpigmentation

Table 17.1 lists drugs that commonly photosensitize. All may cause hyperpigmentation of the exposed skin. Psoralens are used in the photochemotherapy of psoriasis (Chapter 6) and, more rarely, of vitiligo.

The term 'Berloque dermatitis' refers to a 'pendant' of hyperpigmentation, often on the side of the neck, where cosmetics have been applied which contain the photosensitizing 5-methoxypsoralen. Cosmetics for men (pre- and after-shaves, etc.) are a thriving source of these.

Arsenic is seldom used medically nowadays. Once it caused 'raindrop' depigmentation within a diffuse bronzed hyperpigmentation.

Busulphan and bleomycin, used to treat some forms of leukaemia, frequently cause diffuse hyperpigmentation. Minocycline can leave blue-black drug deposits in inflamed acne spots, or on the mucosae.

Post-inflammatory hyperpigmentation

This is common after lichen planus (p. 55). It is also a feature of systemic sclerosis (p. 108) and some types of cutaneous amyloidosis, and is often an unwelcomed sequel of cryotherapy.

Poikiloderma

Poikiloderma is the name given to a triad of signs: reticulate pigmentation, atrophy, and telangiectasia. It is not a disease but a reaction pattern with many causes including X-irradiation, photocontact reactions, and connective tissue and lymphoreticular disorders. Congenital variants (Rothmund–Thomson syndrome, Bloom's syndrome and Cockayne's syndrome), associated with photosensitivity, dwarfism, and mental retardation, also occur.

CHAPTER 19

SKIN TUMOURS

This chapter will deal both with skin tumours arising from the epidermis and its appendages, and with those arising from the dermis (Table 19.1).

Prevention

Actinic keratoses, lentigines, keratoacanthomas, basal cell carcinomas, squamous cell carcinomas, malignant melanomas and, arguably, acquired melanocytic naevi would all become less common if Caucasoids, especially those with a fair skin, protected themselves against exposure to too much sunlight. Education of those living in sunny climates or holidaying in the sun has already reaped great rewards here. Successful campaigns have focussed on regular self-examination and the ways in which sun exposure can be reduced by avoidance, clothing and

Table 19.1 Skin tumours.

Derived from	Benign	Premalignant	Malignant
Epidermis and appendages	Viral wart	Kerato-acanthoma	Basal cell carcinoma
	Squamous cell papilloma	Intra-epidermal carcinoma	Squamous cell carcinoma
	Seborrhoeic keratosis	Actinic keratosis	Malignant melanoma
	Skin tags		Paget's disease of the nipple
	Milium		
	Melanocytic naevus		
	Epidermoid/pilar cysts		
	Chondrodermatitis nodularis helicis		
Dermis	Haemangioma		Kaposi's sarcoma
	Lymphangioma		Lymphoma
	Glomus tumour		Dermatofibrosarcoma protuberans
	Pyogenic granuloma		Secondary deposits
	Dermatofibroma		
	Keloid		
	Lipoma		
	Lymphocytoma cutis		

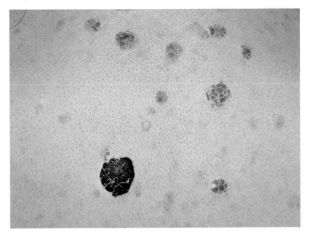

Fig. 19.1 Typical multiple seborrhoeic warts of the back.

Fig. 19.2 Numerous ugly seborrhoeic warts of the face.

sunscreen preparations. Public awareness and compliance has been encouraged by imaginative and gimmicky slogans like the Australian 'slip, slap and slop' advice (slip on the shirt, slap on the hat and slop on the sunscreen).

Tumours of the epidermis and its appendages

Benign

Viral warts

These are discussed in Chapter 15, but are mentioned here for two reasons: first, they are sometimes misdiagnosed if solitary on the face or hands of the elderly; and, second, warts are one of the few tumours in humans which are, without doubt, caused by a virus.

Squamous cell papilloma

This common tumour, arising from keratinocytes, may resemble a viral wart clinically. Sometimes an excessive hyperkeratosis produces a horn-shaped excrescence. Excision, or curettage with cautery to the base, is the treatment of choice. The histology should be checked.

Seborrhoeic keratosis (basal cell papilloma, seborrhoeic wart)

This is a common, benign, epidermal tumour, unrelated to sebaceous glands. The term senile wart should be avoided as it offends many patients.

Cause
Usually unexplained but:
- Multiple lesions may be inherited (autosomal dominant).
- Occasionally follow an inflammatory dermatosis.
- Very rarely the sudden eruption of hundreds of itchy lesions is associated with an internal neoplasm (sign of Leser–Trélat).

Presentation
Seborrhoeic keratoses usually arise after the age of 50, but flat inconspicuous lesions are often visible earlier. They are often multiple (Figs. 19.1 and 19.2) but may be single. Lesions are most common on the face and trunk. The sexes are equally affected.

The physical signs include:
- A distinctive 'stuck-on' appearance.
- May be flat, raised or pedunculated.
- Colour varies from yellow to dark brown.
- Surface may have greasy scaling and scattered keratin plugs ('currant bun' appearance).

Clinical course
Lesions may multiply with age but remain benign.

Differential diagnosis
Seborrhoeic keratoses are easily recognized. Occasional confusion arises with a pigmented cellular naevus, a pigmented basal cell carcinoma and, most importantly, with a malignant melanoma (Fig. 19.3).

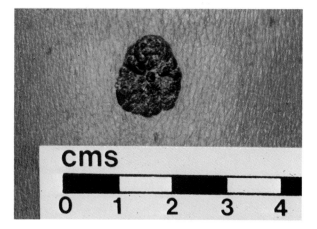

Fig. 19.3 Darkly pigmented seborrhoeic wart needing biopsy to exclude a malignant melanoma.

Warty surface   Horn cyst

Proliferating basal cells above the general level of surrounding epidermis   Basal cells

Fig. 19.4   Histology of basal cell papilloma.

Investigations

Biopsy is needed only in rare dubious cases. The histology is diagnostic (Fig. 19.4). The lesion lies above the general level of the surrounding epidermis and consists of proliferating basal cells and horn cysts.

Treatment

Seborrhoeic keratoses may be left alone, but ugly or easily traumatized ones can be removed by curetting them off under local anaesthetic (this has the advantage of providing histology), or by cryotherapy.

LEARNING   POINT

If you cannot tell a seborrhoeic wart from a melanoma you will send too many old people to the pigmented lesion clinic.

Skin tags (acrochordon)

These common benign outgrowths of skin affect mainly the middle-aged and elderly.

Cause

This is unknown but the trait is sometimes familial. Skin tags are most common in obese women, and rarely are associated with tuberous sclerosis (p. 226), acanthosis nigricans (p. 212) or acromegaly, and diabetes.

Presentation and clinical course

Skin tags occur around the neck and within the major flexures. They look ugly and may catch on clothing and jewellery. They are soft, skin-coloured or pigmented, pedunculated papules (Fig. 19.5).

Differential diagnosis

The appearance is unmistakable. Tags are rarely confused with small melanocytic naevi (p. 191).

Treatment

Small lesions can be snipped off with fine scissors, frozen with liquid nitrogen, or destroyed with a hyfrecator without local anaesthesia. There is no way of preventing new ones from developing.

Fig. 19.5   A cluster of pigmented skin tags in the supraclavicular fossa.

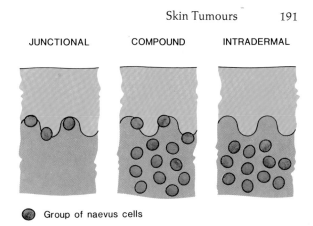

JUNCTIONAL   COMPOUND   INTRADERMAL

Group of naevus cells

Fig. 19.6 Types of acquired melanocytic naevi.

Melanocytic naevi

The term 'naevus' refers to a lesion, often present at birth, which has a local excess of one or more normal constituents of the skin. Melanocytic naevi (moles) are localized benign proliferations of melanocytes. Their classification is shown in Table 19.2 and depends on where the aggregations of naevus cells lie (Fig. 19.6).

Cause and evolution

The cause is unknown. A genetic factor is likely in many families.

With the exception of congenital melanocytic naevi, most appear in early childhood, often with a sharp increase in numbers during adolescence. Further crops may appear during pregnancy or oestrogen therapy, but new lesions come up less often after the age of 20.

Melanocytic naevi in childhood are usually of the 'junctional' type, with proliferating melanocytes in clumps at the dermo-epidermal junction. Later, the melanocytes round off and 'drop' into the dermis. A 'compound' naevus has both dermal and junctional components. With maturation the junctional component disappears so that the melanocytes in an 'intradermal' naevus are all in the dermis (Fig. 19.6).

Presentation

Congenital melanocytic naevi (Fig. 19.7)
These are present at birth and are seldom less than 1 cm in diameter. Their colour varies from brown to black or blue-black. With maturity some become protruberant and hairy, with a cerebriform surface. Such lesions can be disfiguring, e.g. a 'bathing trunk' naevus, and carry an increased risk of malignant transformation.

Junctional melanocytic naevi (Fig. 19.8)
These are roughly circular macules. Their colour

Table 19.2 Classification of melanocytic naevi

1	Congenital melanocytic naevi
2	Acquired melanocytic naevi
	Junctional naevus
	Compound naevus
	Intradermal naevus
	Spitz naevus
	Blue naevus
	Dysplastic naevus

Fig. 19.7 Congenital melanocytic naevus measuring 5 x 2 cm. Smaller and paler than most.

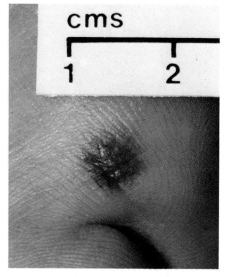

Fig. 19.8   Junctional melanocytic naevus at the base of the little toe.

Fig. 19.9   Compound melanocytic naevus. No recent change.

Fig. 19.10   Intradermal melanocytic naevus with numerous shaved hairs.

Fig. 19.11   Spitz naevus. Rapid evolution and red colour cause diagnostic confusion.

ranges from mid to dark brown and may vary even within a single lesion. Most naevi of the palms, soles and genitals are of this type.

Compound melanocytic naevi (Fig. 19.9)
These are domed pigmented nodules of up to 1 cm in diameter. They may be light or dark brown but their colour is more even than that of junctional naevi. Most are smooth, but larger ones may be cerebri-

form, or even hyperkeratotic and papillomatous; many bear hairs.

Intradermal melanocytic naevi (Fig. 19.10)
These look like compound naevi but are less pigmented and often skin-coloured.

Spitz naevus (juvenile melanoma) (Fig.19.11)
These are usually found in children. They develop

over a month or two as solitary pink or red nodules of up to 1 cm in diameter and are most common on the face and legs. Though benign, they are often excised because of their rapid growth.

Blue naevus

So-called because of their striking slate grey-blue colour, blue naevi usually appear in childhood and adolescence, on the limbs, buttocks and lower back. They are usually solitary.

Mongolian spots

Pigment in dermal melanocytes is responsible for these bruise-like greyish areas seen on the lumbosacral area of most mongoloid and many Negroid babies. They usually fade during childhood.

Dysplastic naevus syndrome (Fig. 19.12)

Clinically and histologically atypical naevi run in some families which are melanoma prone. The many large irregularly pigmented naevi are most obvious on the trunk but some may be present on the scalp. Their edges are irregular and they vary greatly in size; many are over 1 cm in diameter. Some are pinkish and an inflamed halo may surround them.

Differential diagnosis

- *Malignant melanoma.* Most important in the differential diagnosis. These are very rare before puberty. Melanomas are single and more variably pigmented and irregularly shaped. Other features are listed below under Complications.
- *Seborrhoeic keratoses.* These may cause confusion in adults but they have a stuck-on appearance and are warty.
- *Lentigines.* May be found on any part of the skin and mucous membranes. More profuse than junctional naevi, they are usually grey-brown rather than black, and develop more often after adolescence.
- *Ephelides (freckles).* These are tan macules less than 5 mm in diameter. They are confined to sun-exposed areas, being most common in blonds or redheads.
- *Haemangiomas.* Benign proliferations of blood vessels, including haemangiomas and pyogenic

Fig. 19.12 Dysplastic naevus syndrome.

granulomas, may be confused with a vascular Spitz naevus or an amelanotic melanoma.

Histology

All excised specimens must be examined histologically. Most acquired lesions fit into the scheme given in Figure 19.6; orderly nests of benign naevus cells are seen in the junctional region, in the dermis, or in both. However, some types of melanocytic naevi have their own distinguishing features. In congenital naevi the naevus cells may extend to the subcutaneous fat, and hyperplasia of other skin components (e.g. hair follicles) may be seen. A Spitz naevus shows dermal oedema and dilated capillaries, and is composed of large epithelioid and spindle-shaped naevus cells, some of which may be in mitosis.

In a blue naevus, naevus cells are seen in the mid and deep dermis.

The main features of a dysplastic naevus are a lengthening of rete ridges, and the presence of junctional nests showing melanocytic dysplasia (nuclear pleomorphism and hyperchromatism). Fibrosis of the papillary dermis and a lymphocytic inflammatory response are also seen.

Complications

- *Inflammation.* Pain and swelling are common but are not features of malignant transformation. They are due to trauma, bacterial folliculitis, or a foreign body reaction to hair after shaving or plucking.

- *Depigmented halo* (Fig. 19.13). This is rare but benign. There may be vitiligo elsewhere. The naevus in the centre often involutes spontaneously before the halo repigments.
- *Malignant change.* This is extremely rare except in congenital melanocytic naevi, where the risk has been estimated at between 3 and 6% depending on their size (Fig. 19.14) and in the dysplastic naevi of melanoma-prone families. It should be considered if the following changes occur in a melanocytic naevus:
  - Itch.
  - Enlargement.
  - Increased or decreased pigmentation.
  - Asymmetry.
  - Irregularity of surface or edge.
  - Inflammation.
  - Ulceration.
  - Bleeding.

If such changing lesions are examined carefully, remembering the 'A B C D E' features of malignant melanoma (Table 19.3), few malignant melanomas should be missed.

Treatment
Excision is needed when:
1 A naevus is deemed ugly.
2 Malignancy is suspected or is a known risk, e.g. in a large congenital melanocytic naevus.
3 A naevus is repeatedly inflamed or traumatized.

LEARNING POINT

Do not be frightened, even if you think they are harmless, to refer moles which have changed to a dermatologist.

Epidermoid and pilar cysts
Often incorrectly called 'sebaceous cysts', epidermoid cysts are common and occur on the scalp, face, behind the ears, and on the trunk. They often have a central punctum; when they rupture, or are squeezed, foul-smelling cheesy material comes out.

Fig. 19.13 Halo naevus. Involuting melanocytic naevus within area of total depigmentation.

Fig. 19.14 Malignant melanoma developing within a congenital melanocytic naevus.

Table 19.3 The A B C D E of malignat melanoma.

*A*symmetry

*B*order irregularity

*C*olour variability

*D*iameter greater than 0.5 cm

*E*levation irregularity

Histologically the lining of a cyst resembles normal epidermis (epidermoid cyst) or the outer root sheath of the hair bulb (pilar cyst). Occasionally an adjacent foreign body reaction is noted. Treatment is by exci-

Fig. 19.15 Milial cysts.

Fig. 19.16 Kerato-acanthoma with its epidermal shoulders and central plug of keratin.

sion, or by incision followed by expression of the contents and removal of the cyst wall.

Milium

Milia are small, subepidermal keratin cysts (Fig. 19.15). They are common on the face in all age groups and appear as tiny, white, millet seed-like papules of from 0.5 to 2 mm in diameter. They are occasionally seen at the site of a previous subepidermal blister (e.g. in epidermolysis bullosa and porphyria cutanea tarda). The contents of milia can be picked out with a sterile needle without local anaesthesia.

Chondrodermatitis nodularis helicis (painful nodule of the ear)

This terminological mouthful is, strictly, not a neoplasm, but a chronic inflammation. A painful nodule develops on the helix or antehelix of the ear, most often in men. It looks like a small corn, is tender, and prevents sleep if that side of the head touches the pillow. Histologically, a thickened epidermis overlies inflamed cartilage. Wedge resection under local anaesthetic is effective if cryotherapy fails.

Premalignant tumours

Kerato-acanthoma

Some argue that this rapidly growing tumour should be classed as benign, but a very few transform into a squamous cell carcinoma.

Cause

Photosensitizing chemicals such as tar and mineral oils may act as co-carcinogens with ultraviolet radiation. They may also follow therapeutic immunosuppression.

Clinical features

They occur mainly on the exposed skin of fair individuals. More than two-thirds are on the face and most of the rest are on the arms. The lesion starts as a pink papule which rapidly enlarges; it may reach a diameter of 1 cm in a month or two. After five or six weeks the centre of the nodule forms either a keratinous plug or a crater (Fig. 19.16). If left, the lesion often resolves spontaneously over 6–12 months but leaves an ugly depressed scar.

Differential diagnosis

Squamous cell carcinoma is the main tumour to be distinguished from a kerato-acanthoma. However, it grows more slowly, and usually lacks symmetry.

Histology

It is not possible to tell a kerato-acanthoma from a squamous cell carcinoma histologically unless the architecture of the whole lesion can be assessed (Fig. 19.17). A typical lesion is symmetrical and composed of proliferating fronds of epidermis which show mitotic activity but retain a well-differentiated squamous appearance with the production of much 'glassy' keratin. The centre of the cup-shaped mass is filled with keratin.

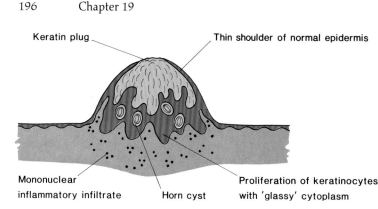

Keratin plug

Thin shoulder of normal epidermis

Mononuclear inflammatory infiltrate

Horn cyst

Proliferation of keratinocytes with 'glassy' cytoplasm

Fig. 19.17   Histology of kerato-acanthoma.

Treatment
Excision or curettage and cautery are both effective. Occasionally a further curetting may be needed but this should be done only once; if this is still ineffective, the lesion must be excised.

Intra-epidermal carcinoma (Bowen's disease)
Usually single, these slowly expanding pink, scaly plaques (Fig. 19.18) take years to reach a diameter of a few centimetres. Their border is sharply defined, with reniform projections and notches. These lesions occasionally change into an invasive squamous cell carcinoma. The presence of several may be a clue to previous exposure to carcinogens (e.g. arsenic in a tonic when young).

Differential diagnosis
Intra-epidermal carcinoma is often mistaken for psoriasis (Chapter 6), discoid eczema (p. 80) or a superficial basal cell carcinoma (*see below*).

Treatment
These lesions are unaffected by local steroids; excision or cryotherapy is therefore needed, though small lesions may be left under observation in the frail and elderly.

Actinic keratoses
These discrete, rough-surfaced lesions crop up on sun-damaged skin. They are premalignant, although only a few turn into a squamous cell carcinoma.

Fig. 19.18   Intra-epidermal carcinoma: a slowly expanding psoriasiform plaque on the thigh. Note the reniform projections and notches so suggestive of an *in situ* malignancy.

Cause
The effects of sun exposure are cumulative. Those with fair complexions living near the equator are most at risk and invariably develop these 'sun warts'. Melanin protects, and actinic keratoses are not seen in black skin. Conversely, albinos are especially prone to develop them.

Fig. 19.19 The back of the hand of a farm worker showing numerous typical rough-surfaced actinic keratoses.

Fig. 19.20 A large neglected actinic keratosis at the angle of the jaw. Already showed transition to a squamous cell carcinoma on biopsy.

Fig. 19.21 Cutaneous horn with a bulbous fleshy base.

Presentation

They affect the middle-aged and elderly in temperate climates, but younger people in the tropics. The pink or grey hyperkeratotic lesions seldom exceed 1.0 cm in diameter. Their surface is rough and sometimes warty, and scales may be removed by minor trauma (Fig. 19.19).

Complications

Transition to a squamous cell carcinoma, although rare, should be suspected if a lesion enlarges, ulcerates or bleeds (Fig. 19.20). Luckily such tumours seldom metastasize. A 'cutaneous horn' is a hard keratotic protrusion based on an actinic keratosis (Fig. 19.21).

Differential diagnosis

There is usually no difficulty in telling an actinic keratosis from a seborrhoeic wart, a viral wart (p. 145), a kerato-acanthoma, an intra-epidermal carcinoma, or a squamous cell carcinoma.

Investigations

A biopsy is needed if there is worry over malignant change.

Histology

Alternating zones of hyper- and parakeratosis overlie a thickened or atrophic epidermis. The normal maturation pattern of the epidermis may be lost and occasional pleomorphic keratinocytes may be seen. Solar elastosis is seen in the superficial dermis.

Treatment

Freezing with liquid nitrogen or carbon dioxide snow is simple and effective. Curettage is best for large lesions and cutaneous horns. Multiple lesions can be treated with 5-fluorouracil cream (Formulary, p. 253) after specialist advice. Lesions which do not respond should be regarded with suspicion, and biopsied.

Malignant epidermal tumours

Basal cell carcinoma (rodent ulcer)

This is the most common form of skin cancer. It

crops up most commonly on the faces of the middle-aged or elderly. Lesions invade locally but, for practical purposes, never metastasize.

Cause

Prolonged sun exposure is the most important factor and these tumours are most common in whites living near the equator. They may also occur in scars caused by X-rays, vaccination or trauma. Photosensitizing pitch, tar and oils can act as co-carcinogens with ultraviolet radiation. Previous treatment with arsenic, once present in many 'tonics', predisposes to multiple basal cell carcinomas often after a lag of many years.

Presentation

Nodulo-ulcerative

This is the most common type. An early lesion is a small, glistening, skin-coloured papule which slowly enlarges. Central necrosis, though not invariable, leaves an ulcer with an adherent crust and a rolled pearly edge (Fig. 19.22). Fine telangiectatic vessels often run across the tumour's surface. Without treatment such lesions may reach 1–2 cm in diameter in 5–10 years.

Cystic

The lesion is at first like the nodular type, but later cystic changes predominate and the nodule becomes tense and translucent, with marked telangiectasia (Fig. 19.23).

Cicatricial (morphoeic)

These are slowly expanding, yellow or white, waxy plaques with an ill-defined edge. Ulceration and crusting, followed by fibrosis, are common, and the lesion may look like an enlarging scar (Fig. 19.24).

Superficial (multicentric)

These arise most often on the trunk. Several lesions may be present, each expanding slowly as a pink or brown scaly plaque with a fine 'whipcord' edge (Fig. 19.25). Such lesions can grow to more than 10 cm in diameter.

Fig. 19.22 Early basal cell carcinoma with rolled opalescent edge and central crusting.

Fig. 19.23 Cystic basal cell carcinoma with marked telangiectasia, on the point of ulcerating.

Fig. 19.24 Poorly defined cicatricial basal cell carcinoma.

Fig. 19.25 Persistent scaly plaque — the whipcord edge gives away the diagnosis of a superficial basal cell carcinoma.

Fig. 19.26 A pigmented tumour on the forehead. The opalescence and telangiectasia point to the diagnosis of a basal cell carcinoma.

Fig. 19.27 A grossly neglected basal cell carcinoma already invading underlying bone.

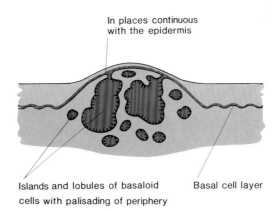

Fig. 19.28 Histology of nodular basal cell carcinoma.

Pigmented

Pigment may be present in all types of basal cell carcinoma (Fig. 19.26).

Clinical course

Slow but relentless growth destroys tissue locally. Untreated, a basal cell carcinoma may invade underlying cartilage or bone (Fig. 19.27) or damage important structures such as the tear ducts.

Histology

Small, darkly staining basal cells grow in well-defined aggregates which invade the dermis (Fig. 19.28). Their outer layer of cells is arranged in a palisade. Numerous mitoses and apoptotic bodies are seen. In the cicatricial type the islands of tumour are surrounded by fibrous tissue.

Differential diagnosis

A nodular basal cell carcinoma may be confused with an intradermal melanocytic naevus, a squamous cell carcinoma, a giant molluscum contagiosum (p. 153) or a kerato-acanthoma. Pigmented basal cell carcinomas should be distinguished from seborrhoeic warts and malignant melanomas. A cicatricial basal cell carcinoma may mimic morphoea (p. 110) or a scar. A superficial basal cell carcinoma may be confused with an intra-epidermal carcinoma, with psoriasis (Chapter 6) or with nummular eczema (p. 80).

Treatment

Excision, with 0.5 cm of surrounding normal skin, is the treatment of choice for patients under 60. Cicatricial tumours, with their ill-defined edges, and lesions near vital structures, should be excised by specialist surgeons. Moh's micrographic surgical technique is highly effective; it includes careful histological checks in all planes of tissue excised during the operation (p. 242). Radiotherapy is also effective but is reserved for biopsy-proven lesions in patients over 60, or when surgery is contra-indicated. Cryotherapy, or curettage and cautery, is sometimes useful for small superficial lesions (p. 242). The five-year cure rate for all types of basal cell carcinoma is over 95%, but regular follow up is necessary to detect local recurrence.

Fig. 19.29 Moderately differentiated squamous cell carcinoma presenting as an ulcerated keratotic nodule on the rim of an ear.

LEARNING POINTS

1 Catch lesions early: small ones are easy to get rid of; large ones leave ugly scars.
2 Do not sit and watch doubtful lesions near the eye.

Squamous cell carcinoma

This is a common tumour in which malignant keratinocytes show a variable capacity to form keratin.

Cause

These tumours often arise in skin damaged by long-term UVR and also by X-rays and infra-red rays. Other carcinogens include pitch, tar, mineral oils, and inorganic arsenic (*see* Basal cell carcinoma). Certain rare genetic disorders, with defective DNA repair mechanisms, such as xeroderma pigmentosum (p. 227), lead to multiple squamous and basal cell carcinomas, and to malignant melanoma; this illustrates the importance of altered DNA in the pathogenesis of malignancy. The DNA of the human papilloma virus (p. 145) may be integrated into the

Fig. 19.30 Persistent nodule of the lower lip of a smoker: squamous cell carcinoma until proved otherwise by biopsy.

nuclear DNA of keratinocytes and cause malignant transformation. Immunosuppression and UVR predispose to this.

Clinical presentation and course

Tumours may arise as thickenings in an actinic keratosis, or, *de novo*, as small keratotic nodules; rapidly growing anaplastic lesions may start as ulcers with a granulating base and an indurated edge (Fig. 19.29). Squamous cell carcinomas are common on the lower

Often hyperkeratotic surface

Proliferating keratinocytes

Adjacent chronic
inflammatory cell infiltrate

Fig. 19.31 Histology of squamous cell carcinoma.

Keratin production
in horn cysts

Invading strands of malignant
keratinocytes ('prickles' between cells)

lip (Fig. 19.30) and in the mouth. Those arising in actinic keratoses seldom mestastasize, but those arising in scars, ulcers, sinus tracks, X-irradiated skin and on mucous membranes often do. All lesions should be treated without delay.

Histology
Keratinocytes disrupt the dermo-epidermal junction and proliferate irregularly into the dermis. Malignant cells usually retain the capacity to produce keratin (Fig. 19.31).

Treatment
After the diagnosis has been confirmed by biopsy, the tumour should be excised with a 0.5 cm border of normal skin. Radiotherapy is effective but should be reserved for the frail and the elderly.

Malignant melanoma
Malignant melanoma attracts a disproportionate amount of attention because it is so often lethal. The public now knows more about its increasing incidence and dangers.

Incidence
The incidence in whites in the U.K. and U.S.A. is increasing, doubling approximately every 10 years. There is a higher incidence in whites living near the equator than in temperate zones. The tumour is rare before puberty and in blacks, although it does occur on their less-pigmented palms and soles, and on mucous membranes.

Cause

Genetic
These tumours are most common in whites with blond hair, fair skin which tans poorly, and many freckles. Those of celtic origin are the most susceptible. Melanoma may affect several members of a single family, in association with dysplastic naevi (p. 193).

Sunlight
Both incidence and mortality increase with decreasing latitude. Tumours occur most often on exposed skin.

Pre-existing melanocytic naevi
The risk of developing a malignant melanoma is highest in those with dysplastic naevi, congenital melanocytic naevi or many banal melanocytic naevi. A pre-existing naevus is seen histologically in about 30% of malignant melanomas.

Trauma
Melanomas are occasionally seen on the bare feet of African Bantus.

Virus
RNA tumour viruses have occasionally been found in metastatic deposits of human melanoma, and in some animal melanomas.

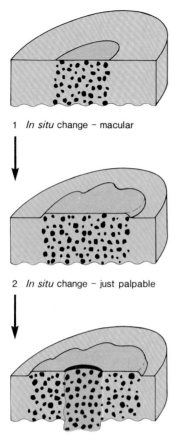

1 *In situ* change – macular

2 *In situ* change – just palpable

3 Invasive, easily palpable nodule
within plaque of *in situ* change

Fig. 19.32   Radial intra-epidermal growth phase of melanoma (1 and 2) precedes vertical and invasive dermal growth phase (3).

Fig. 19.33   This elderly patient had ignored for too long the slowly spreading macule of a lentigo maligna: now she has a frankly invasive melanoma within it.

Fig. 19.34   Superficial spreading melanoma: this lesion has been present for two years and, as yet, has invaded only the superficial dermis. Clearly malignant because of its colour variation, scalloped and notched outline.

Clinical features

Two-thirds of invasive melanomas are preceded by a superficial and radial growth phase, shown clinically as an expanding, irregularly pigmented macule or plaque (Fig. 19.32). Most are multicoloured mixtures of black, brown, tan and pink. Their margins are irregular with reniform projections and notches (Table 19.3). Malignant cells are confined to the epidermis and this phase is an '*in situ*' melanoma. A nodule coming up within the expanding macule signals dermal invasion.

There are four main types of malignant melanoma:

- *Lentigo maligna melanoma* occurs on the exposed skin of the elderly. An irregularly pigmented, irregularly shaped, macule (lentigo maligna) may have been enlarging slowly for many years before an invasive nodule (lentigo maligna melanoma) appears (Fig. 19.33).
- *Superficial spreading melanoma* is the most common type in Caucasoids. Its radial growth phase shows varied colours and is often palpable (Fig. 19.34). A nodule coming up within such a plaque signifies dermal invasion and a poor prognosis.
- *Acral lentiginous melanoma* occurs on the palms and soles and, although rare in Caucasoids, is the most common type in the Chinese and Japanese.

The invasive phase is again signalled by a nodule coming up within the irregularly pigmented macule of the *in situ* phase.

- *Nodular melanoma* (Fig. 19.35) appears as a pigmented nodule with no preceding *in situ* phase. It is the most rapidly growing and aggressive type.

Fig. 19.35 A neglected nodular malignant melanoma: a thick tumour with a poor prognosis.

Totally amelanotic melanomas are rare, and flecks of pigment can usually be seen with a lens. Subungual melanomas are painless areas of pigmentation expanding under the nail and onto the nail fold.

Malignant melanoma is staged clinically into:

- Stage I: primary lesion only.
- Stage II: regional nodal disease.
- Stage III: distant disease (visceral or nodes).

Histology (Fig. 19.36)

- *Lentigo maligna*. Numerous atypical melanocytes, many in groups, are seen along the basal layer extending downwards in the walls of hair follicles.
- *Lentigo maligna melanoma*. Dermal invasion occurs, with a breach of the basement membrane region. *In situ* changes are seen in the adjacent epidermis.
- *Superficial spreading melanoma in situ*. Large epithelioid melanoma cells permeate the epidermis.

IN SITU MELANOMA   INVASIVE MELANOMA

Often years

Lentigo maligna

6 months to 2 years

Superficial spreading

6 months to 2 years

Acral lentiginous

No *in situ* phase

Nodular

Fig. 19.36 Histology of the different types of melanoma.

- Normal melanocyte
- Malignant melanocyte

- *Superficial spreading melanoma.* The dermal nodule may be composed of epithelioid cells, spindle cells or naevus-like cells. *In situ* changes are seen in the adjacent epidermis.
- *Acral lentiginous melanoma in situ.* Atypical melanocytes are seen in the base of the epidermis and permeating the mid-epidermis.
- *Acral lentiginous melanoma.* Melanoma cells invade the dermis. *In situ* changes are seen in the adjacent epidermis.
- *Nodular melanoma.* The tumour comprises epithelioid, spindle and naevoid cells and there is no *in situ* melanoma in the adjacent epidermis.

Microstaging

Histology can help to assess prognosis. Breslow's method is to measure, with an ocular micrometer, the vertical distance from the granular cell layer to the deepest part of the tumour. Clark's method is to assess the depth of penetration of the melanoma (Fig. 19.37) in relation to the different layers of the dermis. The thicker and more penetrating a lesion, the worse is its prognosis (*see below*).

Differential diagnosis

This includes a melanocytic naevus, a seborrhoeic keratosis, a pigmented actinic keratosis, a pigmented basal cell carcinoma, and sclerosing haemangioma; all are discussed in this chapter. A malignant melanoma may also be confused with a subungual or peri-ungual haematoma. A history of trauma will help here, as may paring. '*Talon noir*' is a pigmented petechial area on the heel following minor trauma from ill-fitting training shoes. An amelanotic melanoma is most often confused with a pyogenic granuloma and with a squamous cell carcinoma.

Prognosis

The prognostic indicators, and their significance, are listed in Table 19.4.

Treatment

Only surgical excision is effective. At present a 3–5 cm clearance is recommended, though a 1 cm clearance is acceptable for shallow (<1.0 mm) tumours. The prognosis is excellent (90% five-year survival) for patients with shallow tumours, but worsens in proportion to their depth. Elective regional node dis-

Table 19.4 Prognostic indicators in malignant melanoma.

Indicator	Significance
Depth of primary tumour	Breslow < 1.5 mm good > 3.5 mm bad
Sex	Females do better than males
Age	Prognosis worsens after 50 years, especially in males
Site	Poor prognosis with tumours on trunk, upper arms, neck and scalp
Ulceration	Signifies poor prognosis
Clinical stage	Stage I: five-year survival 75% Stage II: five-year survival 25% Stage III: five-year survival 0–5%

Fig. 19.37 Schematic representation of Breslow's and Clark's methods of microstaging malignant melanoma.

section may benefit patients with tumours of intermediate thickness (2–3.5 mm). Chemotherapy, rarely curative, is palliative in 25% of patients with stage III melanoma. Campaigns to educate doctors and the public to recognize melanoma early, in its superficial and curable phase, must be worthwhile.

LEARNING POINTS

1 Prevention is better than cure; remember 'slip, slap and slop' advice to patients.
2 Do not forget the A B C D and E rules when querying a melanoma.
3 Excise all doubtful lesions and check their histology.
4 If excision biopsy shows that a melanoma is less than 1 mm thick, the only question to be asked is whether it has been excised with a 1 cm clearance in all directions.

Paget's disease of the nipple

A well-defined red, scaly plaque spreads slowly over and around the nipple due to the invasion of the epidermis by cells from an underlying intraductal carcinoma of the breast (Paget cells). It is unilateral, whereas eczema usually affects both nipples. A skin biopsy should be carried out first and if the diagnosis is confirmed mastectomy will be necessary. Extramammary Paget's disease involves sites bearing apocrine glands (Chapter 2) and is due to an underlying ductal carcinoma of these.

Tumours of the dermis

Benign

Vascular naevi

These are either present at birth or appear soon after. They can be classified clinically (Table 19.5) but there is no good clinicohistological correlation. A capillary haemangioma is composed of a network of capillaries in the upper and mid dermis. A capillary-cavernous haemangioma has multiple ectatic channels of

Table 19.5 Common vascular naevi.

Telangiectatic
'Salmon' patch
Capillary haemangioma (port-wine stain)
Angiomatous
Capillary-cavernous haemangioma (strawberry naevus)

varying calibre distributed throughout the dermis and even the subcutaneous fat.

'Salmon' patches

These are the commonest vascular naevi, present in about 50% of all babies. They are dull red, often telangiectatic macules, most commonly on the nape of the neck ('erythema nuchae'), the forehead and the upper eyelids. Nuchal lesions may remain unchanged, but patches in other areas usually disappear within a year.

Capillary haemangioma

'Port-wine' stains are also present at birth. They are pale, pink to purple macules, and vary from the barely noticeable (Fig. 19.38) to the grossly disfiguring.

Fig. 19.38 Port-wine stain of the right cheek. No neurological problems in this patient.

Fig. 19.39 Lifelong vascular naevus of the cheek showing no tendency to resolve. Note port-wine appearance of the upper pole contrasting with the nodular elements elsewhere.

Fig. 19.40 Classic strawberry naevus, occurred and enlarged rapidly shortly after birth.

Fig. 19.41 Strawberry naevus above the ear showing the whitening of the surface which is a sign of spontaneous remission.

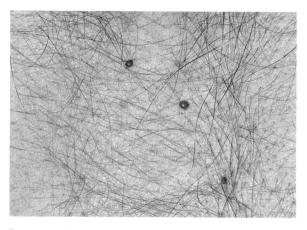

Fig. 19.42 Campbell de Morgan spots (cherry angiomas) of the chest.

Most occur on the face or trunk. They persist, and in middle age may darken and become studded with angiomatous nodules (Fig. 19.39). Occasionally a port-wine stain of the trigeminal area is associated with a vascular malformation of the leptomeninges on the same side, which may cause epilepsy or hemiparesis (the Sturge–Weber syndrome), or with glaucoma.

Treatment is unsatisfactory but encouraging results have been obtained with careful (and time-consuming) laser therapy.

Capillary cavernous haemangioma (strawberry naevus)

Strawberry naevi appear within a few weeks of birth, and grow for a few months, forming a raised, compressible swelling with a bright red surface (Fig. 19.40). Spontaneous regression then follows; the surface whitens centrally (Fig. 19.41) and regression is complete by the age of five in 50% of children and in 90% by the age of nine, leaving only an area of slight atrophy. Bleeding may follow trauma, and ulceration is common in the napkin (nappy) area.

Most lesions should be left untreated. Serial photographs of the way they clear up in other children help parents to accept this. Firm pressure may be needed to stop bleeding. If lesions interfere with feeding, or with vision, or if giant lesions sequestrate platelets (the Kasabach–Merritt syndrome), high doses of systemic steroids or plastic surgery should be considered.

Campbell de morgan spots (cherry angiomas)

These benign angiomas are common on the trunks of the middle-aged and elderly. They are small, bright red papules and of no consequence (Fig. 19.42).

Lymphangiomas

The commonest type is lymphangioma circumscriptum which appears as a cluster of vesicles resembling frog spawn. If treatment is needed, excision has to be wide and deep as dilated lymphatic channels and cisterns extend to the subcutaneous tissue.

Glomus tumour

These are derived from the cells surrounding small arteriovenous shunts. Solitary lesions are painful and most common on the extremities and under the nails. Multiple lesions are seldom painful and may affect other parts of the body. Painful lesions can be removed; others may be left.

Pyogenic granuloma

This badly named lesion is in fact a common benign

Fig. 19.43 Pyogenic granuloma of the thumb: soggy after elastoplast dressing and bleeding easily.

acquired haemangioma, often seen in children and young adults. It develops at sites of trauma, over the course of a few weeks, as a bright red, raised, sometimes pedunculated and raspberry-like lesion which bleeds easily (Fig. 19.43).

The important differential is from an amelanotic malignant melanoma and, for this reason, the histology should always be checked. It shows leashes of vessels of varying calibre invested by a thin, often ulcerated, epidermis.

Lesions should be removed by curettage under local anaesthetic with cautery to the base. Rarely this is followed by recurrence or an eruption of satellite lesions around the original site.

Dermatofibroma (histiocytoma)

These benign tumours are firm, discrete, usually solitary, dermal nodules, often on the extremities of young adults. The lesions have an 'iceberg' effect in that they feel larger than they look. The overlying epidermis is often lightly pigmented and dimples when the nodule is squeezed. Some lesions seem to follow minor trauma or an insect bite. Histologically, the proliferating fibroblasts merge into the sparsely cellular dermis at the margins. A straightforward lesion may be left but, if there is any diagnostic doubt, it should be excised.

Keloid

This is an overgrowth of dense fibrous tissue in the skin, arising in response to trauma, however trivial. Keloid formation is encouraged by infection, foreign material and by wounds (including surgical ones) which are not made along the lines of least tension or the skin creases. Keloids are common in Negroids and may be familial. In Caucasoids they are seen often enough on the presternal area, the neck, upper back and deltoid region of young adults to make doctors think twice before removing benign lesions there. Intralesional steroid injections are the treatment of choice.

Lipoma

Lipomas are common benign tumours of mature fat cells in the subcutaneous tissue. There may be one or many and lipomas are, rarely, a familial trait. They are most common on the proximal parts of the limbs but may occur at any site. They have an irregular lobular shape and a characteristic rubbery consistency. They are rarely painful. They need to be removed only if there is doubt about the diagnosis or if they are painful or ugly.

Malignant

Kaposi's sarcoma
This malignant tumour of proliferating capillaries and lymphatics may be multifocal. There are two types; the classical, and that associated with immunosuppression.

Classical Kaposi's sarcoma is seen most often in Africans and in elderly Jews of European origin. The tumours are usually on the feet and ankles but may be seen on the hands and on parts of the skin which are cold (e.g. ears and nose). Initially they are dark blue to purple macules progressing to plaques and large tumours (Fig. 19.44) which ulcerate and fungate. The rate of spread is variable but often slow. Tumours may metastasize to lymph nodes and spread to internal organs; oedema of the legs may be severe. The tumours are very sensitive to radiother-

apy which is the treatment of choice during the early stages; chemotherapy, with chlorambucil or vinblastine, helps when there is systemic involvement.

Kaposi's sarcoma and immunosuppression. Smaller and more subtle (e.g. bruise-like) lesions may occur in an immunodeficient host. The tumour has recently become well known because of its association with AIDS (p. 154) due to the human immunodeficiency virus (HIV-1). Interestingly, HIV-positive intravenous drug abusers do not develop Kaposi's sarcoma as often as do HIV-positive homosexuals. The prognosis of AIDS patients with Kaposi's sarcoma is poor as most will develop opportunistic infections. Single lesions respond to radiotherapy or intralesional vinblastine; systemic treatment with α-interferon has helped some with multiple lesions.

> LEARNING POINT
> Kaposi's sarcomas often look trivial but odd in those with immunosuppression. Keep HIV in mind.

Fig. 19.44 Kaposi's sarcoma: the larger classical type of tumour.

Lymphomas and leukaemias

Skin involvement falls into two broad categories:
1 Disorders which arise in the skin or preferentially involve it. These include:
  • T cell lymphomas (mycosis fungoides).
  • Sézary syndrome.
  • Lymphoma associated with HIV infection.
2 Those arising extracutaneously, which sometimes involve the skin. These include:
  • Hodgkin's disease.
  • B cell lymphomas.
  • Leukaemia.

Cutaneous T cell lymphoma (mycosis fungoides)
This lymphoma of skin-associated helper T lymphocytes usually evolves slowly. There are three clinical phases: the patch, plaque and tumour stages with in-

volvement of lymph nodes and other tissues occurring late in the disease.

The *premycotic plaque phase* may last for years. Most commonly it consists of scattered, barely palpable, erythematous, slightly pigmented, scaly plaques rather like psoriasis or seborrhoeic dermatitis (Fig. 19.45). They often have a bizarre outline (e.g. arciform, or horseshoe shape) and, on close inspection, atrophy with surface wrinkling is usually evident. Less commonly, the premycotic phase is a widespread poikiloderma, with atrophy, pigmentation and telangiectasia (Fig. 19.46). As the lymphoma develops, some plaques become indurated and palpable — *the infiltrated plaque stage*. Some then turn into frank tumours which may ulcerate (Fig. 19.47).

The first two phases of the disease may take as long as 20 years, but the *tumour stage* is often short, with spread and death usually within three years.

The *Sézary syndrome* is related to mycosis fungoides and is also due to a proliferation of helper T lymphocytes. Generalized erythema and oedema of the skin is associated with pruritus and lymphadenopathy. Abnormal T lymphocytes, with large convoluted nuclei, are found circulating in the blood ('Sézary cells').

Histology

The histological hallmarks of established mycosis fungoides are:

- Intra-epidermal lymphocytic micro-abscesses (Pautrier micro-abscesses).
- A band of lymphoid cells in the upper dermis which infiltrates the epidermis.
- Atypical lymphocytes.

The histology of the premycotic phase poses more problems and may differ little from dermatitis. Many biopsies, over several years, may be needed to prove that a suspicious rash has transformed into mycosis fungoides.

Differential diagnosis

The premycotic patch phase may be mistaken for psoriasis (Chapter 6), seborrhoeic dermatitis (p. 79) or tinea corporis (p. 157). However, it responds poorly to treatment for these disorders; the bizarre patterns often raise suspicion. In the early stages skin scrapings may be needed to exclude tinea.

Fig. 19.45 Premycotic stage of mycosis fungoides with scattered, barely palpable, erythematous, atrophic, scaly patches.

Fig. 19.46 Poikiloderma vasculare atrophicans may be a precursor of mycosis fungoides.

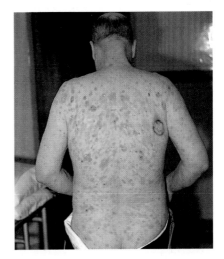

Fig. 19.47 Established mycosis fungoides with ulceration of a plaque.

Treatment

Moderately potent or potent local steroids, and UVB treatment, may offer prolonged palliation in the premycotic phase. As lesions become infiltrated, PUVA or electron beam therapy may be tried. Topical nitrogen mustard paint has also been used with success in this stage. Individual tumours respond well to low dose radiotherapy. Systemic chemotherapy for advanced disease is disappointing.

Lymphomas arising extracutaneously

Hodgkin's disease

This is of interest to dermatologists because it may present with severe generalized pruritus (p. 216). Patients with unexplained pruritus must be examined for lymphadenopathy and hepatosplenomegaly. Only rarely does Hodgkin's disease affect the skin directly, as small nodules and ulcers.

Leukaemia

Rarely the first sign of leukaemia is leukaemic infiltrate in the skin. Clinically, this shows as plum-coloured plaques or nodules or, less often, a thickening and rugosity of the scalp (cutis verticis gyratum) (Fig. 19.48). More often, the rashes associated with leukaemias are non-specific red papules ('leukaemid'). Other non-specific manifestations include pruritus, herpes zoster, acquired ichthyosis and purpura.

Fig. 19.49   B cell lymphoma of the skin.

B cell lymphomas

B lymphocytic lymphomas presenting with skin lesions are rare. They appear as scattered plum-coloured nodules (Fig. 19.49). Histologically, a B cell lymphoma infiltrates the lower dermis in a nodular or diffuse manner. Immunophenotyping shows a monoclonal expansion of B lymphocytes. Treatment is with radiotherapy and systemic chemotherapy.

Dermatofibrosarcoma protuberans

Dermatofibrosarcoma protuberans is a slowly growing malignant tumour of fibroblasts, arising usually on the upper trunk. At first it seems like a dermatofibroma or keloid but, as it slowly expands, it turns into a plaque of red or bluish nodules with an irregular, protuberant surface. It seldom metastasizes. It should be removed with extra wide margins, and even then will sometimes recur.

Cutaneous metastases

About 3% of patients with internal cancers have cutaneous metastases. Usually they arise late and indicate a grave prognosis. Occasionally a solitary cutaneous metastasis is the first sign of the occurrence of a tumour.

The most common cutaneous metastases come

Fig. 19.48   Leukaemic infiltration of the skin.

from breast cancer. The skin of the breast is also most often involved by the direct extension of a tumour. This may show up as a sharply demarcated and firm area of erythema (carcinoma erysipeloides), firm telangiectatic plaques and papules (carcinoma telangiectoides) or as skin like orange peel (*peau d'orange*) due to blocked and dilated lymphatics. Carcinoma of the breast may also send metastases to the scalp causing patches of alopecia (Fig. 19.50), or to other areas as firm and discrete dermal nodules.

Other common primaries metastasizing to the skin are tumours of the lung, GI tract, uterus, prostate and kidney. The most frequent sites are the umbilicus and the scalp.

Fig. 19.50 An indurated patch of alopecia due to a solitary metastasis from a breast carcinoma.

CHAPTER 20

THE SKIN IN SYSTEMIC DISEASE

This subject touches on most of general medicine: only selected aspects are covered here.

The skin and internal malignancy

Obvious and easily explicable skin signs may occur when a tumour invades the skin, or sends metastases to it; but there are other, more subtle, ways in which tumours can affect the skin. Sometimes tumours act physiologically, causing, for example, acne with some adrenal tumours, flushing in the carcinoid syndrome, or jaundice with a bile duct carcinoma. These

cast-iron associations need no further discussion here.

However, the presence of some rare but important conditions should alert the clinician to the possibility of an underlying neoplasm:

1 *Acanthosis nigricans* is a velvety thickening and pigmentation of the major flexures (Figs. 20.1, 20.2, and 20.3). Setting aside those cases due to obesity, or to diabetes, and characterized by insulin resistance, the chances are high of a tumour being present, usually within the abdominal cavity.

2 *Erythema gyratum repens* is a shifting pattern of waves of erythema covering the skin surface and looking like the grain on wood.

3 *Acquired hypertrichosis lanuginosa* ('malignant down') is an excessive and widespread growth of fine lanugo hair.

4 *Necrolytic migratory erythema* is a figurate erythema with a moving crusted edge. When present, usually with anaemia, stomatitis, weight loss, and diabetes, it signals the presence of a glucagon-secreting tumour of the pancreas.

5 *Basex's syndrome* is a papulosquamous eruption of the toes, fingers, ears, and nose, seen with some tumours of the upper respiratory tract.

6 *Dermatomyositis*, other than in childhood (p. 107).

7 *Generalized pruritus*. One of the long list of causes is an internal malignancy, usually a lymphoma (p. 216).

8 *Superficial thrombophlebitis*. The migratory type has traditionally been associated with carcinomas of the pancreas.

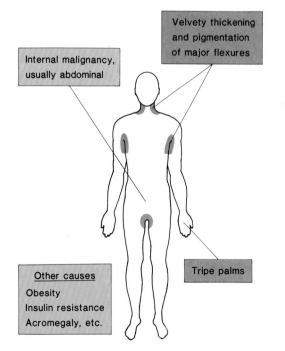

Internal malignancy, usually abdominal

Velvety thickening and pigmentation of major flexures

Tripe palms

Other causes
Obesity
Insulin resistance
Acromegaly, etc.

Fig. 20.1 Acanthosis nigricans.

Fig. 20.2 Acanthosis nigricans: velvety thickening of armpit skin associated with skin tags.

Fig. 20.3 Acanthosis nigricans — pigmentation and thickening of back of neck. Seborrhoeic wart-like lesions on back.

Fig. 20.4 Necrobiosis lipoidica: shiny, yellowish patch with redder edge. Scars have followed indolent ulcers secondary to minor trauma.

Fig. 20.5 Necrobiosis lipoidica: close-up to show atrophy with telangiectasia.

The skin and diabetes mellitus

The following are more common in those with diabetes than in others:

1 *Necrobiosis lipoidica*. Less than 1% of diabetics have necrobiosis, but most patients with necrobiosis will have diabetes: the other few should have a glucose tolerance test followed by regular urine tests as some will become diabetic later. The lesions appear as one or more plaques on the fronts of the shins (Fig. 20.4); they are shiny, atrophic and brown-red or slightly yellow. The underlying blood vessels are easily seen through the atrophic skin (Fig. 20.5) and the margin may be erythematous or violet. Minor knocks may lead to slow-healing ulcers; biopsy may do the same. No treatment is reliably helpful.

2 *Granuloma annulare*. The association with diabetes applies only to a few adults with extensive lesions. Children with standard lesions on the hands need a single urine check for sugar but no more elaborate tests. The cause is not known. Lesions often lie over the knuckles (Fig. 20.6) and are composed of dermal nodules fused into a rough ring shape. On the hands the lesions are skin-coloured or slightly pink; elsewhere a

Fig. 20.6   Granuloma annulare: classic lesions on the knuckles.

Fig. 20.7   Erythema nodosum: large, painful, dusky, plaques on the shins.

purple colour may be seen. Although a biopsy is seldom necessary, the histology shows a diagnostic palisading granuloma like that of necrobiosis lipoidica. Lesions tend to go away over the course of a year or two. Stubborn lesions respond to intralesional triamcinolone injections.

3 *Diabetic dermopathy.* In about 50% of diabetics multiple small (0.5–1 cm in diameter), slightly sunken, brownish scars can be found on the limbs, most obviously over the shins.

4 *Candidal infections* (p. 160).

5 *Staphylococcal infections* (p. 136).

6 *Vitiligo* (p. 182).

7 *Eruptive xanthomas* (p. 219).

8 *Tight waxy skin* on the fingers and hands.

9 *Atherosclerosis* with ischaemia or gangrene of feet.

10 *Neuropathic foot ulcers.*

The skin in sarcoidosis

About one-third of patients with systemic sarcoidosis have skin lesions; in addition it is possible to have cutaneous sarcoidosis without systemic abnormalities. The most important skin changes are as follows:

1 *Erythema nodosum* (Fig. 20.7). This occurs in the early stages of sarcoidosis, especially in young women.

2 *Scar sarcoidosis.* Granulomatous lesions arising in long-standing scars should raise suspicions of sarcoidosis.

3 *Lupus pernio.* Dusky infiltrated plaques appear on the nose and fingers, often in association with sarcoidosis of the upper respiratory tract.

4 *Papular, nodular and plaque forms.* These brownish-red, violaceous, or hypopigmented lesions are indolent though often symptom-free. Sometimes they are annular. They vary in number, size and distribution. Chronic lesions respond poorly to any line of treatment short of systemic steroids which are usually best avoided.

The skin in liver disease

Some of the abnormalities are:

1 *Pruritus.* This is related to obstructive jaundice and may precede it (p. 216).

2 *Pigmentation.* With bile pigments and sometimes melanin (Chapter 18).

3 *Spider naevi.* These are often multiple in chronic liver disease (p. 114).

4 *Palmar erythema* (p. 114).

5 *White nails.* These associate with hypo-albuminaemia.

6 *Porphyria cutanea tarda* (p. 217).

7 *Xanthomas.* In primary biliary cirrhosis (p. 219).

The skin in renal disease

The main changes are:

1 *Pruritus* and a generally dry skin.
2 *Pigmentation.* A yellowish sallow colour and pallor from anaemia.
3 *Half-and-half nail.* The proximal half is white and the distal half is pink or brownish.
4 *The skin changes of the conditions leading to renal disease.* For example, leucocytoclastic vasculitis (p. 93), connective tissue disorders (Chapter 12), Fabry's disease (p. 220).

Pyoderma gangrenosum

An inflamed nodule or pustule breaks down centrally to form an expanding ulcer with a polycyclic or serpiginous outline, and a characteristic undermined bluish edge. The condition is not bacterial in origin but its pathogenesis, presumably immunological, is not fully understood. It may arise in the absence of any underlying disease, but tends to associate with the following conditions:

1 Ulcerative colitis.
2 Crohn's disease.
3 Rheumatoid arthritis.
4 Monoclonal gammopathies.
5 Leukaemia (with a bullous form of pyoderma).

Lesions may be single or multiple. If gut disease is present then control of this will help the pyoderma. Otherwise the condition responds to systemic steroids but not to antibiotics, and lesions heal leaving papery scars.

Graft-versus-host (GVH) disease

Marrow grafting is now used for several disorders including aplastic anaemia and leukaemia. Immunologically competent donor lymphocytes, however, may cause problems by reacting against host tissues, especially the skin, liver and gut.

Acute GVH disease appears within four weeks. Fever accompanies malaise and a worsening morbilliform rash which may progress to a generalized desquamation or even toxic epidermal necrolysis.

Chronic GVH disease occurs later: its skin changes are variable but may be like those of lichen planus or a pigmented scleroderma. The skin changes may be severe enough to need treatment with systemic prednisolone or cyclosporin A.

Malabsorption and malnutrition

Some of the commonest skin changes are listed in Table 20.1.

Table 20.1 Skin changes in malabsorption and malnutrition.

Condition	Skin changes
Malnutrition	Itching Dryness Symmetrical pigmentation Brittle nails and hair
Protein malnutrition (kwashiorkor)	Dry, red-brown hair Pigmented 'cracked skin'
Iron deficiency	Itching Diffuse hair loss Koilonychia Smooth tongue
Vitamin A deficiency	Dry skin Follicular hyperkeratoses Xerophthalmia
Vitamin B$_1$ (aneurin) deficiency	Beri-beri oedema
Vitamin B$_2$ (riboflavine) deficiency	Angular stomatitis Smooth purple tongue Seborrhoeic dermatitis-like eruption
Vitamine B$_6$ (pyridoxine) deficency	Ill-defined dermatitis
Vitamin B$_7$ (niacin) deficiency	Pellagra with dermatitis, dementia and diarrhoea Dermatitis on exposed areas, pigmented
Vitamin C deficiency (scurvy)	Skin haemorrhages especially around follicular keratoses containing coiled hairs Bleeding gums Oedematous 'woody' swellings of limbs in elderly

Generalized pruritus

Pruritus is a symptom with many causes, but not a disease in its own right. Itchy patients fall into two groups: those whose pruritus is due simply to surface causes (e.g. eczema, lichen planus, and scabies), which seldom need much investigation; and the others, who may or may not have an internal cause for their itching, such as:

1 *Liver disease.* Itching signals biliary obstruction. It may be an early symptom of primary biliary cirrhosis. Cholestyramine often helps cholestatic pruritus, possibly by promoting the elimination of bile salts.

2 *Chronic renal failure.* Urea itself seems not to be responsible for this symptom which plagues about one-third of patients undergoing renal dialysis.

3 *Iron deficiency.* Treatment with iron may help the itching.

4 *Polycythaemia.* The itching here is usually triggered by a hot bath; it has a curious pricking quality and lasts about an hour.

5 *Thyroid disease.* Itching and urticaria may occur in hyperthyroidism: the dry skin of hypothyroidism may also be itchy.

6 *Diabetes.* Generalized itching may be a rare presentation of diabetes.

7 *Internal malignancy.* The prevalence of itching in Hodgkin's disease may be as high as 30%. It may be unbearable, yet the skin often looks normal. Pruritus may occur long before other manifestations of the disease. Itching is uncommon in carcinomatosis.

8 *Neurological disease* Paroxysmal pruritus has been recorded in multiple sclerosis and in neurofibromatosis. Brain tumours infiltrating the floor of the fourth ventricle may cause a fierce persistent itching of the nostrils.

9 The skin of the elderly may itch because it is too dry.

The search for a cause has to be tailored to the individual patient, and must start with a thorough history and physical examination. Unless a treatable cause is found, therapy is symptomatic and consists of sedative antihistamines, and the avoidance of rough clothing, overheating and vasodilatation, including that brought on by alcohol. Local applications include calamine and mixtures containing small amounts of menthol or phenol (Formulary, p. 247). Sometimes lubricating the skin with emollients may help.

LEARNING POINTS

1 Learn how to spell pruritus (not pruritis) but do not accept it as a diagnosis in its own right.

2 Ponder underlying causes in those with no primary skin disease.

Fig. 20.8 Congenital erythropoietic porphyria — perhaps the origin of the term 'werewolf'.

The porphyrias

An important multistage metabolic pathway leads from glycine and succinyl CoA, through a sequence of porphyrins, to the formation of haem and thence of haemoglobin, myoglobin, cytochromes and various haem-containing enzymes. Each step of the pathway is regulated by enzymes, and deficiencies of these lead to the accumulation of intermediate metabolites, some of which may cause photosensitivity to UVR of wavelength 400 nm (capable of penetrating through window glass).

Porphyrias are rare and most types are inherited. They can be separated on clinical grounds, aided by the biochemical investigation of urine, faeces and blood. Only the following five varieties will be mentioned here.

Congenital erythropoietic porphyria

This is very rare. Severe photosensitivity is noted soon after birth, and leads to blistering, scarring and mutilation of the exposed parts which become increasingly hairy. The urine is pink, and the teeth are brown, though fluorescing red under Wood's light. A haemolytic anaemia is present. Treatment is unsatisfactory. The hairy appearance, discoloured teeth, and the tendency to avoid daylight may have given rise to legends about werewolves (Fig. 20.8).

Erythrohepatic protoporphyria (erythropoietic protoporphyria)

In this commoner, autosomal dominant condition, a less severe photosensitivity develops during childhood. A burning sensation occurs within minutes of exposure to sunlight. Soon the skin becomes swollen and crusted vesicles sometimes appear, leading to pitted scars. Liver disease and gallstones occur. In addition to sun avoidance and the use of sunscreens (Formulary, p. 247), beta-carotene may be given orally.

Cutaneous hepatic porphyria (porphyria cutanea tarda)

Perhaps occurring against a background of genetic susceptibility, this condition is usually seen in men who have damaged their livers by taking too much alcohol. Blisters and milia form on the exposed parts of the face, and on the backs of the hands (Fig. 20.9), in response to sunlight or to minor trauma. These areas become scarred and hairy (Fig. 20.10). The urine is pink and fluoresces a bright coral-pink under Wood's light (p. 31) due to excessive uropor-

Fig. 20.9 Cutaneous hepatic porphyria (porphyria cutanea tarda).

Fig. 20.10 Blisters on the backs of the hands and fingers in a patient with cutaneous hepatic porphyria.

Fig. 20.11 Cutaneous hepatic porphyria. Coral-red fluorescence of urine under Wood's light denoting excessive uroporphyrins.

phyrins (Fig. 20.11). Treatment is based on avoiding alcohol and oestrogens, but other measures are usually needed too, including regular venesection or very low-dose chloroquine therapy (e.g. 125 mg twice weekly). Higher doses cause toxic hepatitis in these patients.

Acute intermittent porphyria

This condition, inherited as an autosomal dominant, is most common in Scandinavia. Skin lesions do not occur. Attacks of abdominal pain, accompanied by neuropsychiatric symptoms and the passage of dark urine, are sometimes triggered by drugs (especially barbiturates, griseofulvin, oestrogens and sulphonamides).

Variegate porphyria

This disorder, inherited as an autosomal dominant trait, is particularly common in South Africa. It shares the skin features of porphyria cutanea tarda and the systemic symptoms and drug provocation of acute intermittent porphyria.

Amyloid

Systemic amyloidosis of the type which is secondary to chronic inflammatory diseae, such as rheumatoid arthritis or tuberculosis, tends not to affect the skin. In contrast, skin changes are prominent in primary systemic amyloidosis and also in the amyloid associated with multiple myeloma. Skin blood vessels infiltrated with amyloid rupture easily, causing 'pinch purpura' to occur after minor trauma. The waxy deposits of amyloid, often most obvious around the eyes, may also be purpuric. Distinct from the systemic amyloidoses are localized deposits of amyloid. These are uncommon and usually take the form of macular areas of rippled pigmentation or of plaques made up of coalescing papules. Both types are itchy.

Mucinoses

The dermis may become infiltrated with mucin in certain disorders:
1 *Myxoedema.* In the puffy hands and face of hypothyroidism.
2 *Pretibial myxoedema.* Pink or flesh coloured mucinous plaques on the lower shins are seen, together with marked exophthalmos, in some patients with hyperthyroidism. They may also occur after the thyroid abnormality has been treated.
3 *Scleromyxoedema.* A diffuse thickening and papulation of the skin may occur in connection with an IgG monoclonal paraproteinaemia.

4 *Follicular mucinosis.* Infiltrated plaques showing loss of hair; some cases are associated with a lymphoma.

Xanthomas

Deposits of fatty material in the skin and subcutaneous tissues (xanthomas) may provide the first clue to important disorders of lipid metabolism.

Primary hyperlipidaemias are usually genetic. They fall into six groups, classified on the basis of an analysis of fasting blood lipids and electrophoresis of plasma lipoproteins. All, save type I, carry an increased risk of atherosclerosis — in this lies their importance and the need for treatment.

Secondary hyperlipidaemia may be found in a variety of diseases including diabetes, primary biliary cirrhosis, the nephrotic syndrome and hypothyroidism.

The clinical patterns of xanthoma correlate well with the underlying cause. The main patterns and their most common associations are shown in Table 20.2.

Fig. 20.12 Xanthelasma: flat, yellow lesions on the eyelids; in this patient the blood lipids were normal.

Fig. 20.13 The nodular form of tuberous xanthoma on the points of the elbows.

Table 20.2 Xanthomas: clinical appearance and associations.

Type	Clinical appearance	Types of hyperlipidaemia and associated metabolic abnormalities
Xanthelasma palpebrarum (Fig 20.12)	Soft yellowish plaques on the eyelids	None or type II
Tuberous xanthomas (Fig 20.13)	Firm yellow papules and nodules, most often on points of knees and elbows	Types II, III and secondary
Tendinous xanthomas	Subcutaneous swellings on fingers or by Achilles tendon	Types II, III and secondary
Eruptive xanthomas (Fig 20.14)	Sudden onset, multiple small yellow papules Buttocks and shoulders	Types I, III, IV, V and secondary (usually to diabetes)
Plane xanthomas	Yellow macular areas at any site Yellow palmar creases	Type II, III and secondary
Generalized plane xanthomas	Yellow macular lesions over wide areas	Myeloma

Fig 20.14   The numerous, small, yellowish papules of eruptive xanthoma. The patient was a diabetic.

Phenylketonuria

Phenylketonuria is a rare metabolic cause of hypopigmentation. Its prevalence is about 1:25 000. It is inherited as an autosomal recessive trait and is due to a deficiency of the liver enzyme phenylalanine hydroxylase, which catalyses the hydroxylation of phenylalanine to tyrosine. This leads to the accumulation of phenylalanine, phenylpyruvic acid and their metabolites.

Affected individuals have fair skin and hair. They often develop eczema, usually of atopic type, and may be photosensitive. The accumulation of phenylalanine and its metabolites damages the brain during the phase of rapid development just before and just after birth. Extrapyramidal manifestations such as athetosis and mental retardation may occur.

Oculocutaneous albinism can usually be distinguished by its eye signs. The Guthrie test, which detects raised blood phenylalanine levels, is carried out routinely at birth in most developed countries.

Treatment with a low-phenylalanine diet should be started as soon as possible to prevent further neurological damage.

Alkaptonuria

In this rare, recessively inherited disorder, based on a homogentisic acid oxidase deficiency, dark urine may be seen in childhood, and in adult life pigment may be deposited in various places including the ears and sclera. Arthropathy may occur.

Fabry's disease
(angiokeratoma corporis diffusum)

A deficiency of the enzyme ceramide trihexosidase is found in this sex-linked disorder: abnormal amounts of glycolipid are deposited in many tissues as a result. The skin lesions are grouped, almost black, small telangiectatic papules especially around the umbilicus and pelvis. Progressive renal failure occurs in adult life. Most patients have attacks of excruciating unexplained pain in their hands.

CHAPTER 21

THE SKIN AND THE PSYCHE

Lay people accept, perhaps too easily, that there are strong links between skin disease and the emotions. Dermatologists vary in their ability to see such associations, and only in a few skin disorders, such as dermatitis artefacta, are emotional factors obviously their direct cause.

The relationships between the mind and the skin are usually more subtle and more complex than this. Skin patients do have a higher prevalence of psychiatric abnormalities than the general population, but specific personality profiles and disorders are not tied to specific skin diseases. Similarly it is still not clear how, or even how often, psychological factors trigger, worsen or perpetuate such everyday problems as atopic eczema or psoriasis.

Each school of psychiatry has its own theories on the subject, but their explanations do not satisfy everyone. Do people really damage their skin to satisfy guilt feelings? Does their skin 'weep' because they have themselves suppressed weeping? Perhaps, until more is known, it may be better to adopt a simple and more pragmatic approach, in which interactions between the skin and psyche are divided into two broad groups: first, the emotional reactions to the presence of skin disease, real or imagined; and, second, the effects of emotions on skin disease (Fig. 21.1).

Reactions to skin disease

The presence of disfiguring skin lesions may distort the emotional development of a child: some become withdrawn, others become aggressive, but many adjust well. The range of individual reactions to skin

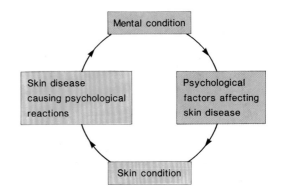

Fig. 21.1 Mind–skin interactions.

disease is, therefore, wide. At one end lies indifference to grossly disfiguring lesions and, at the other, lies an obsession with skin which is quite normal. Between these extremes are reactions ranging from natural anxiety over ugly skin lesions to disproportionate worry over minor blemishes. The concept of 'body image' is useful here.

Body image
All of us think we know how we look, but our ideas may not tally with those of others. The nose, face, hair and genitals tend to rank high in a person's 'corporeal awareness', and trivial lesions in those areas may generate much anxiety. For example, the facial lesions of acne, may lead to an excessive loss of self-esteem.

Dysmorphophobia
This is the term applied to distortions of the body image. Minor and inconspicuous lesions are magnified in the mind to grotesque disfiguring images.

Dermatological 'non-disease'

This is a form of dysmorphobia: no skin abnormality can be found by the clinician, but the distress felt by the patient may lead to anxiety, depression, or even suicide. Such patients are not uncommon. They expect dermatological solutions for complaints such as hair loss, or burning, itching and redness of the face or genitals. The dermatologist, who can see nothing wrong, cannot solve matters and no treatment seems to help. Such patients are reluctant to see a psychiatrist though some may suffer from a monosymptomatic hypochondriacal psychosis.

Monosymptomatic hypochondriacal psychosis

Patients may sustain, for long periods, single hypochondriacal delusions in the absence of other recognizable psychiatric disease. Some are eccentric and live in social isolation. In dermatology many of these patients have the delusion that their skin is infested with parasites. Others believe that they have syphilis, AIDS or skin cancer.

Delusions of parasitosis (Fig. 21.2)

This term is better than 'parasitophobia' which implies a fear of becoming infested. Patients with delusions of parasitosis are unshakably convinced that they are already infested. No rational argument can

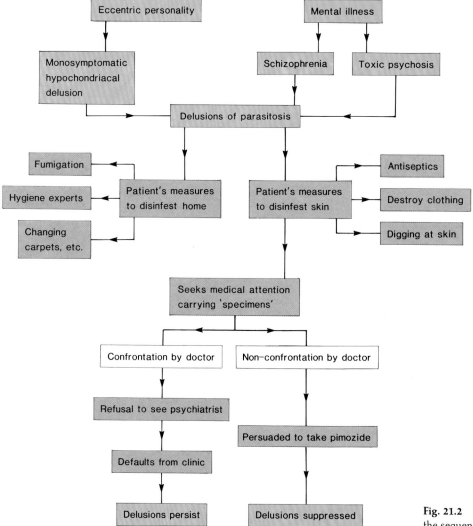

Fig. 21.2 Delusions of parasitosis — the sequence of events.

convince them that they are not; their physician then must be wrong. Their symptoms include odd sensations of crawling and biting, and they often bring to the clinic with them, in a box, specimens of the 'parasite' at different stages of its supposed life cycle. These must be examined microscopically but usually turn out to be fragments of skin, hair, clothing, or unclassifiable debris.

Such patients become angry if doubts are cast on their ideas or if they are referred to a psychiatrist. Direct confrontations are best avoided, and much tact is needed to secure any co-operation with treatment.

The delusions of a few of these patients are based on an underlying depression or schizophrenia, and of a further few on organic problems such as vitamin deficiency or cerebrovascular disease. These disorders must be treated on their own merits. Most patients, however, suffer from monosymptomatic hypochondriacal delusions which can often be suppressed by treatment with pimozide, accepting that this will be needed long-term. Otherwise the outlook for resolution is poor.

Their skin changes may include gouge marks and scratches, but it is convenient to consider these patients separately from dermatitis artefacta.

Dermatitis artefacta

Here the skin lesions are caused and kept going by the patient's own actions, but parasites are not held to be to blame. Patients with dermatitis artefacta continue to deny self-trauma but, naturally, if treatment is left to them to carry out; their problems do not improve. Lesions will heal under occlusive dressings, but these do not alter the underlying psychiatric problems, and lesions may recur or crop up outside the bandaged areas. Different types of dermatitis artefacta are listed in Table 21.1.

The lesions (Fig. 21.3) favour accessible areas, and do not fit with known pathological processes. The diagnosis is often difficult to make but an experienced clinican will suspect it because there are no primary lesions and because of the bizarre shape or grouping of the lesions, which may be rectilinear or oddly grouped and are often limited to accessible parts (Fig. 21.4). Areas damaged by burning, corrosive chemicals, or by digging have their own special appearance.

Apart from frank malingerers, the patients are often young women with some medical knowledge, perhaps a nurse. Some form of 'secondary gain' from having skin lesions may be obvious. The psychological problems may be superficial and easily resolved,

Table 21.1 Types of dermatitis artefacta.

Type	Personality
Minor habits, e.g. excoriated acne	Relatively normal
More obvious lesions	Hysterical or neurotic (secondary gain)
Bizarre	Psychotic
Malingering	Criminal

Fig. 21.3 Look for a trickle effect in self-inflicted corrosive injuries.

Fig. 21.4 Obvious dermatitis artefacta: back your own judgement against the patient's here.

but sometimes psychiatric help is needed and the artefacts are part of a prolonged psychiatric illness. Direct confrontation and accusations are usually best avoided, and the condition may last for some years.

L E A R N I N G   P O I N T S

1 Try pimozide for those with delusions of parasitosis.
2 Direct confrontations with patients with dermatitis artefacta or delusions of parasitosis may make you feel better but do little for them.

Neurotic excoriations

Patients with neurotic excoriations differ from those with other types of dermatitis artefacta in that they admit to picking and digging at their skin. This habit affects women more often than men and is most active at times of stress. The clinical picture is mixed, with crusted excoriations and pale scars, often with a hyperpigmented border, mainly on the face, neck, shoulders and arms. The condition may last for years and psychiatric treatment is seldom successful.

Acne excoriée

Here the self-inflicted damage is based to some extent on the lesions of acne vulgaris which may, in themselves, be mild but become disfiguring when dug and squeezed to excess (Fig. 14.7). The patients are usually young girls who may leave themselves with ugly scars. A psychiatric approach is often unhelpful and a daily ritual of attacking the lesions, helped by a magnifying mirror, may persist for years.

Localized neurodermatitis (lichen simplex)

This term refers to areas of itchy lichenification, perpetuated by bouts of scratching in response to stress. The condition is not uncommon and may occur on any area of skin. In men the lesions are often on the calves; women favour the nape of the neck where the redness and scaling may look like psoriasis.

Some examples of persistent itching in the anogenital area are due to lichen simplex there.

Patients with localized neurodermatitis develop conditioned scratch responses to minor itch stimuli more readily than controls. Local therapy does not alter the underlying cause, but topical steroids, sometimes only the most potent ones, may ameliorate the symptoms. Occlusive bandaging of suitable areas may clear the lesions which are covered.

Hair-pulling habit

Trichotillomania is too dramatic a word for what is usually only a minor comfort habit in children, ranking alongside nail-biting and lip-licking. Perhaps it should be dropped now. The matter is usually of little consequence and children who twist and pull their hair, often as they are going to sleep, seldom have major psychiatric disorders. The habit may go away more quickly if it is ignored. However, more severe degrees of hair pulling are sometimes seen in disturbed adolescents and in the mentally deficient. Here the outlook for full regrowth is less good, even with formal psychiatric help.

The diagnosis can usually be made on the history, but some parents do not know what is going on. The areas of hair loss do not show the exclamation mark hairs of alopecia areata, or the scaling and inflammation of scalp ringworm. The patches are irregular in outline and hair loss is never complete. Those hairs that remain tend to be bent or broken, and of variable length.

Dermatoses precipitated or perpetuated by emotional factors

Fancy rather than fact rules here. Popular candidates for inclusion in this group of diseases are psoriasis, urticaria, atopic eczema, pompholyx, discoid eczema, alopecia areata, and lichen planus. Every dermatologist will have seen associations between external stress and exacerbations of most of the conditons listed here, but proof that stress causes the diseases is hard to find. For example, some studies suggest that even hyperhidrosis of the palms and soles, once thought to be an accentuated response to stress, may have no relationship to chronic anxiety at all.

CHAPTER 22

OTHER GENETIC DISORDERS

Inheritance is important in many of the conditions discussed in other chapters and this has been highlighted in the sections on aetiology. This chapter includes some genetic disorders not covered elsewhere.

Neurofibromatosis

This relatively common disorder affects about one in 3000 people and is inherited as an autosomal dominant trait. There are two main types: von Recklinghausen's neurofibromatosis (which accounts for over 90% of all cases) and bilateral acoustic neurofibromatosis; these are phenotypically and genetically distinct.

Cause

A gene deletion on chromosome 22 has been found in bilateral acoustic neurofibromatosis but not in the von Recklinghausen type.

Clinical features

The physical signs include:

Von Recklinghausen's neurofibromatosis

- Six or more *café au lait* patches (light brown oval macules) (Fig. 22.1), developing usually in the first year of life.
- Axillary freckling (Fig. 22.2) in two-thirds of affected individuals.
- Variable numbers of skin neurofibromas, some small and superficial, others larger and deeper, ranging from flesh-coloured to pink, purple or brown (Fig. 22.1). Most are dome-like nodules, but others are irregular raised plaques. Some are firm, some soft and compressible through a deficient

Fig. 22.1 Neurofibromatosis: one large, but benign, neurofibroma has ulcerated over the sacrum. Several *café au lait* patches are visible.

Fig. 22.2 Freckling of the axilla and *café au lait* patches imply that this child has neurofibromatosis though surface nodules have not yet appeared.

dermis ('button-hole' sign); others feel 'knotty' or 'wormy'. Neurofibromas may not appear until puberty and become larger and more numerous with age.

- Small circular pigmented hamartomas of the iris (Lisch nodules), appear in early childhood.

Bilateral acoustic neurofibromatosis
- Bilateral acoustic neuromas.
- Few, if any, cutaneous manifestations.
- No Lisch nodules.

Diagnosis

The *café au lait* marks, axillary freckling and Lisch nodules should be looked for, as they appear before the skin neurofibromas. Isolated neurofibromas are not uncommon in individuals without neurofibromatosis and are of little consequence unless they are painful.

Complications

Von Recklinghausen's neurofibromatosis
A neurofibroma will occasionally change into a neurofibrosarcoma. Other associated features may include kyphoscoliosis, mental deficiency, epilepsy, renal artery stenosis and an association with phaeochromocytoma. 'Forme-fruste' variants occur, for example segmental neurofibromatosis.

Bilateral acoustic neurofibromatosis
Other tumours of the central nervous system may occur, especially meningiomas and gliomas.

Management

Affected adults may ask about the risk of their children developing the disorder; the chances are one in two. Ugly or painful lesions, and any suspected of undergoing malignant change, should be removed.

Tuberous sclerosis

This uncommon condition is also inherited as an autosomal dominant trait, with variable expressivity even within the same family. As fertility is reduced, transmission through more than two generations is rare.

Clinical features
The skin changes include:
- *Small oval white patches* ('ash leaf macules'). These are important as they may be the only manifestation at birth.
- *Adenoma sebaceum.* Develop at puberty as pink or yellowish acne-like papules on the face, often around the nose (Fig. 22.3).
- *Peri-ungual fibromas.* Develop in adult life as small pink sausage-like lesions emerging from the nail folds (Fig. 22.4).
- *Connective tissue naevi.* Cobblestone, somewhat yellow plaques often arise in the skin over the base of the spine.

Fig. 22.3   Tuberous sclerosis. Adenoma sebaceum.

Fig. 22.4   The peri-ungual fibromas of tuberous sclerosis are found in adult patients.

Other features may include:
- Epilepsy.
- Mental retardation.
- Ocular signs, including retinal phacomas and pigmentary abnormalities, in 50 % of patients.
- Hyperplastic gums.
- Gliomas, renal tumours, and calcification of the basal ganglia.

Diagnosis and differential diagnosis

Any baby with unexplained epilepsy should be examined with a Wood's light (p. 31) to look for ash leaf macules. Skull X-rays and CT scans help to exclude involvement of the central nervous system and kidneys. The lesions of adenoma sebaceum (a misnomer, as histologically they are angiofibromas) may be mistaken for acne.

Management

Affected families need genetic counselling. Apparently unaffected parents with an affected child will wish to know the chances of further children being affected. Before concluding that an affected child is the result of a new mutation, the parents should be examined with a Wood's light and by an ophthalmologist to help exclude the possibility of genetic transmission from a subtly affected parent.

Adenoma sebaceum improves cosmetically after electrodesiccation or destruction by laser but tends to recur.

Xeroderma pigmentosum

Xeroderma pigmentosum is a heterogeneous group of autosomal recessive disorders, characterized by the defective repair of DNA after its damage by ultraviolet radiation.

Cause

When a strand of DNA is damaged by UVR, thymine dimers are formed. A normal individual has the necessary enzymes (endonucleases and DNA polymerases) to remove the damaged segment of DNA, including the thymine dimer, to synthesize a new nucleotide sequence using the non-damaged complementary strand of DNA as a template, and to close the gap by rejoining the new sequence to the

Fig. 22.5 Xeroderma pigmentosum: obvious freckling on neck. Scars on nose mark the spots where tumours have been removed.

adjacent DNA. Deficiences or absence of these enzymes cause the various types of xeroderma pigmentosum.

Clinical features

There are many variants but all follow the same pattern:
- The skin is normal at birth.
- Multiple freckles, roughness and keratoses on exposed skin appear between the ages of six months and two years (Fig. 22.5). Photosensitivity increases thereafter.
- The atrophic facial skin shows telangiectases and small angiomas.
- Many tumours develop on light-damaged skin: these include basal cell carcinomas, squamous cell carcinomas, kerato-acanthomas and malignant melanomas.
- The eyes are affected in most patients. Problems include photophobia, conjunctivitis, and ectropion.
- The condition may be associated with microcephaly, mental deficiency, dwarfism, deafness and ataxia (de Sanctis–Caccione syndrome).

Diagnosis

This becomes evident on clinical grounds, though variants with minor signs may cause difficulty. The DNA repair defect can be detected in a few laboratories after the ultraviolet irradiation of cultured fibroblasts or lymphocytes from the patient.

Treatment

Skin cancers can be prevented by strict avoidance of sunlight, and the use of reflectant sunscreens and dark glasses. Early and complete removal of all tumours is essential. Radiotherapy should be avoided.

Incontinentia pigmenti

This rare condition is probably inherited as an X-linked dominant trait which is usually lethal in males. Ninety-five per cent of patients are female.

Clinical features

There are three stages in the evolution of the skin signs.

- *Vesicular.* Linear groups of blisters occur more on the limbs than trunk.
- *Warty.* After a few weeks the blisters dry up and the predominant lesions are papules with a verrucous hyperkeratotic surface.
- *Pigmented.* A whorled or 'splashed' macular pigmentation, ranging from slate-grey to brown, replaces the warty lesions. Its bizarre patterning is a strong diagnostic pointer.

Occasionally the vesicular and warty stages occur *in utero*; warty or pigmented lesions may therefore be the first signs of the condition. There is also a variant in which pale rather than dark whorls and streaks are seen.

Associated abnormalities are common. A quarter of the patients have defects of their central nervous system, most commonly mental retardation, epilepsy or microcephaly. Skull and palatal abnormalities may also be found. Delayed dentition, and even a total absence of teeth, are recognized features. The incisors may be cone- or peg-shaped. Ocular defects occur in a third of patients, the most common being strabismus, cataract and optic atrophy.

Diffential diagnosis

Diagnosis is usually made in infancy when bullous lesions predominate so the differential diagnosis includes bullous impetigo (p. 136), candidiasis (p. 160), and the rarer linear IgA bullous disease of childhood (p. 100) and epidermolysis bullosa (*see below*).

Investigations

There is frequently an eosinophilia in the blood. Biopsy of an intact blister reveals an intra-epidermal vesicle filled with eosinophils.

Management

This is symptomatic and includes measures to combat bacterial and candidal infection during the vesicular phase. Family counselling should be offered.

Epidermolysis bullosa

There are several types of epidermolysis bullosa; the five main ones are listed in Table 22.1. All are characterized by an inherited tendency to develop blisters after minimal trauma (Fig. 22.6). Acquired epidermolysis bullosa is not inherited and is discussed on p. 102.

Simple epidermolysis bullosa

This is the most common type; it may be so mild that medical advice is not sought or needed. Blisters appear on the feet and, less often, on the hands and other areas subject to friction. The problem is made

Table 22.1 Simplified classification of epidermolysis bullosa.

Type	Mode of inheritance
Simple epidermolysis bullosa	Autosomal dominant
Junctional epidermolysis bullosa (epidermolysis bullosa letalis)	Autosomal recessive
Dystrophic epidermolysis bullosa	Autosomal dominant
Dystrophic epidermolysis bullosa	Autosomal recessive
Acquired epidermolysis bullosa	Not inherited

Fig. 22.6 Level of blister in epidermolysis bullosa at the epidermal–dermal junction.

Fig. 22.7 Junctional epidermolysis bullosa; a baby with numerous large raw areas. The condition was fatal.

Fig. 22.8 Autosomal recessive dystrophic epidermolysis bullosa: note large-blood filled blister. Scarring has led to fixed deformity of the fingers and loss of nails.

worse by hyperhidrosis and ill-fitting footwear. The blisters heal like ordinary friction blisters, without scarring. The nails and oral mucosa are unaffected. Blisters are prevented by avoiding trauma, wearing soft, well-fitting shoes and reducing friction by using foot powders. Large blisters should be pricked with a sterile needle and dressed; their roofs should not be removed. Local antibiotics may be needed for infection.

Junctional epidermolysis bullosa
This rare and often lethal form is evident at birth. The newborn child shows large raw areas and flaccid blisters which are slow to heal (Fig. 22.7). The perioral and peri-anal skin is usually involved, as are the nails and oral mucous membrane. There is no effective treatment though systemic steroids and phenytoin are usually tried.

Autosomal dominant dystrophic epidermolysis bullosa
Blisters in this type appear in late infancy. They are most common on friction sites, e.g. knees, elbows and fingers. They heal with scarring, and with milia formation. The nails may be deformed or even lost. The mouth is not affected. The only treatment is to avoid trauma and to dress the blistered areas.

Autosomal recessive dystrophic epidermolysis bullosa
In this tragic form of epidermolysis bullosa, blisters

start in infancy. They are subepidermal, and may be filled with blood. They heal with scarring and this may be so severe that the nails are lost and webs form between the digits (Fig. 22.8). The hands and feet may become useless balls which have lost all of the fingers and toes. The teeth, mouth and upper part of the oesophagus are all affected; oesophageal strictures may form. Treatment is unsatisfactory but phenytoin, which reduces the raised dermal collagenase levels found in this variant, sometimes helps. Systemic steroids are disappointing. It is especially important to minimize trauma, to prevent contractures and web formation between the digits, and to combat secondary infection. Referral to centres with expertise in mangement of these patients is strongly recommended.

Ehlers–Danlos syndrome
Several collagen defects are responsible for this group of disorders: at least 10 types are now known.

Cause
There is clinical, genetic, and biochemical heterogeneity. Inheritance may be autosomal dominant, autosomal recessive or X-linked recessive. Single enzyme defects (e.g. deficiency of lysyl hydroxylase) are responsible for some types but the biochemical abnormality is not known in the majority.

Clinical features
• Elasticity of the skin.

Fig. 22.9 Ehlers–Danlos syndrome: showing hyperextensible joints and easy bruising.

- Hyperextensibility of the joints (Fig. 22.9).
- Fragility of skin and blood vessels.
- Easy bruising.
- Ugly ('papyraceous') scars.

Complications

These depend on the type. They include subluxation of joints, varicose veins in early life, an increased liability to develop hernias, kyphoscoliosis, aortic aneurysms, and ruptured large arteries, and intraocular haemorrhage. Affected individuals may be born prematurely as a result of early rupture of fragile fetal membranes.

Diagnosis and treatment

The diagnosis is made on the clinical features and family history. The frequent skin lacerations and prominent scars may suggest child abuse. The diagnosis and type can sometimes be confirmed by enzyme studies on isolated fibroblasts. There is no effective treatment but genetic counselling is needed.

Pseudo-xanthoma elasticum

Various defects in elastin, and probably collagen, are responsible for this condition of which at least four types are known.

Cause and pathology

Inheritance may be dominant or recessive. As yet no specific enzyme defects have been detected. The elastic fibres in the mid-dermis become swollen and fragmented; their calcification is probably a secondary feature. The elastic tissue of blood vessels and of the retina may also be affected.

Clinical features

The skin of the neck and axillae, and occasionally of other body folds, is loose and wrinkled. Groups of small yellow papules give these areas a 'plucked chicken' appearance. Breaks in the retina show as angioid streaks, which are grey, poorly defined areas radiating from the optic nerve head. Arterial involvement may lead to peripheral, coronary, or cerebral arterial insufficiency.

Complications

The most important are hypertension, recurrent gut haemorrhages, ischaemic heart disease and cerebral haemorrhage.

Diagnosis and treatment

The diagnosis is made clinically and confirmed by the histology. There is no effective treatment.

LEARNING POINT

The decision to have children, or not to do so, must lie with the family concerned. Make sure they have all the facts before them.

CHAPTER 23

DRUG ERUPTIONS

Drugs work by changing metabolic events. Sometimes they alter them for the worse: such an unwanted effect is a drug reaction. Sometimes these affect the skin and produce a rash. Almost any drug can cause a cutaneous reaction, and many inflammatory skin conditions can be caused or exacerbated by drugs. A drug reaction can reasonably be included in the differential diagnosis of most skin diseases.

Cause (Table 23.1)

Non-allergic drug reactions

Not all drug reactions are allergic. Some are due to overdosage, others to the accumulation of drugs, or to unwanted pharmacological effects, e.g. stretch marks from systemic steroids (Fig. 23.1). Other reactions are idiosyncratic (i.e. an odd reaction peculiar to one individual), or due to alterations of ecological balance (*see below*).

Cutaneous reactions can be expected from the very nature of some drugs. These are normal but unwanted responses. Patients show them when a drug is given in a high dose or even in a therapeutic dose. For example, mouth ulcers frequently occur as a result of the cytotoxicity of methotrexate. Silver-based preparations, given for prolonged periods, can lead to a slate-grey colour of the skin (argyria). Acute vaginal candidiasis occurs when antibiotics remove the normal resident bacteria from the female genital tract and foster colonization by yeasts. Dapsone or rifampicin, given to patients with lepromatous leprosy, may cause erythema nodosum leprosum as the immune response to the bacillus is re-established.

Non-allergic reactions are often predictable. They affect many, or even all, patients taking the drug at a sufficient dose for a sufficient time. Careful studies before marketing should indicate the types of reaction that can be anticipated.

Allergic drug reactions

Allergic drug reactions are less predictable. They occur in only a minority of patients receiving a drug and can do so even with low doses. Allergic reac-

Table 23.1 Some mechanisms involved in drug reactions.

Pharmacological
Due to overdosage or failure to excrete or metabolize
Cumulative effects
Altered skin ecology
Allergic
Idiosyncratic
Exacerbation of pre-existing skin conditions

Fig 23.1 Gross striae due to systemic steroids.

tions are not a normal biological effect of the drug and usually appear after the latent period required for an immune response. Chemically related drugs may cross-react.

Fortunately allergic drug reactions take up only a limited number of forms, namely urticaria and angioedema, vasculitis, erythema multiforme, or a morbilliform erythema. Rarer allergic reactions include bullae, erythroderma, pruritus, and toxic epidermal necrolysis.

Presentation

Some drugs and their reactions

Antibiotics
Penicillins and sulphonamides are among the most common drugs causing allergic reactions. These are often morbilliform (Fig. 23.2), but urticaria and erythema multiforme are common too. Viral infections are often associated with exanthems, and many rashes are incorrectly blamed on an antibiotic when, in fact, a virus was responsible. Most patients with infectious mononucleosis develop a morbilliform rash if ampicillin is administered. Penicillin is a common cause of severe anaphylactic reactions which may be life-threatening. Minocycline can accumulate in the tissues and produce a brown or grey colour in the mucosa, sun-exposed areas, or at sites of inflammation, as in the lesions of acne.

Penicillamine
Like penicillin itself, this can cause morbilliform

Fig 23.2 Symmetrical erythematous maculopapular rash due to ampicillin.

eruptions or urticaria, but the drug has also been incriminated as a cause of haemorrhagic bullae at sites of trauma, of the extrusion of elastic tissue through the skin, and of pemphigus.

Oral contraceptives
The frequency of reactions to these is less now that their hormonal content is small. The hair fall which may follow stopping the drug is like that seen after pregnancy (telogen effluvium) (p. 64). Hirsutism, erythema nodosum, acne, chloasma, and photosensitivity are other reactions.

Gold
This frequently causes rashes. Its side effects range from pruritus to morbilliform eruptions, to curious papulosquamous eruptions like pityriasis rosea, or lichen planus. Erythroderma, erythema nodosum, hair fall, and stomatitis may also be provoked by gold.

Steroids
Cutaneous side effects from systemic steroids include a ruddy face, cutaneous atrophy, striae (Fig. 23.1), hirsutism, and a susceptibility to cutaneous infections, which may be atypical.

Some common reactions and their causes

Toxic erythema
This vague term describes the most common type of drug eruption, sometimes looking like measles or scarlet fever, and sometimes with prominent urticarial (Fig. 23.3) or erythema multiforme-like elements. Itching and fever may accompany the rash. Culprits include antibiotics (especially ampicillin), sulphonamides and related compounds (diuretics and hypoglycaemics), barbiturates, phenylbutazone, and PAS.

Urticaria (Chapter 10)
Many drugs may cause this: salicylates are the most common, working non-immunologically as histamine releasers. Antibiotics are also often to blame. Dairy products may contain enough penicillin to affect patients known to be allergic to it. Insect repellants and nitrogen mustards can cause urticaria on contact. Urticaria may be part of a severe and gen-

Fig 23.3 Toxic erythema with urticarial features.

eralized reaction (anaphylaxis) which includes bronchospasm and collapse (Fig. 23.4).

Allergic vasculitis (Chapter 10)

The clinical changes range from urticarial papules, through palpable purpura, to necrotic ulcers. Erythema nodosum may occur. Sulphonamides, phenylbutazone, indomethacin, phenytoin, and oral contraceptives are among possible causes.

Erythema multiforme (Chapter 10)

Target-like lesions appear mainly on the extensor aspects of the limbs, and bullae may form. In the Stevens–Johnson syndrome the patients are often ill and the mucous membranes are severely affected. Sulphonamides, barbiturates, and phenylbutazone are known offenders.

Purpura

Clinical features are seldom distinctive apart from the itchy, brown petechial rash on dependent areas that was characteristic of carbromal reactions. Thrombocytopenia and coagulation defects should be excluded (Chapter 13). Thiazides, sulphonamides, phenylbutazone, sulphonylureas, barbiturates, and quinine are among the drugs reported to cause purpura.

Bullous eruptions

Some of the reactions noted above may become bullous. Bullae may also develop at pressure sites in drug-induced coma.

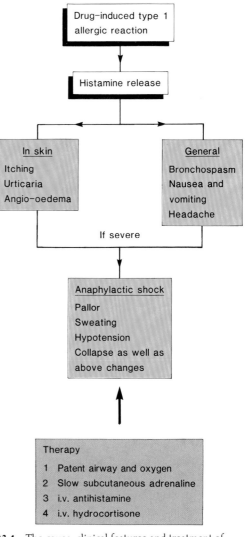

Fig 23.4 The cause, clinical features and treatment of anaphylaxis.

Eczema

This is not a common pattern and occurs mainly when patients sensitized by topical application are given the drug systemically. Penicillin, sulphomamides, neomycin, phenothiazines, and local anaesthetics should be considered.

Exfoliative dermatitis

The entire skin surface becomes red and scaly. This can be caused by drugs (particularly phenylbutazone, PAS, isoniazid and gold), but can also be due to a widespread attack of skin diseases such as psoriasis and eczema.

Fig 23.5 Fixed drug eruption due to barbiturates; unusually severe bullous reaction.

Fig 23.6 Note sparing of skin creases and area shielded by spectacle frames in this patient with pigmentation from a phenothiazine drug.

Fixed drug eruptions

Round, erythematous or purple and sometimes bullous plaques recur at the same site each time the drug is taken (Fig. 23.5). Phenolphthalein (in some purgatives), barbiturates, sulphonamides, quinine or tetracycline may be responsible. Pigmentation persists between acute episodes.

Acneiform eruptions

Lithium, iodides, bromides, oral contraceptives, androgenic or glucocorticosteroids, antituberculosis and anticonvulsant therapy may cause an acneiform rash (Chapter 14).

Lichenoid eruptions

These resemble lichen planus (Chapter 7), but not always very closely, as mouth lesions are uncommon and as scaling and eczematous elements may be seen. Consider antimalarials, gold, phenothiazines, and PAS.

Toxic epidermal necrolysis (p. 139)

In adults this 'scalded skin' appearance is usually drug-induced (e.g. barbiturates, phenylbutazone, oxyphenbutazone, phenytoin, or penicillin).

Hair loss

This is a predictable side effect of etretinate and cytotoxic agents, an unpredictable response to some anticoagulants, and sometimes seen with antithyroid drugs. Diffuse hair loss may occur during, or just after, the use of an oral contraceptive.

Hypertrichosis

This is a dose-dependent effect of diazoxide, minoxidil, and cyclosporin A.

Pigmentation

Chloasma (p. 186) may follow an oral contraceptive plus sun exposure. Large doses of phenothiazines impart a blue-grey colour to exposed areas (Fig. 23.6); heavy metals can cause a generalized browning; and mepacrine turns the skin yellow.

Photosensitivity

This is dealt with in Chapter 17. Always exclude the common drug causes (thiazides, tetracyclines, phenothiazines, sulphonamides, psoralens, or nalidixic acid).

Xerosis

The skin can become rough and scaly in patients receiving oral retinoids, nicotinic acid or lithium.

Exacerbation of pre-existing skin conditions

Psoriasis and acne are good examples of this. Psoriasis may be made worse by giving beta-blockers, antimalarials, or lithium. Acne may be exacerbated by androgens, anticonvulsants, and lithium.

Course

The different types of reaction vary so much that a

brief summary is not possible. In previously exposed patients the common toxic erythema reaction may start 2–3 days after the administration of the drug. If such a reaction occurs during the first course of treatment, the eruption characteristically begins later, often coming up at about the ninth day or even after the drug has been stopped. The speed with which a drug eruption clears depends on the type of reaction and the rapidity with which the drug is eliminated.

Differential diagnosis

The differential diagnosis ranges over the whole subject of dermatology depending on which disease is mimicked. For instance, toxic erythema reactions can look very like measles, pityriasis rosea, or even secondary syphilis. The general rule is never to forget the possibility of a drug eruption when an atypical rash is seen. Six vital questions should be asked (Table 23.2).

Table 23.2 The six vital questions to be asked when a drug eruption is suspected.

1. Can you exclude a simple dermatosis (such as scabies or psoriasis) and known skin manifestations of an underlying disorder (e.g. systemic lupus erythematosus)?

2. Does the rash itself suggest a drug eruption (e.g. symmetrical, perhaps with unusual features)?

3. Does a past history of drug reactions correlate with current prescriptions?

4. Was any drug introduced a few days before the eruption appeared?

5. Which of the current drugs most commonly cause drug eruptions, e.g. penicillins, sulphonamides, thiazides, allopurinol, phenylbutazone, etc?

6. Does the eruption fit with a well-recognized pattern caused by one of the current drugs?

Treatment

The first approach is to withdraw the suspected drug, accepting that several drugs may need to be stopped at the same time. This is not always easy. Sometimes a drug is necessary and there is no alternative available. At other times the patient may be taking many drugs and it is difficult to know which one to stop. The decision to stop or continue a drug depends upon the nature of the drug, the severity of the reaction, its potential reversibility, and the probability that the drug is actually causing the reaction.

Assessment depends upon clinical detective work (Table 23.2). Judgements must be based on probabilities and common sense. Every effort must be made to correlate the onset of the rash with prescription records. Often, but not always, the latest drug to be introduced is the most likely culprit. Prick tests and *in vitro* tests for allergy are still too unreliable to be of value. Re-administration, as a diagnostic test, is usually unwise except when no suitable alternative drug exists.

Non-specific therapy depends upon the type of eruption. In urticaria, antihistamines are helpful. In some reactions, topical or systemic corticosteroids can be used, and applications of calamine lotion may be soothing.

Anaphylactic reactions require special treatment to ensure that the airway is not compromised (e.g. oxygen, assisted respiration or even emergency tracheostomy). One or more subcutaneous injections of adrenaline (epinephrine) (1:1000) 0.3–0.5 ml should be given slowly subcutaneously in adults before the slow (over 1 minute) intravenous injection of chlorpheniramine maleate (10–20 mg diluted in syringe with 5–10 ml of blood). Although the action of intravenous hydrocortisone (100 mg) is delayed for several hours it should be given to prevent further deterioration in severely affected patients.

To re-emphasize, the most important treatment is to stop the responsible drug.

LEARNING POINTS

1. This whole chapter is a warning against polypharmacy. Do your patients really need all the drugs they are taking?
2. Avoid provocation tests unless there are very strong indications for them.

CHAPTER 24

DERMATOLOGICAL THERAPY

An accurate diagnosis, based on a proper history and examination (Chapter 4), must come before rational treatment can be chosen; and even when a firm diagnosis has been reached, each patient must be treated as an individual. For some, no treatment may even be the best treatment especially when the disorder is cosmetic or if the treatments are dangerous. A patient with minimal psoriasis, for example, may be helped more by careful explanation and reassurance than by prescriptions.

If a diagnosis cannot be reached, the doctor has to decide whether a specialist opinion is needed, or whether it is best to observe the rash for a while and treat it perhaps with a bland application. In either case, the indiscriminate use of topical steroids or other medications, in the absence of a working diagnosis, often confuses the picture and may render the future diagnosis more difficult.

Usually, however, a firm diagnosis can be made, and a sensible course of treatment can be planned; but even then results are often better when patients understand their disease and the reason behind their treatment. The cause and nature of their disease should be explained carefully, in language which they can understand, and they must be told what can realistically be expected of their treatment. False optimism or undue pessimism, by patients or doctors, leads only to an unsound relationship. Too often patients become discontented, not because they do not know the correct diagnosis but because they have not been told enough about its cause or prognosis. Even worse, they may have little idea of how to use the treatment and what to expect of it; poor compliance often follows poor instruction. As treatment may be complex,

instruction sheets are helpful; they reinforce the spoken word and answer unasked questions.

The principal steps in diagnosis and management are:
- History.
- Examination.
- Investigations.
- Diagnosis.
- Explanation of condition, its cause and prognosis.
- Choice of treatment and instructions about it.
- Discussion of expectations.
- Follow-up, if necessary.

LEARNING POINT

One correct diagnosis is worth a hundred therapeutic trials.

Therapeutic options

Some of the treatments used in dermatology are listed in Table 24.1.

Topical versus systemic therapy

The great advantage of topical therapy is that drugs are delivered directly where they are needed at an optimum concentration to the target organ. Systemic side effects from absorption are less than those expected from the same drug given systemically: with topical treatment vital organs such as the marrow,

Table 24.1 Therapeutic options in dermatology.

Drugs	Topical
	Systemic
Physical	Surgical
	excision
	curettage
	Electrodesiccation
	Cryotherapy
	Radiotherapy
	Phototherapy
	Destruction by laser

liver and kidneys are exposed to lower drug concentrations than is the skin. However, topical treatment is often messy, time-consuming and incomplete, and takes time to apply, whereas systemic treatment is clean and quick and uniform over the entire skin surface. Cost must also be considered.

Some drugs can only be used topically (e.g. gamma-benzene hexachloride for scabies and mupirocin for bacterial infections), while others work only systemically (e.g. dapsone for dermatitis herpetiformis and griseofulvin for fungal infections).

When a choice exists, and both possibilities are equally effective, then local treatment is usually preferred. Most cases of pityriasis versicolor, for example, respond to topical antifungals alone so systemic ketoconazole is not the treatment of choice.

Topical treatment

Percutaneous absorption
Drugs used on the skin must be dissolved or suspended in bases (vehicles). The choice of drug and of the base are both important and depend on the diagnosis and the state of the skin. For a drug to be effective topically it must pass the barrier to diffusion presented by the horny layer (Chapter 2). This requires the drug to be transferred from its base to the horny layer, from which it will diffuse through the epidermis into the papillary dermis. Passage through the horny layer is the rate-limiting step.

The transfer of a drug from its base to the horny layer depends on its relative solubility in each (measured as the 'partition co-efficient'). Movement across the horny layer depends upon both the concentration gradient and on restricting forces (its 'diffusion constant'). In general, non-polar substances penetrate more rapidly than polar ones. A rise in skin temperature and in hydration, both achieved by covering a treated area with polyethylene occlusion, encourages penetration.

Some areas of skin present less of a barrier than do others. Two extreme examples are palmar skin, with its impermeable, thick horny layer, and scrotal skin, which is thin and highly permeable. The skin of the face is more permeable than the skin of the body. Body fold skin is more permeable than nearby unoccluded skin. In humans, absorption through the hair follicles and sweat ducts is of little significance and the amount of hair on the treated site is no guide to its permeability.

In many skin diseases the horny layer becomes abnormal, and loses some of its barrier function. The abnormal nucleated (parakeratotic) horny layer of psoriasis and chronic eczema, though thicker than normal, has lost much of its protective qualities. Water loss is increased and therapeutic agents penetrate more readily. Similarly, breakdown of the horny layer by chemicals (e.g. soaps and detergents), and by physical injury, will allow the more rapid penetration of drugs.

In summary, the penetration of a drug through the skin depends on the following factors:
- Its concentration.
- The base.
- Its partition co-efficient.
- Its diffusion constant.
- The thickness of the horny layer.
- The state, including hydration, of the horny layer.
- Temperature.

Active ingredients
These include corticosteroids, tar, dithranol, antibiotics, antifungal and antiviral agents, benzoyl peroxide, retinoic acid and many others (Formulary, p. 245). The choice depends on the action required, and the prescriber should know how each works. As topical steroids are the mainstay of much local

Table 24.2 The pharmacology of topical steroid applications.

Active constituents	Include hydrocortisone and synthetic halogenated derivatives Halogenation increases activity	
Bases	Available in lotions, creams, ointments, sprays and tapes	
Penetration	Readily penetrate via the horny layer and appendages Form a reservoir in the horny layer Polyethylene occlusion and high concentrations increase penetration	
Metabolism	Some minor metabolism in epidermis and dermis (e.g. hydrocortisone conversion to cortisone and other metabolites) Leave skin via dermal vascular plexus and enter general metabolic pool of steroids Further metabolism in liver	
Excretion	As sulphate esters and glucuronides	
Actions	Anti-inflammatory	1 Vasoconstrict 2 Decrease permeability of dermal vessels 3 Decrease phagocytic migration and activity 4 Decrease fibrin formation 5 Decrease kinin formation 6 Inhibit phospholipase A_2 activity and decrease products of arachidonic acid metabolism 7 Depress fibroblastic activity 8 Stabilize lysosomal membranes
	Immunosuppressive	Antigen–antibody interaction unaffected but inflammatory consequences lessened (above mechanisms and by inhibiting release of cytokines) Lympholytic
	Decrease epidermal proliferation	
Side effects	1 Thinning of epidermis 2 Thinning of dermis 3 Telangiectasia and striae (due to **1** and **2**) 4 Bruising (due to **2** and vessel wall fragility) 5 Hirsutism 6 Folliculitis and acneiform eruptions 7 May worsen or disguise infections (bacterial, viral and fungal) 8 Systemic absorption (rare but may be important in infants, when applied in large quantities under polyethylene pants) 9 Tachyphylaxis — lessening of clinical effect with the same preparation 10 Rebound — worsening, sometimes dramatic on withdrawing treatment	
Uses	Eczema, psoriasis in a few instances (facial, flexural, and palms/soles) Many non-infective pruritic dermatoses	

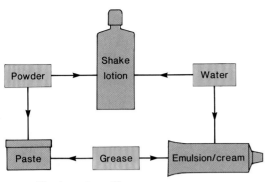

Fig. 24.1 The derivation of bases.

dermatological therapy their pharmacology is summarized in Table 24.2.

Bases (vehicles)

Most bases are a mixture of powders, water and greases (usually obtained from petroleum). Figure 24.1 shows that blending these bases together produces preparations which retain the characteristics of each of their components.

A base should maximize the delivery of topical drugs but it may also have useful properties in its own right. Used carelessly bases may even do harm. Suggested indications are shown in Table 24.3. The choice of base depends upon the action desired, availability, messiness, ease of application, and cost.

Table 24.3 Bases and their properties.

Base	Used on	Effect	Points of note
Dusting powders	Flexures (may be slightly moist)	Lessen friction	If too wet clump and irritate
Alcohol-based applications	Scalp	Clean vehicle for steroid application	Cosmetically elegant, does not gum up hair May sting raw areas
Watery and shake lotions	Acutely inflamed skin (wet and oozing)	Drying, soothing and cooling	Tedious to apply Frequent changes (lessened by polyethylene occlusion) Powder in shake lotions may clump
Creams	Both moist and dry skin	Cooling, emollient and moisturizing	Short shelf life Fungal and bacterial growth in base Sensitivities to preservatives and emulsifying agents
Ointments	Dry and scaly skin	Occlusive and emollient	Messy to apply, soils clothing Removed with an oil
Pastes	Dry, lichenified and scaly skin	Protective and emollient	Messy and tedious to apply (linen or calico needed) Most protective if applied properly
Sprays	Weeping, acutely inflamed skin Scalp	Drying, non-occlusive	Vehicle evaporates rapidly No need to touch skin to treat it
Gels	Face and scalp	Vehicle for steroids, salicylic acid and tretinoin	May sting when applied to inflamed skin Can be covered by make-up

Individual bases

Dusting powders are used in the folds to lessen friction between opposing surfaces. They may repel water (for example, talc) or absorb it (for example, starch); zinc oxide powder has an absorptive power midway between these extremes. Powders ought not to be used in moist areas where they tend to cake and abrade.

Watery lotions evaporate and cool inflamed areas. This effect is hastened by adding an alcohol, but glycerol or arachis oil slow evaporation and retain skin moisture. Substances which precipitate protein (astringents), for example silver nitrate, lessen exudation.

Shake lotions are watery lotions to which powder has been added so that the area for evaporation is increased. These lotions dry wet, weeping skin. When water has evaporated from the skin, the powder particles clump together and may become abrasive. This is less likely if an oil such as glycerol has been added.

Creams are used for their cooling, moisturizing, and emollient effects. They are either oil-in-water emulsions (e.g. aqueous cream [U.K.], acid mantle cream [U.S.A.]) or water-in-oil emulsions (e.g. oily cream [U.K.], cold cream [U.S.A.]). Emulsifying agents are added to increase the surface area of the dispersed phase and that of any therapeutic agent in it.

Ointments are used for their occlusive and emollient properties. They allow the skin to remain supple by preventing the evaporation of water from the horny layer. There are three main types: those which are water-soluble (macrogols, polyethylene glycols); those which emulsify with water; and those which repel water (mineral oils, and animal and vegetable fats).

Pastes are used for their protective and emollient properties and usually are made of powder added to a mineral oil or grease. The powder lessens the oil's occlusive effect.

Variations on these themes have led to the numerous topical preparations available today. Rather than use them all, and risk confusion, doctors should limit their choice to one or two from each category; Table 24.3 summarizes the properties and uses of some common preparations.

Methods of application

Ointments and creams are usually applied sparingly twice daily, but the frequency of application will depend on many factors including the nature, severity and duration of the rash, the sites involved, convenience and, most important, common sense.

Three techniques of application are more specialized: immersion therapy by bathing, wet dressings (compresses), and occlusive therapy.

Baths

Once-daily bathing helps to remove crusts, scales and medications. After soaking for about ten minutes, the skin should be rubbed gently with a sponge, flannel or soft cloth; cleaning may be made easier by soaps, oils, or colloidal oatmeal.

Medicated baths are occasionally helpful, the most common ingredients added to the bath water being bath oils, antiseptics, and solutions of coal tar.

After cleaning, the most important function of a bath is hydration. The skin absorbs water and this can be held in the skin for some time if an occlusive ointment is applied after bathing.

Older patients may need help to get into a bath and should be warned about falling if the bath contains an oil or another slippery substance.

Wet dressings (compresses)

These are used to clean the skin or to deliver a topical medication. They are especially helpful for weeping, crusting, and purulent conditions. Five or six layers of soft cloth (e.g. cotton gauze) are soaked in the solution to be used; this may be tap water, saline, an astringent or antiseptic solution, and the compress is then applied to the skin. Open dressings allow the water to evaporate and the skin to cool. They should be changed frequently, for example every 15 minutes for an hour.

Closed dressings are covered with a plastic (usually polyethylene) sheet; they do not dry out so quickly and are usually changed twice daily. They are especially helpful for debriding adherent crusts and for draining exudative and purulent ulcers.

Occlusive therapy

Sometimes steroid-sensitive dermatoses (e.g. psoriasis) will respond to a steroid only when it is applied under a plastic sheet to encourage penetration. This technique is best reserved for the short-term treatment of stubborn, localized rashes. The drawback of this treatment is that the side effects of topical steroid treatment (Table 24.2) are highly likely to occur. The most important is systemic absorption if a large surface area of skin, relative to body weight, is treated (e.g. when steroids are applied under polyethylene pants to infants).

Monitoring local treatment

One common fault is to underestimate the amount required. The guidelines given in Table 24.4 and Figure 24.2 are based on twice daily applications. Lotions go further than creams, which go further than ointments and pastes.

LEARNING POINT

You know how much digoxin your patients are taking, but do you know how much local steroid they are applying? Keep a check on this.

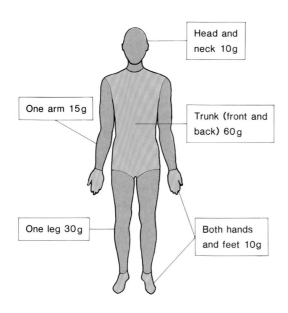

Fig. 24.2 The minimum amount of a cream required in one week by an adult applying it twice daily.

Table 24.4 Minimum amount of cream (g) required for twice-daily application for one week.

Age	Whole body	Trunk	Both arms and legs
6 months	35	15	20
4 years	60	20	35
8 years	90	35	50
12 years	120	45	65
Adult (70 kg male)	170	60	90

Systemic therapy

Systemic treatment is needed if a skin condition is associated with systemic disease, or if the medicament of choice is inactive topically (for example, griseofulvin). The principles of systemic therapy in dermatology are no different from those in other branches of medicine. Some drugs act specifically; others non-specifically. For example, antihistamines (H1 blockers) act specifically in urticaria, and non-specifically, by a sedative effect, on the most common skin symptom — itch.

Systemic disease co-exists with skin disease in several ways (Chapter 20). Sometimes a systemic disease such as systemic lupus erythematosus may cause a rash; at other times, a skin disease causes a systemic upset. Examples of this are the depression, which occurs in some patients affected with severe rashes, and high-output cardiac failure, which may occur in exfoliative dermatitis from the shunting of blood through the skin. A systemic upset due to skin disease can be treated with drugs designed for such problems while the skin is being treated in other ways.

Physical forms of therapy

The skin is also accessible to treatment by surgery, freezing, burning, ultraviolet radiation, and laser cautery. As the population grows older, and more concerned by appearance, requests for minor surgery become more common. Some broad principles will be discussed here.

Surgical

The indications for biopsy, and the techniques employed, are described in Chapter 4.

Shave excision. Many small lesions are removed by simply shaving them off at their bases with a scalpel under local anaesthesia. Although simple, the procedure may leave some cells at the base and these, in the case of tumours, may lead to recurrence.

Excision under local anaesthetic, using an aseptic technique, is another way to remove small tumours. The lesion must be examined carefully and important underlying structures (e.g. the temporal artery) noted. If possible the incision should run along the line of a skin crease, especially on the face. If necessary, charts or pictures of standard skin creases should be consulted. After injection of the local anaesthetic (usually 1 or 2% lignocaine [lidocaine, U.S.A] with or without 1 in 200 000 adrenaline [epinephrine]), the lesion is excised as an ellipse with a margin of normal skin which varies with the nature of the lesion and the site. The scalpel should be held perpendicular to the skin surface and the incision should reach the subcutaneous fat. The ellipse of skin is carefully removed with the help of a skin hook or fine-toothed forceps. Larger wounds, and those where the scar is likely to stretch (e.g. on the back), are closed in layers with absorbable sutures (e.g. dexon) before apposing the skin edges with non-absorbable interrupted or continuous subcuticular sutures such as nylon or prolene. Stitches are removed from the face in 4–5 days and from the trunk and limbs in 7–14 days. Artificial sutures (e.g. Steristrip) may be used to take the tension off the wound edges after the stitches have been taken out.

Curettage under local anaesthetic is used to treat benign exophytic lesions (e.g. seborrhoeic keratoses) and, combined with electrodesiccation (*see below*), to treat some basal cell carcinomas. Its main advantage over purely destructive treatment is that histological examination can be carried out on the curettings. A sharp curette is used to scrape off the lesion and haemostasis is achieved by electrocautery or electrodesiccation. The wound heals by secondary intention over 2–3 weeks, with good cosmetic results in most cases.

When a basal cell carcinoma is treated, the curette is scraped carefully and firmly along the sides and bottom of the tumour (the surrounding dermis is tougher and more resistant to curettage than the carcinoma) and the bleeding wound bed is then electrodesiccated. The process is repeated once or twice at the same session to ensure that all of the tumour has been removed or destroyed. With experience and regular follow up the cure rate is good.

Microscopically controlled excision is useful to treat:
- A basal cell carcinoma with a poorly defined edge.
- A recurrent basal cell carcinoma.
- A basal cell carcinoma lying where excessive margins of skin cannot be sacrificed to achieve complete removal of the tumour (e.g. one near the eye).
- Basal cell carcinomas in areas with a high incidence of recurrence such as the nose, glabella, or nasolabial folds.
- Occasional tumours other than basal cell carcinomas.

This form of surgery is time-consuming and expensive, but the probability of cure is greater than with excision or curettage. First the tumour is removed with a narrow margin. The excised specimen is then marked at the edges, mapped, and, after rapid histological processing, is immediately examined in horizontal and vertical section. If the tumour extends to any margin, further tissue is removed from the appropriate place, based on the markings and mappings, and again checked histologically. This process is repeated until clearance has been proved histologically at all margins. The resulting wound may then be closed directly, covered with a split skin graft or allowed to heal by secondary intention.

Electrosurgery

This is often combined with curettage, under local anaesthesia, to treat skin tumours. The main types are shown in Figure 24.3.

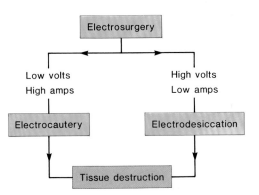

Fig. 24.3 Types of electrosurgery.

Cryotherapy

Liquid nitrogen (-196°C) is now used more often than carbon dioxide snow ('dry ice', -79°C). It is effective for viral warts, seborrhoeic keratoses, actinic keratoses and some superficial skin tumours (e.g. intra-epidermal carcinoma and lentigo maligna). It is applied either on a cotton bud or with a special spray gun. The lesion is frozen until it turns white, with a 1–2 mm halo of freezing around. Two freeze–thaw cycles kill tissue more effectively than one but are usually unnecessary for warts and keratoses. Standard freeze–thaw times have been established for superficial tumours but temperature probes in and around deep tumours are needed to gauge the degree of freezing for their effective treatment. A single application of a very potent local steroid, after thawing, lessens post-treatment pain and may prevent blistering. A crust, including the necrotic tumour, should slough off after about two weeks.

Radiotherapy

Superficial radiation therapy (50–100 kV) is often used to treat biopsy-proven skin cancers in those over 60 years old or who are too frail to tolerate surgery. Three thousand cGy is the usual dose, given in fractions over 5–10 days. The scars from radiotherapy worsen with time, in contrast to surgical scars which improve. Nowadays radiotherapy is seldom used for inflammatory conditions.

Phototherapy

UVR helps some conditions, for example psoriasis, parapsoriasis, pityriasis rosea, mycosis fungoides, and acne. For psoriasis, UVB may be given 3–5 times weekly, for 3–8 weeks, on its own or combined with tar (Goeckerman) treatment or dithranol (anthralin) (Ingram) treatment (Chapter 6). After tests to establish a starting dose, irradiance is increased by small increments, aiming to produce minimal erythema only after 24 hours. UVA is combined with psoralens in PUVA treatment (p. 52). Close supervision is needed to avoid side effects such as severe erythema. A careful record should be kept of the cumulative UVR dose.

Laser therapy

Lasers, *L*ight *A*mplification by the *S*timulated *E*mission of *R*adiation, are now being used to treat many skin lesions including capillary haemangiomas, tattoos, epidermal naevi, seborrhoeic keratoses, warts, and tumours. Although laser technology is advancing rapidly and many types of laser are available for clinical use, the full potential of laser therapy has not yet been exploited.

FORMULARY:
1. TOPICAL TREATMENTS

Our selection has been determined by personal preferences and we accept that we have left out many effective remedies. However, the preparations listed here are those which we use most often. As a result some products appear only in the U.K. column but not in the U.S.A. one, and vice versa.

Type of preparation and general comments	U.K. preparations	U.S.A. preparations
Emollients These are used to make dry scaly skin smoother. Most are best applied after a shower or bath	Soft white paraffin Emulsifying ointment Aqueous cream — can be used as a soap substitute E45 cream (Crookes Products) — contains lanolin Oilatum cream (Stiefel) Unguentum merck (E. Merck) — a useful diluent: contains propylene glycol and sorbic acid, which may sentitize Aquadrate cream (Norwich Eaton) — contains urea Calmurid cream (Pharmacia) — contains urea	Petrolatum alba (USP) Aquaphor (Beiersdorf) Eucerin (Beiersdorf) Lubriderm (Warner-Lambert) Cold Cream (USP) Complex 15 (Baker/Cummins) Carmol range (Syntex) — contains urea Nutraplus (Owen) — contains urea Lacticare (Stiefel) — contains lactic acid LacHydrin lotion (Westwood) — contains ammonium lactate
Bath additives These are a useful way of ensuring application to the whole skin. Most contain emollients which help dry itchy skin. Others contain tar (*see* section on psoriasis) or antibacterials	Balneum bath oil (E. Merck) Oilatum emollient (Stiefel) Ster-Zac concentrate (Hough) — contains antibacterial triclosan	Alpha Keri (Westwood) Lobana (Ulmer) Oilated Aveeno (Rydelle) — contains colloidal oatmeal, mineral oil
Shampoos All contain detergents which help to remove debris and scales; some have added ingredients to combat psoriasis, seborrhoeic eczema and bacterial infections. Most work best if their lather is left on the scalp for five minutes before being rinsed off	*Containing tar* Alphosyl shampoo (Stafford-Miller) Polytar liquid (Stiefel) T-Gel shampoo (Neutrogena)	*Containing tar* Pentrax (GenDerm) Sebutone (Westwood) T-Gel (Neutrogena) Denorex (Whitehall) Ionil-T (Owen)

Type of preparation and general comments	U.K. preparations	U.S.A. preparations
Shampoos continued	*Others* Betadine shampoo solution (Napp) — contains antibacterial povidone iodine Ceanel concentrate shampoo (Quinoderm) — contains cetrimide, undecenoic acid Selsun shampoo (Abbott) — contains selenium sulphide and can be used to treat pityriasis versicolor (p. 162) Nizoral shampoo – contains ketoconazole and is useful for seborrhoeic dermatitis	*Others* Capitrol (Westwood) — contains chloroxine (may stain hair yellow) Ionil Plus (Owen) — contains salicylic acid Head and Shoulders (Procter & Gamble) — contains zinc pyrithione Selsun shampoo (Abbott) — contains selenium sulphide
Cleansing agents These are used to remove debris and to combat infection. Some are astringents which precipitate protein and in doing so help to seal the moist surface of a weeping eczema or a stasis ulcer	Normasol (Schering) — 0.9% solution of sodium chloride used to clean wounds and ulcers Permitabs (Bioglan) — one tablet in four litres water makes 0.01% solution of potassium permanganate (will stain clothing and skin) Aluminium acetate lotion — use at 0.65% in water. Mildly astringent and used as wet dressing Cetavlon solution (ICI) — contains 40% cetrimide (detergent/antibacterial) and has to be diluted to 1% Hibitane 5% concentrate (ICI) — use diluted to one in 100, i.e. a 0.05% solution of chlorhexidine in water for skin disinfection Roccal (Winthrop) — contains 1% benzalkonium chloride. Use diluted one in 10 or one in 100	Normal saline Cetaphil lotion (Owen) — a non-lipid soap substitute Domeboro tablets or powder (Miles) — contains aluminium sulphate, calcium acetate Acetic acid — 0.125–0.25% or one part white vinegar to 20 parts water Sodium hypochlorite — 0.25% in water (Dakin's solution)
Barrier preparations These are used to protect the skin from iritants and are of value in the napkin or nappy area and around stomas. Many contain the silicone, dimethicone. The choice of barrier creams for use at work depends upon individual circumstances: recommendations are not given here	Dimethicone cream Zinc and castor oil ointment Conotrane cream (Boehringer-Ingelheim) — contains dimethicone, benzalkonium Siopel cream (Care) — contains dimethicone and cetrimide Thovaline ointment (Ilon) — contains zinc oxide, kaolin, talc Timodine cream (R & C) — contains dimethicone, hydrocortisone, nystatin, benzalkonium Vasogen cream (Pharmax) — contains dimethicone, calamine, zinc oxide	Zinc oxide paste (USP) Kerodex range (Ayerst) pH Stabil (Hermal) Desitin ointment (Leeming) — contains zinc oxide, vitamins A and D, cod liver oil

Type of preparation and general comments	U.K. preparations	U.S.A. preparations
Camouflaging preparations Blemishes which cannot be removed can often be made less obvious by covering them: expert cosmetic advice may be needed to obtain the best colour match	Boots Covering cream (Boots) Covermark range of products (Stiefel) Keromask masking creams and finishing powder (Innoxa)	Covermark range (O'Leary) Dermablend (Dermablend Cosmetics) Liquimat acne coverup (Owen/Allercreme) Vitadye (Elder) — vitiligo stain

Sunscreens and sunblocks
These help the light-sensitive but are not a substitute for sun avoidance and sensible protective clothing. The sun protection factor (SPF) is a measure of their effectiveness, which is greater against UVB than UVA
 	
Allergic contact dermatitis from the sunscreen ingredients (usually PABA esters) may be missed and the rash put down to a deterioration of the original photosensitivity
	Contains PABA:
	    Spectroban 15 lotion (Stiefel)
	Contains cinnamate:
	    RoC Total Sunblock cream 15 A + B
	Contains cinnamate and oxybenzone:
	    Piz Buin cream No 12 (Colson & Key)
		Contain PABA or PABA ester:
		    PreSun (Westwood)
		    Sundown (Johnson & Johnson)
		    Supershade (Plough)
		    Eclipse (Dorsey)
		Contains benzophenone:
		    Solbar (Person & Covey)
		Sunblock creams:
		    RVPaque (Elder)
		    Zinc oxide paste
		Lip sunscreens:
		    Chapstick Sunblock (Robins)
		    PreSun Stick (Westwood)

Antipruritics Remember that these are of limited value: try to make a firm diagnosis which will lead to an effective line of treatment	Calamine lotion Calamine lotion, oily — contains arachis oil Menthol (0.5%) or phenol (1.0%) in aqueous cream Eurax cream and lotion (Ciba Consumer) — contains crotamiton; also used to treat scabies	Calamine lotion Prax (Ferndale) — contains pramoxine Sarna lotion (Stiefel) — contains menthol, phenol, camphor Tucks (Parke - Davis) — contains glycerin, witch hazel Eurax cream and lotion (Westwood)
Antiperspirants The most effective preparations for excessive sweating in the armpits are those which contain aluminium chloride hexahydrate in an alcohol base (p. 133). They also help palmar sweating but to a lesser extent	Anhydrol forte solution (Dermal) — contains 20% aluminium chloride hexahydrate Driclor solution (Stiefel) — contains 20% aluminium chloride hexahydrate	Xerac AC (Person & Covey) — contains 6.5% aluminium chloride hexahydrate Drysol (Person & Covey) — contains 20% aluminium chloride hexahydrate
Keratolytics These are used to counter an excessive production of keratin. Salicylic acid preparations should be used for limited areas only and not above 6%, as absorption and toxicity may follow their prolonged and extensive application, especially in infants	Salicylic acid, 2–4% in emulsifying ointment or soft white paraffin Keralyt gel (Bristol Myers) — contains 6% salicylic acid; used mostly for scalp psoriasis Urea preparations (*see* Emollients)	Salicylic acid, 2–4% in petrolatum alba (USP) Keralyt gel (Westwood) Urea preparations (*see* Emollients)

Type of preparation and general comments	U.K. preparations	U.S.A. preparations
Steroids Our selection here has had to be ruthless as so many brands and mixtures are now on the market. Conventionally, they are classified according to their potency: your aim should be to use the least potent preparation which will cope with the skin disorder being treated. Side effects and dangers are listed in Table 24.2 (p. 238) Nothing stronger than 1% hydrocortisone should be used on the face (except in special circumstances, e.g. discoid LE) or in infancy. Be reluctant to prescribe more than 200 g of a mildly potent, 50 g of a moderately potent, or 30 g of a potent preparation per week for any adult for more than a month Most of the preparations listed are available as lotions, creams, oily creams, and ointments; your choice of vehicle will depend upon the condition under treatment (p. 239)	*Mildly potent* Hydrocortisone 0.5%, 1.0%, 2.5% (numerous manufacturers) Modrasone (Kirby-Warrick) Mildison Lipocream (Brocades) *Moderately potent* Eumovate (Glaxo) Stiedex L.P. (Stiefel) Ultradil (Schering) *Potent* Betnovate (Glaxo) Locoid (Brocades) Synalar (ICI) *Very potent* Dermovate (Glaxo) Halciderm (Squibb) Nerisone forte (Schering)	*Mildly potent* Hydrocortisone 0.5%, 1.0%, 2.5% (numerous manufacturers) Tridesilon 0.05% (Miles) *Moderately potent* Kenalog (Squibb) Aristocort (Lederle) Valisone (Schering) Westcort (Westwood) *Potent* Lidex (Syntex) Halog (Princeton) Diprosone (Schering) *Very potent* Diprolene (Schering) Temovate (Glaxo)

Steroid combinations:

With clioquinol (antiseptic)	*Mildly potent* Barquinol HC (Fisons) Vioform hydrocortisone (Zyma) *Potent* Betnovate-C (Glaxo) Locoid-C (Brocades) Synalar-C (ICI)	*Mildly potent* Vioform-HC (Ciba)
With antibiotics	*Mildly potent* Terra-Cortril (Pfizer) — with oxytetracycline Hydroderm (M.S.D.) — with neomycin *Moderately potent and potent* Propaderm-A (A & H) — with chlortetracycline Betnovate-N (Glaxo) — with neomycin Adcortyl (Squibb) — with graneodin Synalar-N (ICI) — with neomycin	*Mildly potent* Neo-Cort-Dome (Miles) — with neomycin, hydrocortisone *Moderately potent and potent* Neo-Synalar (Syntex) — with neomycin Cordran-N (Dista) — with neomycin

Type of preparation and general comments	U.K. preparations	U.S.A. preparations
Steroid combinations continued		
With antifungals	*Mildly potent* Canestan HC (Bayer) Daktacort (Janssen) Econacort (Squibb)	
	Moderately potent and potent Nystadermal (Squibb)	*Moderately potent and potent* Lotrisone (Schering) Mycolog II (Squibb)
With antibacterials and antifungals	*Mildly potent* Nystaform HC (Bayer) Terra-Cortril Nystatin (Pfizer) Timodine (Lloyds)	No U.S.A. equivalents
	Moderately potent Trimovate (Glaxo)	
With tar	*Mildly potent only* Alphosyl HC (Stafford - Miller) Tarcortin (Stafford - Miller)	No U.S.A. equivalents
With salicylic acid	*Potent only* Diprosalic (Kirby - Warrick)	No U.S.A. equivalents
Preparations for use in the mouth		
Useful mouth washes	Difflam oral rinse (Riker) — an analgesic for painful inflammation in the mouth Corsodyl mouth wash (ICI) — contains chlorhexidine	Diphenhydramine elixir (Roxane) — anaesthetic Chloraseptic (Richardson - Vicks) — contains phenol Amosan (Oral B) — liberates oxygen upon contact with mouth fluids or blood
Topical steroids	Adcortyl in orabase paste (Squibb) — adheres to mucous membranes Corlan pellets (Glaxo) — dissolve slowly in mouth near lesion	Kenalog in Orabase (Squibb) — adheres to mucous membranes Lidex gel (Syntex)
For yeast infections	Daktarin oral gel (Janssen) — contains miconazole Fungilin lozenges (Squibb) — contain amphotericin Nystatin oral suspension (Squibb)	Mycelex troche (Miles) — contains clotrimazole Mycostatin pastilles (Squibb) — contain nystatin Nystatin oral suspension (numerous manufacturers)
Preparations for otitis externa		
Otitis externa, essentially an eczema, is often complicated by bacterial or yeast overgrowth — hence the combinations listed here	Aluminium acetate ear drops 8% — an effective astringent for the weeping phase: best applied on ribbon gauze Otosporin drops (Calmic) — hydrocortisone with neomycin and polymyxin	Otic Domeboro solution (Miles) — contains aluminium sulphate, acetic acid Corticosporin otic suspension (Burroughs Wellcome) — contains polymixin B, neomycin, hydrocortisone

Type of preparation and general comments	U.K. preparations	U.S.A. preparations
Preparations for otitis externa continued	Terracortril drops (Pfizer) — hydrocortisone with oxytetracycline and polymyxin Canesten solution (Bayer) — contains clotrimazole	Otic-HC ear drops (Hauck) — contains chloroxylenol, hydrocortisone, pramoxine, acetic acid Vo-Sol-HC (Wallace) — contains acetic acid, hydrocortisone
Antibacterial preparations The ideal preparation should have high antibacterial activity, low allergenicity, and the drug should not be available for systemic use; this combination is hard to find. Some compromises are given here	Graneodin ointment (Squibb) — contains neomycin (a sensitizer), gramicidin Chlortetracycline — may be used systemically Bactroban ointment (Beecham) — contains mupirocin To eliminate nasal carriage of staphylococci: Naseptin cream (ICI) — contains neomycin Bactroban-N cream (Beecham)	Polysporin ointment, powder, or spray (Burroughs Wellcome) — contains polymixin B, bacitracin Bacitracin ointment (Fougera) Bactroban ointment (Beecham) — contains mupirocin Betadine ointment (Purdue - Fredrick) — contains povidone iodine
Antifungal preparations In our view imidazole creams have now supplanted their messier, more irritant, and less effective rivals, e.g. Whitfield's ointment. They have the added advantage of combating yeasts as well as dermatophytes Systemic therapy will be needed for tinea of the scalp, of the nails, and of widespread or chronic skin infections which prove resistant to topical treatment	Canesten cream (Baypharm) — contains clotrimiazole Daktarin cream (Janssen) — contains miconazole Ecostatin cream (Squibb) — contains econazole Trosyl nail solution (Pfizer) — contains tioconazole. Applied locally it may increase the success rate of griseofulvin. Used by itself it may also cure or improve some nails	Naftin cream (Herbert Laboratories) — contains naftifine, not an imidazole Lotrimin cream and solution (Schering) — contains clotrimazole Monistat-derm cream (Ortho) — contains miconazole Spectazole cream (Ortho) — contains econazole Nizoral cram (Janssen) — contains ketoconazole Loprox cream (Hoechst) — contains ciclopirox, not an imidazole
Antiviral preparations These have little part to play in the management of herpes zoster. However, if used early and frequently, they may help with recurrent herpes simplex infections	Zovirax cream (Wellcome) — contains acyclovir Herpid application (Boehringer - Ingelheim) — contains idoxuridine in dimethyl sulphoxide. Absorption of dimethyl sulphoxide may cause a garlic taste	Zovirax cream (Burroughs - Wellcome) — contains acyclovir
Wart treatments (p. 148)		
Palmoplantar warts	Salactol paint (Dermal) Glutarol solution (Dermal) Cuplex gel (S & N Pharm) Veracur gel (Typharm)	Duofilm paint (Stiefel) Occlusal range (GenDerm)
Anogenital warts	Podophyllin paint compound — contains 15% podophyllin resin (use with care (p. 149)	Podophyllin, 15% in tincture of benzoin (use with care, p. 149)

Type of preparation and general comments	U.K. preparations	U.S.A. preparations
Preparations for treatment of scabies Poor results follow inefficient usage rather than ineffective preparations. We prefer precipitated sulphur in young children, and pregnant and lactating women. Written instructions are helpful (p. 171)	Ascabiol application (M & B) — contains benzyl benzoate Eurax Cream (Geigy) — contains crotamiton Quellada lotion (Stafford - Miller) — contains lindane (gamma benzene hexachloride) Precipitated sulphur 6% in soft white paraffin	Kwell lotion and cream (Reed & Carnrick) — contains lindane Scabene lotion (Stiefel) — contains lindane Eurax lotion and cream (Westwood) — contains crotamiton Precipitated sulphur 6% in petrolatum alba
Preparations for treatment of pediculosis Resistance to lindane has limited its usefulness for scalp lice. Lotions left on for a minimum of 12 hours are perhaps more effective, though less convenient than shampoos	Prioderm lotion and cream shampoo (Napp) — contains malathion Derbac-M lotion and shampoo (International Labs) — contains carbaryl Quellada lotion (*see above*)	Nix cream rinse (Burroughs Wellcome) — contains permethrin R & C spray (Reed & Carnrick) — contains pyrethroids RID lotion (Leeming) — contains pyrethrin Kwell shampoo (Reed & Carnrick) — contains lindane
Preparations for acne Active ingredient:		
Benzoyl peroxide (an antibacterial agent) induces dryness during the first few weeks; this usually settles even with continued use	Panoxyl and Acetoxyl ranges (Stiefel) 2.5%, 5%, 10% Quinoderm cream (Quinoderm) — contains potassium hydroxyquinolone	PanOxyl range (Stiefel) Desquam X range (Westwood) — contains laureth-4 Sulfoxyl 5%, 10% (Dermik) — contains 2% sulphur
Tretinoin	Retin-A preparations (Ortho - Cilag)	Retin-A gel, cream, and solution (Ortho)
Antibiotics	Dalacin-T solution (Upjohn) — contains clindamycin Stiemycin solution (Stiefel) — contains erythromycin Topicycline solution (Norwich Eaton) — contains tetracycline. May stain yellow and fluoresce at discos	Cleocin-T (Upjohn) — contains clindamycin EryDerm (Abbott) — contains erythromycin Topicycline (Norwich Eaton) — contains tetracycline
Abrasives	Brasivol paste Nos 1–3 (Stiefel) Ionax scrub (Alcon)	Bravisol (Stiefel) Ionax scrub (Owen)
Sulphur	2–10% sulphur in calamine lotion	Liquimat (Owen - Allercreme) Rezamid (Dermik) — contains resorcin

Type of preparation and general comments	U.K. preparations	U.S.A. preparations
Preparations for psoriasis **Tar**: these clean refined tar preparations are suitable for home use. Messier, though more effective, formulations exist but are best used in treatment centres		
Bath additives	Polytar emollient (Stiefel) Psoriderm bath emulsion (Dermal)	Polytar (Stiefel) Balnatar (Westwood)
Applications	Alphosyl cream (Stafford Miller) Carbo-Dome cream (Lagap) Meditar wax stick (Brocades)	Estar gel (Westwood)
Scalp applications	Alphosyl lotion (Stafford - Miller)	
Dithranol/anthralin stains normal skin and clothing. May be irritant, therefore start with low concentration. For 30-minute regimen *see* p. 50	Anthranol ointment range (Stiefel) Dithrocream range (Dermal) Psoradrate cream range (Norwich Eaton) — contains urea	Dithrocreme (American Dermal) Lasan cream and ointment (Stiefel)
Steroids: routine long-term treatment with potent or very potent steroids is not recommended. For indications *see* p. 50		
Scalp applications	Betnovate scalp application (Glaxo) Synalar gel (ICI) Diprosalic scalp lotion (Kirby - Warrick) — also contains salicylic acid	Diprolene ointment (Schering) Lidex gel solution (Syntex) Valisone solution (Schering) Synalar solution (Syntex)
For use elsewhere	*See* section on topical steroids above	*See* section on topical steroids above
Tar–steroid combinations are helpful		
Salicylic acid: used mostly for scalp psoriasis	*See* Keratolytics	*See* Keratolytics
Tar–salicylic acid combinations	Pragmatar cream (Bioglan) — also contains sulphur Gelcosal (Quinoderm)	T-gel scalp solution (Neutrogena) P & S plus gel (Baker Cummins) Pragmatar ointment (Smith Kline) — also contains sulphur

Type of preparation and general comments	U.K. preparations	U.S.A. preparations
Preparations for venous ulcers Regardless of topical applications, venous ulcers will heal only if local oedema is eliminated. Remember that the surrounding skin is easily sensitized. To choose treatment for an individual ulcer *see* p. 121		
For cleansing	Saline, potassium permanganate, *see* Cleansing agents Hydrogen peroxide solution (3%)	Prolonged soaks in tap water or saline Hydrogen peroxide solution (3%) Acetic acid aqueous solution (0.25%)
Antibacterial gauze dressings	Bactigras tulle dressing (S & N) Softratulle (Roussel) Fucidin Intertulle (Leo)	
Other applications	Variclene gel (Dermal) — contains brilliant green Flamazine cream (S & N Pharm) — contains silver sulphadiazine active against *Pseudomonas* Silver nitrate aqueous solution (0.5%) Iodosorb (Stuart) — contains cadexomer iodine	Silvadene cream (Marion) Bactroban ointment (Beecham)
Medicated bandages: beware of allergic contact reactions to parabens preservatives which are in most bandages	Calaband (Seton) Ichthopaste (S & N) Viscopaste PB7 (S & N) Cortacream (S & N) — contains hydrocortisone and is useful for eczema around venous ulcers	
Other dressings	Granuflex (Squibb Surgicare) Kaltostat (Cair) – contains calcium alginate	Duoderm (Squibb) Vigilon (Bard) Tegaderm (3M) Opsite (American Hospital Co.)
Miscellaneous **5-flourouracil** The treatment of individual lesions in patients with multiple actinic keratoses is tedious or impossible. For such cases a 5% cream containing 5-fluorouracil is useful. It should be applied twice daily for two weeks. Patients should be warned about the inevitable inflammation and soreness which appears after a few days. Lesions on the scalp and face do better than those on the arms and hands	Efudix cream (Roche)	Efudex cream and solution (Roche) Fluoroplex cream and solution (Herbert)

Type of preparation and general comments	U.K. preparations	U.S.A. preparations
Minoxidil May be used as a possible treatment for early male-pattern alopecia. The response is slow, and only a small minority of patients will obtain a dense regrowth even after 12 months. Hair regained will fall out when treatment stops — warn patients about this	Regaine (Upjohn) — only private prescription	Regaine (Upjohn)

FORMULARY:
2. SYSTEMIC MEDICATION

We list here only preparations we use commonly for our patients with skin disease. The doses given are the usual oral doses for adults. We occasionally use some of these drugs for uses not approved by federal regulatory agencies. We have included some, but not all, of the side effects and interactions; these are more fully covered in the *British National Formulary* (U.K.) and *Physicians' Desk Reference* (U.S.A.). Physicians prescribing these drugs should read about them in more detail before treating their patients. If possible, systemic medications should be avoided in pregnant women.

Main dermatological uses and usual adult dosage	Adverse effects	Interactions	Cautions
Antibacterials			
Amoxycillin A broad-spectrum penicillin for cellulitis and Gram-negative folliculitis (250 mg three times daily)	Gut upsets Candidiasis Pseudomembranous colitis (rarely) 10% of patients develop a morbilliform eruption	Probenecid increases blood levels Rashes with allopurinol	Accumulates in renal failure Rashes commonly arise in infectious mononucleosis and leukaemia
Cephradine For Gram-positive and negative infections resistant to penicillin, erythromycin and co-trimoxazole (250–500 mg four times daily)	Candidiasis Rarely nephrotoxic Cross-reacts with penicillin in 10% of those allergic to penicillin	Ethacrynic acid and frusemide/furosemide may enhance nephrotoxicity	Not usually indicated as first line or 'blind' therapy
Ciprofloxacin For Gram-negative infections, especially *Pseudomonas*, and for Gram-positive infections (500 mg twice daily)	Gut upsets Raised liver enzymes	Antacids reduce absorption Potentiates action of theophylline	Crystalluria if fluid intake is inadequate Care if renal impairment Avoid in pregnancy, breast feeding, children, and epileptics
Co-trimoxazole (trimethoprim plus sulphamethoxazole) 1 Gram-positive and negative infections	Gut upsets Stomatitis	Folate antagonists (e.g. methotrexate) may	Blood effects most severe in the elderly and in those

Main dermatological uses and usual adult dosage	Adverse effects	Interactions	Cautions
Co-trimoxazole continued **2** Reserve therapy for acne and rosacea Two tablets (equivalent to trimethoprin 160 mg and sulphamethoxyzole 800 mg) twice daily	Megaloblastic, aplastic and haemolytic anaemia Neutropenia Thrombocytopenia Rashes including erythema multiforme and photosensitivity, exfoliative dermatitis, and toxic epidermal necrolysis	potentiate its marrow toxicity Co-trimoxazole potentiates antifolate effects of folate antagonists (e.g. methotrexate), enhances anticoagulant effects of warfarin, prolongs the half-life of phenytoin and potentiates the hypoglycaemic effects of oral hypoglycaemic drugs	treated with high doses, e.g. for *Pneumocystis carinii* pneumonia Avoid in pregnancy
Erythromycin **1** Acne vulgaris (250–500 mg twice daily) **2** Gram-positive infections, particularly staphylococcal and streptococcal (250–500 mg four times daily)	Gut upsets Rashes Cholestatic hepatitis if treatment prolonged (reversible and most common with estolate salt)	Increased risk of toxicity if given with theophylline or carbamezapine Potentiates effects of warfarin, ergotamine, and cyclosporin A	Avoid estolate in liver disease
Flucloxacillin **Dicloxacillin** **Cloxacillin** Penicillins used for infections with penicillinase-forming staphylococci (250 mg four times daily)	Gut upsets Morbilliform eruptions Arthralgia Anaphylaxis		Accumulate in renal failure Atopics may be at increased risk of hypersensitivity reactions
Metronidazole **1** Anaerobic infections (200–400 mg three times daily) **2** Stubborn rosacea (200 mg twice daily) **3** Trichomoniasis (200 mg three times daily for seven days)	Gut upsets Metallic taste Candidiasis Ataxia and sensory neuropathy	Drugs that induce liver enzymes (e.g. rifampicin, barbiturates, griseofulvin, phenytoin, carbamezapine, and smoking), increase destruction of metronidazole in liver and necessitate higher dosage May have disulfiram-like effect with alcohol (headaches, flushing, vomiting, abdominal pain)	Use lower dose in presence of liver disease Neurotoxicity more likely if CNS disease
Minocycline A tetracycline used for acne and rosacea (50 mg daily or twice daily)	Gut upsets Dizziness and vertigo Candidiasis Deposition in bones and teeth of fetus and children	May impair absorption of oral contraceptives	Avoid in pregnancy and in children under 12 years

Main dermatological uses and usual adult dosage	Adverse effects	Interactions	Cautions
Minocycline continued	Deposition in skin causes grey pigmentation Benign intracranial hypertension		
Tetracycline and oxytetracycline Acne and rosacea (250–500 mg twice daily)	Gut upsets Candidiasis Rashes Deposition in bones and teeth of fetus and children Rare phototoxic reactions Benign intracranial hypertension	Absorption impaired when taken with food, antacids, and iron May impair absorption of oral contraceptives	Avoid in pregnancy and in children under 12 years Should not be used if renal insufficiency
Penicillin V **(phenoxymethylpenicillin)** 1 For infections with Gram-positive cocci (250–500 mg four times daily) 2 Prophylaxis of erysipelas (250 mg daily)	Gut upsets Morbilliform rashes Urticaria Athralgia Anaphylaxis		Accumulates in renal failure Atopics at increased risk of hypersensitivity reactions

Antifungals

Main dermatological uses and usual adult dosage	Adverse effects	Interactions	Cautions
Griseofulvin Dermatophyte infections of skin, nails, and hair. Not for *Candida* or pityriasis versicolor (500 mg microsize daily)	Gut upsets Headaches, rashes, photosensitivity	Induces microsomal liver enzymes and so may increase elimination of drugs such as warfarin and phenobarbitone	Not for use in pregnancy, liver failure, porphyria or systemic LE Absorbed better when taken with fatty foods
Ketoconazole 1 Systemic mycoses and their prophylaxis in immunosuppressed patients 2 Serious chronic mucocutaneous candidiasis 3 Rarely for dermatophyte infections not responsive to other treatment (200–400 mg daily)	Abnormal liver function and hepatitis Gut upsets Rashes Headache Thrombocytopenia Gynaecomastia (rare)	Absorption decreased by antacids, anticholinergic drugs, cimetidine, and ranitidine Plasma concentration reduced by phenytoin and rifampicin Potentiates effect of phenytoin, cyclosporin A, and warfarin	Check liver function tests after first 10 days and then twice every month Avoid if liver impairment and in pregnancy
Nystatin 1 Recurrent vulval and perineal candidiasis 2 Persistant GI candidiasis in immunosuppressed patients (500 000 units three times daily)	Unpleasant taste Gut upsets		Not absorbed and when given by mouth, acts only on bowel yeasts

Main dermatological uses and usual adult dosage	Adverse effects	Interactions	Cautions
Antivirals			
Acyclovir			
1 Severe herpes simplex infections — primary or recurrent (200 mg five times daily for five days) 2 Severe herpes zoster infections (800 mg five times daily for seven days) 3 Prophylaxis for recurrent herpes simplex especially in the immunocompromised and to treat eczema herpeticum (for dosages see specialist literature)	Transient rise in urea and creatinine in 10% of patients after intravenous use	Excretion may be delayed by probenicid	Risk in pregnancy unknown Reduce dose in severe renal impairment No effect on virus in latent phase Must be given early in acute infections
Antihistamines All those listed here are H$_1$-blockers though some dermatologists combine these with H$_2$-blockers in recalcitrant urticaria			
Non-sedative Used for urticaria and type I hypersensitivity reactions			
● Terfenadine (60 mg twice daily) ● Astemizole (10 mg daily)	Hair loss Weight gain rarely		Little or no antipruritic effect save in urticaria Avoid in pregnancy
Sedative Urticaria, type I hypersensitivity including intravenous use in anaphylaxis (p. 233). Also used as antipruritic agents in, e.g. atopic eczema, lichen planus ● Chlorpheniramine (4 mg three or four times daily) ● Diphenhydramine (25–50 mg four times daily) ● Hydroxyzine (10–50 mg four times daily) ● Cyproheptadine (4 mg four times daily) ● Promethazine (10–25 mg daily to three times daily) ● Trimeprazine (2.5–10 mg once or twice daily)	Sedation (promethazine > trimeprazine > hydroxyzine > chlorpheniramine = diphenhydramine = cyproheptadine) Anticholinergic effects: ● dry mouth ● blurred vision ● urinary retention ● tachycardia	Potentiate effect of alcohol and CNS depressants Potentiate effect of other anticholinergic drugs	Increased rate of elimination in children Sedation may be useful in an excited, itchy patient Warn of risk of drowsiness when driving or operating dangerous machinery

Main dermatological uses and usual adult dosage	Adverse effects	Interactions	Cautions

Antiandrogens

Cyproterone acetate and ethinyl oestradiol
(U.K.: Dianette;
U.S.A.: not available)
1 Acne vulgaris, in women only, unresponsive to systemic antibiotics
2 Idiopathic hirsutism
One tablet (cyproterone acetate 2 mg, ethinyl oestradiol 35 μg) daily for 21 days, starting on fifth day of menstrual cycle and repeated after a seven-day interval. Treat for six months at least

	Adverse effects	Interactions	Cautions
	As for combined oral contraceptives	Should not be given with other oral contraceptives	Contra-indicated in pregnancy. Cyproterone acetate is an antiandrogen and if given to pregnant women may feminize a male fetus. For women of childbearing age, therefore, it must be given combined with a contraceptive (the ethinyl oestradiol component) Also contra-indicated in liver disease, disorders of lipid metabolism, and with past or present endometrial carcinomas Not for use in males or children

Immunosuppressants

Azathioprine
For auto-immune conditions, e.g. systemic LE, pemphigus, and bullous pemphigoid — often used to spare dose of systemic steroids
(1–2.5 mg/kg daily)

	Adverse effects	Interactions	Cautions
	Gut upsets Bone marrow suppression, usually leucopenia or thrombocytopenia Hepatotoxicity Predisposes to infections, including warts	Increased toxicity if given with allopurinol	Regular blood checks are necessary Reduce dose if severe renal impairment Avoid in pregnancy

Methotrexate
Severe psoriasis unresponsive to local treatment
(initially, 2.5 mg test dose and observe for one week, then 5–15 mg once every *week* orally or intramuscularly)

	Adverse effects	Interactions	Cautions
	Gut upsets Stomatitis Bone marrow depression Liver or kidney dysfunction	Aspirin, probenicid, and some non-steroidal anti-inflammatory drugs delay excretion and increase toxicity Anti-epileptics, co-trimoxazole, and pyrimethamine increase antifolate effect	Regular blood checks are necessary Avoid in pregnancy Reduce dose if renal or hepatic impairment Folinic acid given concomitantly prevents bone marrow depression Many insist on a liver biopsy before treatment and periodically thereafter as this is the best way of detecting hepatic fibrosis Elderly may be more sensitive to the drug

Main dermatological uses and usual adult dosage	Adverse effects	Interactions	Cautions

Corticosteroids

Prednisone and prednisolone

Acute and severe allergic reactions, severe erythema multiforme, connective tissue disorders, pemphigus, pemphigoid and vasculitis (5–80 mg daily or on alternate days)	Impaired glucose tolerance Redistribution of fat (centripetal) Muscle wasting, proximal myopathy Osteoporosis and vertebral collapse Aseptic necrosis of head of femur Growth retardation in children Peptic ulceration Euphoria, psychosis and depression Cataract formation Precipitation of glaucoma Increase in blood pressure Sodium and water retention Potassium loss Skin atrophy and capillary fragility Spread of infection Iatrogenic Cushing's syndrome	Liver enzyme inducers (e.g. phenytoin, griseofulvin, rifampicin) reduce effect of corticosteroids Carbenoxolone and most diuretics increase potassium loss due to corticosteroids Corticosteroids reduce effect of many antihypertensive agents Corticosteroids will interact with drugs that affect glucose metabolism	1 Before long-term treatment screen: ● Chest X-ray ● Blood pressure ● Weight ● Glycosuria ● Electrolytes ● Tuberculin skin test (U.S.A.) ● Past history of peptic ulcer, cataracts/glaucoma, and affective psychosis 2 During treatment check BP, weight, glycosuria, and electrolytes regularly Patients should carry a steroid treatment card or wear a labelled bracelet Always bear in mind the possibility of masked infections and perforations 3 Long-term treatment has to be tapered off slowly to avoid adrenal insufficiency 4 Do not use for psoriasis or long-term for atopic eczema

Retinoids

Etretinate

Severe psoriasis, resistant to other forms of treatment (may be used with PUVA, p. 51), palmoplantar pustulosis, severe ichthyoses, Darier's disease, pityriasis rubra pilaris (0.2–1.0 mg/kg daily)	1 *Mucocutaneous* (common) Rough, scaly, dry-appearing skin and mucous membranes Chafing Atrophy of skin and nails Diffuse thinning of scalp and body hair Curly hair Exuberant granulation tissue (especially toe nail folds) Disease flare-up Photosensitivity 2 *Systemic* Teratogenesis	Avoid concomitant high doses of vitamin A	All women of childbearing age must use effective oral contraception for one month before treatment, during treatment and for at least two years after treatment. They should sign a consent form indicating that they know about the danger of teratogenicity Regular screening should be carried out to exclude: 1 Abnormalities of liver function 2 Hyperlipidaemia

Main dermatological uses and usual adult dosage	Adverse effects	Interactions	Cautions
Etretinate continued	Diffuse interstitial skeletal hyperostosis Arthralgia, myalgia, and headache Benign intracranial hypertension **3** *Laboratory abnormalities* Haematology: ↓WBC ↑ESR Liver function tests: ↑Bilirubin ↑AST/ALT ↑Alkaline phosphatase (abnormal in 20% of patients) Serum lipids: ↑Cholesterol ↑Triglycerides ↓High-density lipoprotein (abnormal in 50% of patients)		**3** Disseminated interstitial skeletal hyperostosis Avoid if renal or hepatic impairment
Isotretinoin (13 *cis*-retinoic acid) Severe acne vulgaris, unresponsive to systemic antibiotics (0.5–1.0 mg/kg daily for 16 weeks)	*See* Etretinate	*See* Etretinate	Females of childbearing age must take effective contraception for one month before treatment is started, during treatment, and for three months after treatment is stopped; check a pregnancy test before starting treatment and monthly. Females should sign a consent form which states the dangers of teratogenicity Avoid in renal or hepatic impairment Blood tests as for etretinate

Drugs acting on the CNS

Amitriptyline **1** Depression secondary to skin disease **2** Post-herpetic neuralgia (50–100 mg at night; start with 10–25 mg in the elderly)	Sedation Anticholinergic effects Cardiac arrhythmias Confusion in the elderly Postural hypertension	Potentially lethal CNS stimulation with monoamine oxidase inhibitors Increases effects of other	Avoid in the presence of heart disease or hypertension Use small doses at first to avoid confusion in the elderly

Main dermatological uses and usual adult dosage	Adverse effects	Interactions	Cautions
Amitriptyline continued			
	Jaundice Neutropenia May precipitate seizures in epileptics	CNS depressants and anticholinergics Metabolism may be inhibited by cimetidine	Warn about effects on skills such as driving
Diazepam Anxiety — often associated with skin disease (2 mg three times daily)	Sedation Impaired skills (e.g. driving) or ataxia Dependence (withdrawal may lead to sleep-lessness, anxiety, tremors)	Potentiates effects of other CNS depressants including alcohol Breakdown inhibited by cimetidine and propranolol Liver enzyme inducers (e.g. phenytoin, griseofulvin, rifampicin) increase elimination	Use for short spells only (to avoid addiction) Avoid in pregnancy and breast feeding Use with care in presence of liver, kidney, or respiratory diseases, and in the elderly

Miscellaneous

Adrenaline (epinephrine) injection Emergency treatment for acute anaphylaxis 0.5 mg (0.5 ml of one in 1000 solution given as a slow subcutaneous or rarely intramuscular injection. May be repeated after 10 minutes if necessary)	Tachycardia Cardiac arrhythmias Anxiety Tremor Headache Hypertension Hyperglycaemia Hypokalaemia	If given with some beta-blockers may lead to severe hypertension	Do not confuse the different strengths Give *slowly*, subcutaneously or intramuscularly, but *not* intravenously, except in cardiac arrest
Dapsone Leprosy, dermatitis herpetiformis, vasculitis, pyoderma gangrenosum (50–150 mg daily)	Haemolytic anaemia Methaemoglobinaemia Headaches Lethargy Hepatitis Peripheral neuropathy Exfoliative dermatitis Toxic epidermal necrolysis Agranulocytosis Aplastic anaemia Hypoalbuminaemia	Reduced excretion and increased side effects if given with probenecid	Regular blood checks necessary (weekly for one month, monthly for five months and then six-monthly) Not felt to be teratogenic, but should not be given during pregnancy and lactation if possible. For dermatitis herpetiformis, a gluten-free diet is preferable at these times Avoid in patients with glucose 6-phosphate dehydrogenase deficiency

Main dermatological uses and usual adult dosage	Adverse effects	Interactions	Cautions
Hydroxychloroquine Systemic and discoid LE, porphyria cutanea tarda, polymorphic light eruption, LE: 200–400 mg daily, maintaining level at lowest effective dose. Must not exceed 6.5 mg/kg body weight/day (based on the ideal/lean body weight and not on the actual weight of the patient) Porphyria cutanea tarda: 50–100 mg twice *weekly*	Retinopathy which may cause permanent blindness Corneal deposits Headaches Gut upsets, pruritus and rashes Worsening of psoriasis	May raise plasma digoxin levels Potential neuromuscular toxicity if taken with gentamycin, kanamycin, or tobramycin Bioavailability decreased if given with antacids	All patients must have an ophthalmic examination (acuity, ophthalmoscopy, visual fields with red target) before treatment and every six months thereafter whilst on it. Discontinue drug if any change occurs Reduce dose with poor renal or liver function Best avoided in the elderly and children Do not give automatic repeat prescriptions Prefer intermittent short courses to continuous treatment if possible Use minute doses to treat porphyria cutanea tarda; ordinary doses cause toxic reactions
8-methoxypsoralen (methoxsalen) Used usually with UVA as PUVA therapy (p. 52) Severe psoriasis, vitiligo, localized pustular psoriasis, cutaneous T cell lymphoma; rarely, lichen planus, atopic dermatitis Tablets: 0.6–0.8 mg/kg body weight taken as a single dose 1–2 hours before exposure to UVA Liquid (Ultra Capsules) (U.S.A.): 0.3 mg/kg body weight taken one hour before exposure to UVA	Nausea Itching Photoxicity Cataracts Lentigines Ageing changes Hyperpigmentation Cutaneous neoplasms	Avoid other photosensitizers (Chapter 17)	Eyes should be protected with polarizing lenses for 24 hours after taking the drug Protective goggles must be worn during radiation If feasible, shield face during treatment Patients must protect skin against additional sun exposure after ingestion Monitor eyes for development of cataracts

INDEX

Page numbers in *italic* refer to tables and/or diagrams

abscess *28*, 29
absorption, percutaneous 237–40
acantholysis 98
acanthosis nigricans 212, *213*
acne excoriée 224
acne vulgaris
    apocrine 134–5
    causes 125–6
    drug-related 234
    presentation 126–8
    prevalence *2*, 125
    treatment 128–31, 251
    variants 126–8
acoustic neurofibromatosis 225, 226
acquired ichthyosis 38
acquired immune deficiency
        syndrome 154–5, 208
acral lentiginous melanoma 202–3
acrochordon 190
acrocyanosis 113
actinic cheilitis 178
actinic elastosis 179
actinic keratoses 196–7
actinic prurigo 178
actinic reticuloid 177
actinomycosis 164
acute intermittent porphyria 218
acyclovir 151, 153, 258
Addison's disease 186, *187*
adenoma sebaceum 226
adrenalin 262
ageing, cutaneous 179
AIDS 154–5, 208
albinism 181–2
    oculocutaneous 181–2
alkaptonuria 220
allergic contact dermatitis 76–7, 247
    patch testing 32
allergic vasculitis 93–4, 233
alopecia
    androgenic 62–3
    diffuse 64, *65*
    localized 60–4
    scarring 63–4
    traction 63
alopecia areata 60–2

nail changes in 68
aluminium chloride 129, 133, 247
amelanotic melanoma 203
amitriptyline 261–2
amoxycillin 225
amphotericin 162
amyloid 218
anagen 12, *13*
anaphylactic reactions 19–20, *21*, 233,
        235
anaphylactoid purpura 93–4, 233
anchoring fibrils 14, *15*
anchoring filaments 14, *15*
androgenic alopecia 62–3
angioedema 87
    definition *28*, 29
    differential diagnosis 73
    hereditary 86, *89*
    immunological basis 20
    see also urticaria
angiokeratoma corporis diffusum 220
angioma, cherry *206*, 207
anhidrosis 134
anhidrotic ectodermal dysplasia 134
annular lesions 30
anogenital warts 147, 148–9
anthralin 49–50, 252
antiandrogens 259
antibiotics
    adverse reactions to 232
    combined with steroids 248, 249
    systemic 129–30, 255–7
    topical 129, 250
antibody-mediated cellular
        cytotoxicity 25
antifungal preparations 250, 257
    combined with steroids 249
antigens
    Class I 25–6
    Class II 26
    presentation 19, *20*
antihistamines 258
    in urticaria 89
antiperspirants 247
antiproteases, in psoriasis 43
antipruritics 247

antiviral preparations 250, 258
apocrine acne 134–5
apocrine sweat glands 14
    disorders 134–5
arachidonic acid metabolism
        in psoriasis 42, *43*
arcuate lesions 30
arrector pili muscles 17
arterial disease 115–16
arteritis, temporal 116
arthritis, rheumatoid 111
arthropd infestation 165–71
arthropathy, psoriatic 48
Arthus reaction 23, 25
aryl sulphatase deficiency 37
ash leaf macules 226
asteatotic eczema 82
atherosclerosis 116
    leg ulcers due to 119
athlete's foot 156–7
atopic eczema 77–9
atrophie blanche 118
atrophy 30
axillary freckling 225
azathioprine 53, 259

B cell lymphomas 210
bacterial infections 136–45
baldness, male-pattern 62–3
    see also alopecia
barrier preparations 246
basal cell carcinoma 197–200
basal cell papilloma 189–90, 193
basal layer 4, *5*, 6
bases 239–40
Basex's syndrome 212
bath additives 245
bathing, therapeutic 240
Bazin's disease 143
Beau's lines 68, *69*
bed bugs 166
bee sting, reactions to 20
Behçet's syndrome 111–12
benzoyl peroxide 129, 251
Berloque dermatitis 187

biopsy, skin   33
bitten nails   67
blastomycosis   164
blisters *see* bullae; bullous diseases
blood vessels, cutaneous   17
Bloom's syndrome   187
blow-out   118
blue naevus   193
blushing   115
body image   221
body lice   167–8
boils   137–9
Borrelia burgdorferi   114, 142
Bowen's disease   196
bullae   *28*, *29*, 96, *97*, 233
bullous diseases   96–102
    linear IgA   100
bullous ichthyosiform erythroderma   38
bullous pemphigoid   99–100
    antigen   15
burrow   29
Buruli ulcers   145
'button-hole' sign   226

café au lait patches   225
calf muscle pump   117
callosities   41
calmodulin, levels in psoriasis   43
camouflage preparations   129, 247
cAMP levels in psoriasis   43
Campbell de Morgan spots   *206*, 207
Candida endocrinopathy syndrome   161
Candida intertrigo   160, *161*
candidiasis   160–2
    chronic mucocutaneous   161
    genital   160
    systemic   162
canities   184
capillary cavernous haemangioma
    206–7
capillary haemangiona   205–6
carbuncle   139
carcinoma
    basal cell   197–200
    intra-epidermal   196
    squamous cell   200–1
carcinoma erysipeloides   211
carcinoma telagdiectoides   211
carotene   180
cat-scratch disease   155
catagen   12, *13*
cell cycle   6
cell-mediated immunity   *24*, 25
cellulitis   140
cephradine   255
cGMP, levels in psoriasis   43
chalone   8
cherry angioma   *206*, 207
chickenpox   149–50
chilblains   113
chloasma   186, *187*

cholinergic urticaria   85
    management   *89*
chondrodermatitis nodularis helicis   195
chronic mucocutaneous candidiasis   161
cicatricial pemphigoid   100
ciprofloxacin   255
circinate lesions   30
13-*cis*-retinoic acid   130, 261
cleansing agents   246
clioquinol   248
cloxacillin   256
clubbing   68
coal tar preparations   49, 249, 251–2
coccidioidomycosis   164
Cockayne's syndrome   187
cold sores   152
cold urticaria   85
    management   *89*
collagen   15–16
collagen injections   130–1
collodion baby   37
comedo   29
common warts   145, *146*, 147
complement
    C3b   21, 33
    C5a   22, *22*, 23
complement activation   21, *22*
compound melanocytic naevi   192
compresses   240
compression bandaging   121
condyloma acuminata   147, *148*–9
condyloma lata   140, 148
configuration of lesions   30–1
congenital erythropoietic porphyria   *216*,
    217
congenital melanocytic naevi   191
congenital syphilis   140
connective tissue
    disorders   103–12
    naevi   226
connective tissue disease, mixed   110–11
contact urticaria   86
contagious pustular dermatitis   154
corns   41
    plantar   148
corticosteroids *see* steroids
cosmetic camouflage   129, 247
co-trimoxazole   255–6
Coxsackie viruses   155
crabs   168
creams   *239*, 240
    amount required   *241*
C R E S T syndrome   110
Cronkhite–Canada syndrome   186
crust   30
cryoglobulinaemia   123–4
cryotherapy   148, 243
curettage   242
Cushing's syndrome   186
cutaneous hepatic porphyria   102,
    217–18
cutaneous horn   197

cutaneous T cell lymphoma   49, 58–9,
    208–10
cuticle   13
cutis marmoras   115
cutis verticis gyratum   210
cysticercosis   172
cysts, epidermoid   194–5
cytotoxic reactions, humoral   21–3
cytology,   32
cytotoxicity, antibody-mediated
    cellular   25

dapsone   101, 262
Darier's disease   39–40
dartos muscle   17
de Sanctis–Caccione syndrome   227
deep vein thrombosis   116, *117*
delusions of parasitosis   222–3
depigmentaton, post-inflammatory   184
dermabrasion   130
dermal papillae   4, *5*, 15
dermatan sulphate   17
dermatitis *see* eczema
dermatitis
    allergic contact   76–7, 247
    contagious pustular   154
    exfoliative   59, 233
    napkin   83–4
dermatitis artefacta   223–4
dermatitis herpetiformis   100–1
dermatofibroma   207
dermatofibrosarcoma protuberans   210
dermatological non-disease   222
dermatological therapy   236–43
dermatomyositis   107–8, 212
dermatophyte infections   63, 69–70,
    156–60
dermatosis
    juvenile plantar   83
    subcorneal pustular   97
dermis   4, 15
    benign tumours   205–8
    blood vessels   17
    cells   15, *16*
    fibres   15–16
    ground substance   16–17
    innervation   17–18
    juction with epidermis   *5*, *7*, 14–15
    lymphatics   17
    malignant tumours   208
    muscles   17
    in psoriasis   44
dermo-epidermal junction   *5*, *7*, 14–15
dermographism   85, *86*
    management   *89*
desmosomes   6, *7*
diabetes mellitus   213–14, 216
diabetic dermopathy   214
    diagnosis   27–35
diaper area *see* napkin dermatitis; napkin
    psoriasis

diascopy   31
diazepam   262
dicloxacillin   256
discoid eczema   49, 80–1
discoid lesions   30
discoid lupus erythematosus   106–7
DISH syndrome   52
distribution of lesions   28
dithranol   49–50, 252
dopa oxidase   9
drugs, cutaneous reactions to   86
    allergic   231–2
    course   234–5
    non-allergic   231
    photo-allergy   175–7
    phototoxicity   174–5, 234
    presentation   232–4
    treatment   235
drug reactions, lichenoid   56, 234
dusting powders   *239*, 240
dysmorphophobia   221–2
dysplasias, ectodermal   65
dysplastic naevus syndrome   193

ecchymoses   *28, 29*, 123–4
eccrine sweat glands   13–14
    disorders   132–4
ecthyma   137
ectodermal dysplasias   65
eczema
    acute   72, 97
    in AIDS   155
    asteatotic   82
    atopic   77–9
    causes   71
    chronic   72, *73*
    classification   71
    clinical features   72
    complications   72–3
    differential diagnosis   49, 73–4
    discoid   49, 80–1
    drug-related   233
    gravitational   82
    herpeticum   152
    histology   72, *73*
    investigations   74
    irritant contact   75–6
    nails in   68
    nummular   49, 80–1
    patterns   75–84
    seborrhoeic   49, 79–80, *81*, 155
    treatment   74–5
    in venous leg ulcers   118, *119*
Ehlers–Danlos syndrome   229–30
elastic fibres   16
electrosurgery   242, *243*
elephantiasis   172
emboli, arterial   116
emollients   245
emotional sweating   14
enteropathy, gluten-sensitive   100–1

eosinophilic fasciitis   110
ephelides   184–5, *186*, 193
epidermal barrier   8
epidermal growth factor   8
epidermal–melanin unit   8, *9*
epidermal ridges   4, *5*
epidermal T cell activating factor   19
epidermis
    appendages   11–14
    barrier function   8
    benign tumours   189–95
    cell cohesion   8
    cell kinetics in psoriasis   42
    cell proliferation   8
    cells in   8–11
    junction with dermis   5, *7*, 14–15
    keratinization   *5, 6*, 8
    malignant tumours   197–205
    premalignant states   195–7
    structure   4–6
    vitamin D synthesis in   8
epidermodysplasia verruciformis   147–8
epidermoid cysts   194–5
epidermolysis bullosa   102, 228–9
    acquisista   102
    junctional   229
    nail loss in   66
epidermolytic hyperkeratosis   38
epinephrine   262
erosion   30
erysipelas   139
    differentila diagnosis   73, 88
erysipeloid   140
erythema   113–14
    necrolytic migratory   212
    palmar   114
    toxic   113, *114*, 232, 233
    urticated   113
erythema ab igne   115
erythema chronicum migrans   114, 142
erythema gyratum repens   212
erythema induratum   143
erythema infectiosum   156
erythema multiforme   *87*, 88, 89–91, *92*, 102, 152, 233
erythema nodosum   91–3, 214
erythema nuchae   205
erythemas
    figurate   113–14
    reactive   85–93, 113, *114*
erythrasma   136
erythrocyanosis   113
erythroderma   59, 233
erythrodermic psoriasis   47–8
erythrohepatic protoporphyria   217
erythromelalgia   113
erythromycin   130, 256
ETAF   19
etretinate   52, 260–1
eumelanin   9
examination   27–8
excision   242

microscopically controlled   242
    shave   242
excoriation   30
    neurotic   224
exfoliative dermatitis   59, 233
exostoses, subungual   70

Fabry's disease   220
facial warts   147, 149
fasciitis
    eosinophilic   110
    necrotizing   140
favus   158
fibroblasts   15, *16*
fibromas
    peri-ungual   70, 226
fifth disease   156
figurate erythemas   113–14
filariasis   171–2
fingerprints   15
fissure   30
fixed drug eruptions   234
flucloxacillin   256
5-fluorouracil   253
flushing   115
follicular mucinosis   218
folliculitis   155
Fordyce spots   14
Fox–Fordyce disease   135
freckles   184–5, *186*, 193
fungal infections   156–63
    age-dependent prevalence   *2*
    deep   163–4
    differential diagnosis   73
    potassium hydroxide test   31
furunculosis   137–9

gap junctions   6
genital candidiasis   160
German measles   156
Gianotti–Crosti syndrome   155
glomus tumour   207
    nails   70
glutathione   10
gluten-sensitive enteropathy   100–1
glycosaminoglycans   17
Goeckerman regimen   51
gold, adverse reactions to   232
'goose pimples'   17
Gottron's papules 107
graft-versus-host disease   215
granular cell layer   4, *5, 6, 7*
granuloma annulare   148, 213–14
granulomas   25
granulomatous reactions   25
gravitational eczema   82
gravitational syndrome   117–23
griseofulvin   159, 257
groin
    candidiasis   160

tinea infection 157
growth fraction 6
gummas 141
gustatory sweating 14
guttate psoriasis 45, *46*
    treatment 51
GVH disease 215
gyrate lesions 30

habit tic nail dystrophy 67
haemangioma 193
    capillary 205–6
    capillary cavernous 206–7
haematoma *28, 29*
    subungual 67
haemorrhages, splinter 67
hair 11–12
    'bambo deformity' 38
    cosmetics 66
    cycle 12, *13, 60*
    disorders of growth 60–6
    drug-related loss 234
    exclamation-mark *61*
    lanugo 12
    pulling habit 224
    white 184
hair follicle *12*
halo naevus 194
hand, foot and mouth disease 155
hands, tinea infection 157
head lice 73, 167
heat bumps 166
heat stroke 134
heat urticaria 85
hemidesmosomes 14
hemiptera 166
Henoch–Schönlein purpura 93–4
herald plaque 54
herpangina 155
herpes gestationis 100
herpes simplex 152–3
    and erythema multiforme 91
herpes zoster 150–1
hidradenitis, suppurative 134–5
hirsutism 65–6
histamine 20
histiocytoma 207
histocompatibility 25–6
histoplasmosis 163–4
history-taking 27
HIV 154–5, 208
Hodgkin's disease 210
Homan's sign 116
hormone therapy 130
horny layer 4, *5, 6, 7*
HPV 145
human immunodeficiency virus 154–5, 208
human papilloma virus 145
humoral cytotoxic ractions 21–3
hyaluronic acid 17

hydatid disease 172
hydroxychloroquine 263
hydroxyurea, in psoriasis 53
hyperhidrosis 132–3
hyperkeratosis 124
    epidermolytic 38
hyperlipidaemias 219, *220*
hyperpigmentation
    nutritional 187
    post-inflammatory 187
hypersensitivity reactions,
        immediate 19–20, *21*, 233, 235
hypersensisitivity urticaria 86
    management *89*
hypersensitivity vasculitis 93–4, 233
hypertension, venous 117
hyperthyroidism, hair loss in *65*
hypertrichosis 66
    drug-related 234
    lanuginosa 212
hypodermis 4, *5*
hypohidrosis 134
hypopigmentation 181–4
hypopituitarism 182
hypotrichosis 65

ichthyoses 36–8
ichthyosiform erythroderma, bullous 38
ichthyosis
    acquired 38
    lamellar 37–8
    sex-linked 37
ichthyosis vulgaris 36–7
IL-1 19, *20*
IL-2 19
imidazole 159, 162
immediate hypersensitivity
        reactions 19–20, *21*, 233, 235
immune complex disease 23, 25
immunity, cell-mediated 24, 25
immunodeficiency 26
immunofluorescent tests *34*
    in bullous diseases 99
immunological reactions 19–25
immunology 19–26
immunosuppressants 259
immunosuppression 208
impetigo 96, 136–7
incontinentia pigmenti 228
infective ulcers 120
infestations 165–72
    delusions of 222–3
Ingram regimen 51
ingrowing nails 67
innervation, cutaneous 17–18
inoculation tuberculosis 142
insect bites 165–6
interleukin 1 19, *20*
interleukin 2 19
intradermal melanocytic naevi 192
intra-epidermal carcinoma 196

iontophoresis 133
iron deficiency *215*, 216
irritant contact eczema 75–6
isotretinoin 130, 261
itch spots 17
itching 17–18
    generalized 212, 216

junctional epidermolysis bullosa 229
junctional melanocytic naevi 191–2
juvenile melanoma 192–3
juvenile plantar dermatosis 83

K cells 25
kala-azar 145
Kaposi's sarcoma 155, 208
Kasabach–Merritt syndrome 207
Kawasaki's disease 155
keloid 207
keratinization *5, 6, 8*
    disorders of 36–41
keratinocytes 6
    in antigen presentation 19
keratinosomes 6
kerato-acanthoma 195–6
keratoderma, palms and soles 40
keratoderma blenorrhagicum 111
keratoderma climactericum 40
keratohyalin *6,7*
keratolysis, pitted 136
keratolytics 247
keratosis, seborrhoeic 189–90, 193
keratosis follicularis 39–40
keratosis pilaris 38–9
kerion 158
ketoconazole 159–60, 257
knuckle pads 40–1
Koebner phenomenon 44, 55, *56*
koilonychia 68, *69*
kwashiorkor 187, *215*

laboratory tests 33, *34*
lamellar bodies 6
lamellar ichthyosis 37–8
lamellar splitting 67
lamina densa 14, *15*
lamina lucida 14, *15*
laminin 14–15
Langerhans cell *7*, 11, 15, *16*
    role in antigen presentation 19, *20*
lanugo hairs 12
larva migrans 172
laser therapy 243
LE 102, 103–7, 178
leg ulcers 119–20
    see also venous leg ulcers
leishmaniasis 145
lentigo 185–6, 193
lentigo maligna melanoma 202

leopard syndrome   186
leprosy   143–5
lesions
    configuration   30–1
    distribution   28
    morphology   28–9
    terminology   28, 29–30
leucocytoclastic vasculitis   93–4, 233
leukaemia   210
leukotrienes   20
lice   73, 167–8, 251
lichen planus   55–7, 73
    nail changes in   68, 69
lichen sclerosus   110
lichen simplex   82–3, 224
lichenoid drug reactions   56, 234
light see ultraviolet radiation
light eruption, polymorphic   177–8
light reaction, persistent   176–7
linear IgA bullous disease   100
lipodermatosclerosis   117, 118
lipoma   207–8
Lisch nodules   226
livedo reticularis   94, 115
liver disease   214, 216
'liver spots'   185, 186
lupus erythematosus   102, 103–7, 178
    discoid   106–7
    subacute cutaneous   105–6
    systemic acute   103–5
lupus pernio   214
Lyell's disease   102, 139, 234
Lyme disease   114, 142
lymphangioma   207
lymphangitis   124
lymphatics, cutaneous   17
    disorders   124
lymphocytes   15, 16
    in immunological reactions   25
lymphoedema   124, 131–2
lymphokines   25
lymphomas
    B cell   210
    cutaneous T cell   49, 58–9, 208–10
    skin involvement   208–10

macrophage activating factor   25
macrophage migration inhibitory
        factor   25
macule   28, 29
Madura foot   164
MAF   25
malabsorption   215
male-pattern baldness   62–3
    see also alopecia
'malignant down'   212
malignant melanoma
    causes   201
    clinical features   202–3
    differential diagnosis   193, 204
    features   194

histology   203–4
incidence   201
microstaging   204
subungual   70
treatment   204–5
malignant ulcers   120
malnutrition   215
'mask of pregnancy'   186
mast cell   15, 16
measles   155–6
mechanoreceptors   17
meibomian glands   14
melanin   180
    decreased pigmentation   181–4
    increased pigmentation   184–7
melanocyte stimulating hormone   10
melanocytes   8–10
melanocytic naevi   191–4
    and malignant melanoma   201
melanogenesis   9–10
melanoma
    acral lentiginous   202–3
    amelanotic   203
    juvenile   192–3
    lentigo maligna   202
    nodular   203
    superficial spreading   202
    see also malignant melanoma
melanosomes   9–10
Menke's syndrome   65
Merkel cells   11
methotrexate   259
    in psoriasis   52–3
8-methoxypsoralen   263
metronidazole   256
mica scales   59
microscopically controlled excision   242
MIF   25
migratory superficial
        thrombophlebitis   117
miliaria   97, 134
milium   195
milker's nodules
minocycline   130, 256–7
minoxidil   254
mixed connective tissue disease   110–11
moles see melanocytic naevi
molluscum contagiosum   148, 153–4
Mongolian spots   193
monilethrix   65
mononuclear phagocytes   15, 16
monosymptomatic hypochondriacal
        psychosis   222
morphoea   110
morphology of lesions   28–9
mosaic warts   146, 147
'mossy foot'   124
mouth
    candidiasis   160, 161
    preparations for use in   249
MSH   10
mucinoses   218–19

mucinosis, follicular   219
mucocutaneous lymph node
        syndrome   155
muscles, cutaneous   17
mycetoma   164
Mycobacterial infections   142–5
Mycobacterium leprae   92, 143–5
Mycobacterium marinum   145
Mycobacterium ulcerans   145
mycosis fungoides   49, 58–9, 208–10
myiasis   166
myxoedema   218
myxoid cysts   70

naevi
    compound melanocytic   192
    congenital melanocytic   191
    intradermal melanocytic   192
    junctional melanocytic   191–2
    melanocytic   191–4
        and malignant melanoma   201
    spider   114
    vascular   205–7
naevus
    blue   193
    dysplastic syndrome   193
    halo   194
    Spitz   192–3
    strawberry   206–7
nail   12–13
    congenital abnormalities   66–7
    in Darier's disease   39
    dermatoses   46, 47, 68
    effects of trauma   67
    'en racquette'   67
    half-and-half   68, 215
    infections   49, 68–70, 156, 157
    ingrowing   67
    in systemic disease   67–8
    tumours   70
nail dystrophy, habit tic   67
nail fold   12, 13
    telangiectasia   68, 69
nail–patella syndrome   66
napkin dermatitis   83–4
napkin psoriasis   47
natural killer cells   25
necrobiosis lipoidica   213
necrolytic migratory erythema   212
necrotizing fasciitis   140
Netherton's syndrome   38, 65
neurodermatitis, localized   82–3, 224
neurofibromatosis   225–6
    von Recklinghausen's   225–6
neuromelanin   9
neurotic excoriations   224
Nikolsky's sign   98, 102
nipple, Paget's disease of the   205
nits   167
NK cells   25
nociceptors   17

nodular melanoma   203
nodular vasculitis   92
nodule   *29, 29*
nummular eczema   49, 80–1
nummular lesions   30
nutritional hyperpigmentation   187
nystatin   162, 257

occlusive therapy   240–1
oculocutaneous albinism   181–2
Odland bodies   6
office tests   31–3
ointments   *239*, 240
onchocerciasis   171
onychogryphosis   67
onycholysis   *46, 47*, 67
oral candidiasis   160,*161*
oral contraceptives, adverse reactions
      to   232
orf   154
oriental sores   145
otitis externa, preparations for   249
oxytetracycline   257

pachyonychia congenita   *66,67*
Paget's disease of the nipple   205
palmar erythema   114
palms
   keratoderma   40
   psoriasis   47
panniculitis   91–3, 112
papilloma   29
   basal cell   189–90, 193
   squamous cell   189
papular urticaria   165–6
papule   *28, 29, 30*
papulosquamous disorders   42–59
parapsoriasis en plaque   58–9
parasite infestation   165–72
   delusions of   222–3
parasitosis, delusions of   222–3
paronychia   68, 69, 161
pastes   *239*, 240
patch tests   32, 74
Pautrier micro-abscesses   209
peau d'orange   211
pediculosis   73, 167–8, 251
pemphigoid   99–100
   cicatricial   100
pemphigus   23, 97–9
penicillamine, adverse reactions to   232
penicillin V   257
percutaneous absorption   237–40
peri-ungual fibromas   226
permanent waving solutions   66
perniosis   113
persistent light reaction   176–7
petechiae   *28, 29*, 123–4
Peutz–Jeghers syndrome   185, *186*
phaeomelanin   9

pharmacological urticaria   86
phenoxymethylpenicillin   257
phenylketonuria   182, 220
photo-allergy   175–6
   persistent   176–7
photochemotherapy (PUVA)   243
   in psoriasis   51, 52
photopatch tests   74, 177
phototoxicity   174–5, 234
phrynoderma   39
physical therapy   241–3
phytophotodermatitis   175
piebaldism   182
pigmentation   30
   disorders   180–7
   drug-related   234
   genetic differences   11
pigments, abnormal   *180*
pilar cyst   194–5
pili torti   65
pimozide   223
pitted keratolysis   136
pityriasis lichenoides   59
pityriasis rosea   49, 54–5, 73
pityriasis rubra pilaris   57–8
pityriasis versicolor   73, 162–3
plane warts   147, 149
plantar corns   148
plantar warts   *146*, 147, 148
plaque   *28, 29*
plaque psoriasis   44–5
podophyllin   148–9
poikiloderma   30, 187, 209
polyamines
   synthesis in psoriasis   43
polyarteritis nodosa   94–5, 112
polychondritis   111
polycythaemia   216
polymorphic light eruption   177–8
pompholyx   81–2, 97
porphyria
   acute intermittent   218
   congenital erythropoietic   *216*, 217
   cutaneous hepatic   102, 217–18
   erythrohepatic proto   217
   variegate   218
porphyrias   102, 187, *216*, 217–18
port-wine stains   205–6
post-herpetic neuralgia   151
post-inflammatory depigmentation   184
post-inflammatory
      hyperpigmentation   187
potassium hydroxide test   31
potassium permanganate   133
prednisolone   260
prednisone   260
pregnancy, pigmentation in   186–7
pressure urticaria   86
pretibial myxoedema   218
prick testing   32–3
prickle cell layer   4, *5*, 6
   cell cohesion in   8

prickly heat   134
primary chancre   140
Propionobacterium acnes   126
proteases, in psoriasis   43
pruritus
   senile   216
   generalized   212, 216
   see also itching
'pseudopelade'   64
pseudo-xanthoma elasticum   230
psoralens   187
psoriasis
   biochemical abnormalities   42–3
   cell kinetics   42
   complications   48
   differential diagnosis   49, 73
   erythrodermic   47–8
   genetics   42
   guttate   45, *46*
   hair loss in   63
   histology   44, *45*
   immunopathology   43–4
   investigations   49
   nail changes in   *46, 47*, 68
   napkin   47
   pathogenesis   42–4
   plaque   44–5
   precipitating factors   44
   presentation   44–8
   prevalence   2
   treatment   49–53, 252
psoriatic arthropathy   48
psychosis, monosymptomatic
      hypochondriacal   222
pterygium   68, *69*
public lice   168
punch biopsy   33
purpura   *28, 29*, 123–4, 233
   anaphylactoid   93–4, 233
   Henoch–Schönlein   93–4
pustular psoriasis   47, *48*
pustule   *28, 29*
PUVA *see* photochemotherapy
pyoderma gangrenosum   120, 215
pyogenic granuloma   207

radiation, ultraviolet (UVR)   173
radiotherapy   243
Raynaud's phenomenon   108, 109–10,
      115, *116*
reactive erythemas   85–93, 113, *114*
Refsum's syndrome   38
Reiter's syndrome   111
relapsing polychondritis   111
renal disease   215
renal failure, chronic   187, 216
Re–PUVA regimen   52
reticulate lesions   30
reticulin   16
retiform lesions   30
retinoic acid   129, 251

retinoids   52, 129, 130, 251, 260–1
rheumatoid arthritis   111
rhinophyma   131
ringworm   63, 69–70, 156–60
rodent ulcer   197–200
rosacea   131–2
Rothmund–Thomson syndrome   187
rubella   156
Rud's syndrome   38

salicylic acid   249, 252
'salmon' patches   205
sarcoidosis   214
satyr's tuft   66
scabies   32, 73, 168–71
    treatment preparations   251
scalded skin syndrome   102, 234
    staphylococcal   96, 102, 139
scale   30
scalp
    involvement in psoriasis   45, 46, 47
        treatment   51
    ringworm   63, 157–8
scalpel biopsy   33
scar   30
    sarcoidosis   214
scarring alopecia   63–4
schistosomes   172
sclerodactyly   108, 109
scleromyxoedema   218
scrofuloderma   142
sebaceous glands   14
    disorders   125–32
seborrhoeic eczema   49, 79–80, 81, 155
seborrhoeic keratosis   189–90, 193
sensitization   19
septicaemia, chronic gonococcal   142
sex-linked ichthyosis   37
Sézary syndrome   209
shake lotions   239, 240
shampoos   245–6
shave excision   242
shellfish, allergy to   20
shingles   150–1
side-room tests   31–3
sign of Leser–Trelat   189
sinus   30
skin
    ageing   179
    biopsy   33
    colour   180
    flora   136
    in internal malignancy   212, 213
    and psyche   221–4
    structure and function   4–18
skin diseases
    causes   3
    emotional reactions to   221–4
    morbidity   2–3
    precipitated by emotional factors   224
    prevalence   2

skin tags   190
small vessel vasculitis   93–4, 233
solar urticaria   85, 178
    management   89
soles, keratoderma   40
spider naevi   114
spinous cell layer see prickle cell layer
spirochaetal infections   140–2
Spitz naevus   192–3
splinter haemorrhages   67
spongiosis   72
sporotrichosis   164
squamous cell carcinoma   200–1
squamous cell papilloma   189
Staphylococcus aureus   136–9
stasis eczema   82
steroids   248
    adverse reactions to   231, 232
    combinations   248–9
    systemic   260
    topical applications   238
        in psoriasis   50, 51
        strength   75
sterol sulphatase   8
Stevens–Johnson syndrome   89–90, 91,
        102
stratum corneum   4, 5, 6, 7
strawberry naevus   206–7
streptococcal infections   136–7,
        139–40
stria   30
Sturge–Weber syndrome   206
subacute cutaneous lupus
        erythematosus   105–6
subcorneal pustular dermatosis   97
subungual exostoses   70
subungual haematoma   67
sulphapyridine   101
sulphur   129
'sun warts'   196–7
sunburn   10, 173–4
sunscreens   247
superficial spreading melanoma   202
suppurative hidradenitis   134–5
surgery   242
sweat glands   13–14
    disorders   132–5
    eccrine   13–14
sweating
    emotional   14
    gustatory   14
    stimuli   14
    thermal   14
swimmer's itch   172
syphilis   49, 55, 140–2
    congenital   140
systemic candidiasis   162
systemic lupus erythematosus,
        acute   103–5
    bullous   102
systemic sclerosis   108–10
systemic therapy   236–7, 241

talon noir   204
tanning   10, 173–4
tapeworms   172
tar see coal tar preparations
target lesions   89, 90
telangiectasia   30, 114
    nail fold   68, 69
telogen   12, 13
telogen effluvium   64, 65
temporal arteritis   116
terminal hairs   12
terminology of lesions   28, 29–30
tetracycline   129–30, 257
therapy, dermatological   236–43
thermal sweating   14
'thimble pitting'   46, 47
threadworms   172
thrombophlebitis   117
    migratory superficial   117
    superficial   212
thrombosis, deep vein   116, 117
    leg ulcers in   120
thyroid disease   216
tinea capitis   63, 157–8
tinea corporis   157, 158
tinea infection, hands   157
tinea incognito   158
tinea pedis   156–7
tinea rubrum   157
'tinker's tartan'   115
tonofibrils   6
topical therapy   236–41
toxic epidermal necrolysis   102, 139, 234
toxic erythema   113, 114, 232, 233
'toxic sock syndrome'   83
traction alopecia   63
Treponema pallidum   140–1
Treponema pertenue   142
tretinoin   129, 251
trichomycosis axillaris   136
trichophytide   158
trichorrhexis nodosa   65
trichotillomania   224
tuberculides   142
tuberculosis   142–3
    inoculation   142
tuberous sclerosis   226–7
tumour, definition   29
tumours, internal, cutaneous effects   212,
        213
tumours, skin
    age-dependent prevalence   2
    dermis
        benign   205–8
        malignant   208
    epidermis
        benign   189–95
        malignant   197–205
        premalignant   195–7
    metastatic   210–11
    prevention   188–9
tylosis   40

tyrosinase   9
Tzank smear   32

ulcer   30
    infective   120
    leg   119–20
    malignant   120
    venous leg
        causes   117
        clinical features   117–18
        differential diagnosis   119–20
        investigations   120–1
        treatment   121–3, 252–3
ultraviolet radiation (UVR)   173
    disorders caused by   173–9
    therapy   243
        in acne   130
        in psoriasis   51
urticaria
    causes   85–6, 87, 88
    cholinergic   85
    cold   85
        management   89
    complications   87
    contact   86
    course   87
    differential diagnosis   87–8
    drug-related   232–3
    heat   85
    hypersensitivity   86
        management   89
    immunological basis   20
    investigations   88
    papular   165–6

pharmacological   86
physical   85–6
presentation   87
solar   85, 89, 178
treatment   89
urticarial vasculitis   88
urticated erythema   113
UVR see ultraviolet radiation

vagabond's disease   167
varicella   149–50
variegate porphyria   218
vascular disorders   113–24
vascular naevi   205–7
vasculitis   23, 25, 88, 92, 93–5
    allergic   93–4, 233
    hypersensitivity   93–4, 233
    leg ulcers in   120
    leucocytoclastic   93–4, 233
    nodular   92
    small vessel   93–4, 233
    urticarial   88
vellus hairs   12
venous disease   116–24
venous hypertension   117
venous leg ulcers
    causes   117
    clinical features   117–18
    differential diagnosis   119–20
    investigations   120–1
    treatment   121–3, 253
vesicle   28, 29
viral infections   145–56
    bullae in   97

vitamin D synthesis   8
vitamin deficiencies   215
vitiligo   182–4
von Recklinghausen's
    neurofibromatosis   225–6

Waardenburg syndrome   182
warts
    anogenital   147, 148–9
    peri-ungual   70
    seborrhoeic   189–90, 193
    'sun'   196–7
    treatment preparations   250
    viral   145–9, 189
watery lotions   239, 240
Wegener's granulomatosis   95
Werner's syndrome   184
wet dressings   240
wheal   28, 29
Wickham's striae   55, 56
Wood's light   31
    in dermatophyte infections   159
worms, parasitic   171–2

xanthomas   219, 220
xeroderma pigmentosum   227–8
xerosis   234

yaws   142
yellow nail syndrome   66–7